Comparative Effectiveness Review
Number 125

Testing of CYP2C19 Variants and Platelet Reactivity for Guiding Antiplatelet Treatment

Prepared for:
Agency for Healthcare Research and Quality
U.S. Department of Health and Human Services
540 Gaither Road
Rockville, MD 20850
www.ahrq.gov

Contract No. 290-2007-10055-I

Prepared by:
Tufts Evidence-based Practice Center
Boston, MA

Investigators:
Issa J. Dahabreh, M.D., M.S.
Denish Moorthy, M.B.B.S., M.S.
Jenny L. Lamont, M.S.
Minghua L. Chen, M.D., M.P.H.
David M. Kent, M.D., M.S.
Joseph Lau, M.D.

AHRQ Publication No. 13-EHC117-EF
September 2013

This report is based on research conducted by the Tufts Evidence-based Practice Center (EPC) under contract to the Agency for Healthcare Research and Quality (AHRQ), Rockville, MD (Contract No. 290-2007-10055-I). The findings and conclusions in this document are those of the authors, who are responsible for its contents; the findings and conclusions do not necessarily represent the views of AHRQ. Therefore, no statement in this report should be construed as an official position of AHRQ or of the U.S. Department of Health and Human Services.

The information in this report is intended to help health care decisionmakers—patients and clinicians, health system leaders, and policymakers, among others—make well-informed decisions and thereby improve the quality of health care services. This report is not intended to be a substitute for the application of clinical judgment. Anyone who makes decisions concerning the provision of clinical care should consider this report in the same way as any medical reference and in conjunction with all other pertinent information, i.e., in the context of available resources and circumstances presented by individual patients.

This report may be used, in whole or in part, as the basis for development of clinical practice guidelines and other quality enhancement tools, or as a basis for reimbursement and coverage policies. AHRQ or U.S. Department of Health and Human Services endorsement of such derivative products may not be stated or implied.

This document is in the public domain and may be used and reprinted without special permission. Citation of the source is appreciated.

Persons using assistive technology may not be able to fully access information in this report. For assistance contact EffectiveHealthCare@ahrq.hhs.gov.

None of the investigators have any affiliations or financial involvement that conflicts with the material presented in this report.

Suggested citation: Dahabreh IJ, Moorthy D, Lamont JL, Chen ML, Kent DM, Lau J. Testing of CYP2C19 Variants and Platelet Reactivity for Guiding Antiplatelet Treatment. Comparative Effectiveness Review No. 125. (Prepared by Tufts Evidence-based Practice Center under Contract No. 290-2007-10055-I.) AHRQ Publication No. 13-EHC117-EF. Rockville, MD: Agency for Healthcare Research and Quality; September 2013. www.effectivehealthcare.ahrq.gov/reports/final/cfm.

Preface

The Agency for Healthcare Research and Quality (AHRQ), through its Evidence-based Practice Centers (EPCs), sponsors the development of systematic reviews to assist public- and private-sector organizations in their efforts to improve the quality of health care in the United States. These reviews provide comprehensive, science-based information on common, costly medical conditions, and new health care technologies and strategies.

Systematic reviews are the building blocks underlying evidence-based practice; they focus attention on the strength and limits of evidence from research studies about the effectiveness and safety of a clinical intervention. In the context of developing recommendations for practice, systematic reviews can help clarify whether assertions about the value of the intervention are based on strong evidence from clinical studies. For more information about AHRQ EPC systematic reviews, see www.effectivehealthcare.ahrq.gov/reference/purpose.cfm

AHRQ expects that these systematic reviews will be helpful to health plans, providers, purchasers, government programs, and the health care system as a whole. Transparency and stakeholder input are essential to the Effective Health Care Program. Please visit the Web site (www.effectivehealthcare.ahrq.gov) to see draft research questions and reports or to join an email list to learn about new program products and opportunities for input.

We welcome comments on this systematic review. They may be sent by mail to the Task Order Officer named below at: Agency for Healthcare Research and Quality, 540 Gaither Road, Rockville, MD 20850, or by email to epc@ahrq.hhs.gov.

Richard G. Kronick, Ph.D.
Director
Agency for Healthcare Research and Quality

Jean Slutsky, P.A., M.S.P.H.
Director, Center for Outcomes and Evidence
Agency for Healthcare Research and Quality

Stephanie Chang, M.D., M.P.H.
Director
Evidence-based Practice Program
Center for Outcomes and Evidence
Agency for Healthcare Research and Quality

Elisabeth Kato, M.D., M.R.P.
Task Order Officer
Center for Outcomes and Evidence
Agency for Healthcare Research and Quality

Acknowledgments

The authors would like to thank C. Michael White, Pharm.D., FCP, FCCP, the Associate Editor for this report, for numerous helpful suggestions.

Key Informants

In designing the study questions, the EPC consulted several Key Informants who represent the end-users of research. The EPC sought the Key Informant input on the priority areas for research and synthesis. Key Informants are not involved in the analysis of the evidence or the writing of the report. Therefore, in the end, study questions, design, methodological approaches, and/or conclusions do not necessarily represent the views of individual Key Informants.

Key Informants must disclose any financial conflicts of interest greater than $10,000 and any other relevant business or professional conflicts of interest. Because of their role as end-users, individuals with potential conflicts may be retained. The TOO and the EPC work to balance, manage, or mitigate any conflicts of interest.

Three Key Informants could not be contacted to obtain permission for listing them here. The list of the other Key Informants who participated in developing this report follows:

Gordon Huggins, M.D.
Associate Professor of Medicine
Tufts University
Faculty, Institute for Clinical Research and Health Policy
Tufts Medical Center
Boston, MA

David Kent, M.D., C.M., M.Sc.
Associate Professor of Medicine and Neurology, Tufts Medical Center and Tufts University School of Medicine
Associate Professor of Clinical and Translational Science
Director, Clinical and Translational Science Program, Sackler School of Graduate Biomedical Sciences, Tufts University
Boston, MA

Mary Ross Southworth, Pharm.D.
Deputy Director for Safety, Office of New Drugs
Division of Cardiovascular and Renal Products
U.S. Food and Drug Administration
Silver Spring, MD

Technical Expert Panel

In designing the study questions and methodology at the outset of this report, the EPC consulted several technical and content experts. Broad expertise and perspectives were sought. Divergent and conflicted opinions are common and perceived as healthy scientific discourse that results in a thoughtful, relevant systematic review. Therefore, in the end, study questions, design, methodologic approaches, and/or conclusions do not necessarily represent the views of individual technical and content experts.

Technical Experts must disclose any financial conflicts of interest greater than $10,000 and any other relevant business or professional conflicts of interest. Because of their unique clinical or content expertise, individuals with potential conflicts may be retained. The TOO and the EPC work to balance, manage, or mitigate any potential conflicts of interest identified.

The list of Technical Experts who participated in developing this report follows:

W. David Dotson, Ph.D.
Health Scientist, Office of Public Health Genomics
Centers for Disease Control and Prevention
Atlanta, GA

Paul A. Gurbel, M.D., FACC
Director, Center for Thrombosis Research, Sinai Hospital of Baltimore
Director, Cardiovascular Research, Life Bridge Health
Associate Chief for Research, Department of Medicine, Sinai Hospital of Baltimore
Professor of Medicine, Johns Hopkins University School of Medicine
Baltimore, MD

Jessica L. Mega, M.D., M.P.H.
Assistant Professor of Medicine
Harvard Medical School
Brigham and Women's Hospital
Boston, MA

Guillaume Paré, M.D., M.Sc., FRCPC
Assistant Professor, Department of Pathology & Molecular Medicine
Joint Member, Department of Clinical Epidemiology & Biostatistics
Director, Genetic and Molecular Epidemiology Laboratory
McMaster University
Ontario, Canada

Alan Shuldiner, M.D.
Director, Program in Personalized and Genomic Medicine
Head, Division of Endocrinology, Diabetes and Nutrition
University of Maryland, School of Medicine
Baltimore, MD

David Veenstra, Pharm.D., Ph.D.
Professor, Pharmaceutical Outcomes Research and Policy Program
Auxiliary Member, Institute for Public Health Genetics
University of Washington
Seattle, WA

Peer Reviewers

Prior to publication of the final evidence report, EPCs sought input from independent Peer Reviewers without financial conflicts of interest. However, the conclusions and synthesis of the scientific literature presented in this report does not necessarily represent the views of individual reviewers.

Peer Reviewers must disclose any financial conflicts of interest greater than $10,000 and any other relevant business or professional conflicts of interest. Because of their unique clinical or content expertise, individuals with potential nonfinancial conflicts may be retained. The TOO and the EPC work to balance, manage, or mitigate any potential nonfinancial conflicts of interest identified.

The list of Peer Reviewers follows:

Mark Hlatky, M.D.
Professor of Health Research and Policy
Professor of Medicine (Cardiovascular Medicine)
Stanford University School of Medicine
Stanford, CA

David R. Holmes Jr., M.D.
Professor of Medicine
Division of Cardiovascular Diseases
Mayo Clinic
Rochester, MN

Michael V. Holmes, M.R.C.P., M.Sc., M.B.B.S., B.Sc.
UK MRC Population Health Scientist Fellow
Institute of Cardiovascular Science
Faculty of Population Health Sciences
University College London (UCL)
London, United Kingdom

Rajnikanth Madabushi, Ph.D.
Team Leader
Division of Cardiovascular and Renal Products, Office of Clinical Pharmacology
U.S. Food and Drug Administration
Silver Spring, MD

Alvin Mushlin, M.D. Sc.M.
Professor and Chair, Department of Public Health
Professor of Medicine
Weill Cornell Medical College
New York, NY

Michael Pacanowski, Pharm.D., M.P.H.
Associate Director for Genomics and Targeted Therapy
Genomics Group, Office of Clinical Pharmacology
U.S. Food and Drug Administration
Silver Spring, MD

Mary Southworth, Pharm.D.
Deputy Director for Safety
Division of Cardiovascular and Renal Products, Office of Clinical Pharmacology
U.S. Food and Drug Administration
Silver Spring, MD

Testing of CYP2C19 Variants and Platelet Reactivity for Guiding Antiplatelet Treatment

Structured Abstract

Objectives. This comparative effectiveness review evaluated the analytic validity, prognostic value, and comparative effectiveness of two types of medical tests (genetic testing for CYP2C19 variants and phenotypic testing to measure platelet reactivity) to identify patients who are most likely to benefit from clopidogrel-based antiplatelet therapy and to guide antiplatelet therapy in patient populations who are eligible to receive or are already receiving clopidogrel treatment.

Data sources. We searched MEDLINE®, the Cochrane Central Trials Registry, the Cochrane Database of Systematic Reviews, the Human Genome Epidemiology Network database, and the National Institutes of Health Genetic Association Database, from inception to July 27, 2012. We also searched the Food and Drug Administration Web site and ClinicalTrials.gov, and contacted test manufacturers and authors of primary studies.

Review methods. We used established systematic review methods to identify English-language articles describing studies performed in all relevant care settings on the basis of predetermined eligibility criteria: adult patients with cardiovascular, cerebrovascular, or peripheral arterial disease who were candidates for or were receiving clopidogrel; use of genetic testing (for CYP2C19 variants) or phenotypic testing (for platelet reactivity). Studies had to report information on the analytic validity, prognostic ability for intermediate (platelet reactivity) or clinical outcomes, use of tests to guide antiplatelet therapy, or adverse events from testing itself or from test-directed treatment.

Results. The literature search yielded 10,475 unique citations, 1,419 of which were obtained in full text and reviewed. A total of 326 publications were judged to have met the inclusion criteria. (Some publications contributed data to multiple analyses.)

Eleven studies provided information for the analytic validity of genotyping assays and 105 for the analytic validity of platelet reactivity assays. Test-retest reliability and interassay agreement for genotyping assays appeared adequate; however, few studies were available. Agreement between assays for measuring platelet reactivity was poor to moderate. Generally, agreement was higher between measurements obtained from the same assay using different agonist concentrations than between different assay types. Only 12 studies provided information on analytic test performance, and they reported variable results.

One hundred six studies provided information on the ability of genetic testing for CYP2C19 variants to predict clinical outcomes or platelet reactivity during followup. The majority of studies were conducted in populations with ischemic heart disease. Under a dominant model, loss-of-function alleles were associated with higher on-clopidogrel platelet reactivity and were statistically significantly associated with stent thrombosis (relative risk [RR] = 1.52; 95% confidence interval [CI], 1.17 to 1.97); major adverse cardiovascular events (RR=1.20; 95% CI, 1.04 to 1.39); and cardiovascular mortality (RR=1.98; 95% CI, 1.13 to 3.46). Associations were nonstatistically significant in meta-analyses of loss-of-function alleles and all-cause mortality, acute coronary syndromes, stroke, and bleeding events. Sensitivity analyses under recessive and additive models for the two outcomes with adequate data (major adverse cardiovascular events and stent thrombosis) produced results in the same direction but with larger effect sizes than the dominant model. Under a dominant model, gain-of-function alleles were significantly associated with reduced risk of major adverse cardiovascular events (RR=0.82; 95% CI, 0.74 to 0.92).

One hundred twenty-eight studies provided information on the ability of baseline on-clopidogrel platelet reactivity to predict clinical outcomes or platelet reactivity during followup. The majority of studies were conducted in populations with ischemic heart disease. Patients with high platelet reactivity at baseline were more likely to be clopidogrel nonresponders during followup. The ability to predict clinical outcomes was reported for various assays; the most commonly assessed were light-transmission aggregometry (55 studies); VerifyNow P2Y12 (38 studies); vasodilator-stimulated phosphoprotein assay (19 studies); Multiplate analyzer (18 studies); and Platelet Function Analyzer-100 (11 studies). Overall, studies suggested that increased on-clopidogrel reactivity was associated with increased rates of adverse cardiovascular outcomes.

Fourteen studies provided information on the use of genetic testing for CYP2C19 variants for guiding treatment choice: 1 randomized trial of testing versus no testing, 12 randomized treatment trials assessing effect modification by CYP2C19 status, 1 randomized treatment trial selecting patients on the basis of CYP2C19 genotype. Twenty-four studies provided information on the use of platelet reactivity measurements to guide antiplatelet therapy: 7 comparative studies of alternative testing strategies (6 with random allocation), 3 randomized treatment trials assessing effect modification by reactivity status, 14 randomized treatment trials selecting patients on the basis of platelet reactivity levels. Studies had heterogeneous designs and compared different treatment strategies. Overall, there was insufficient evidence regarding the use of genotyping CYP2C19 variants or phenotypic testing for platelet reactivity to guide treatment selection.

Conclusions. We found evidence to support an association between loss-of-function CYP2C19 variants and increased risk of adverse cardiovascular outcomes. Similarly, we found evidence that high on-clopidogrel platelet reactivity is associated with an increased risk of adverse cardiovascular outcomes, at least for some of the available assays. The strength of evidence regarding these prognostic effects was judged to be low or moderate because of concerns regarding selective outcome reporting and publication bias, and the relatively small number of studies reporting data on most clinical outcomes. The strength of evidence regarding the use of genetic or platelet reactivity testing to guide antiplatelet treatment selection was judged to be insufficient because studies reporting on clinical outcomes were few, had diverse designs, and included heterogeneous populations. Comparative data on alternative test strategies (genetic versus phenotypic) are lacking.

Contents

Tables

xiii

Figures

Appendixes

Executive Summary

Background

Burden of Disease and Clinical Setting

Approximately 82 million Americans currently suffer from some form of cardiovascular disease.[1] In the United States, coronary heart disease alone is the cause of 1 of every 6 deaths, and stroke, 1 of every 18 deaths.[2] There were approximately 7 million inpatient cardiovascular operations and procedures in the United States in 2007, of which 1 million were either percutaneous coronary intervention (PCI) or coronary artery bypass graft (CABG) surgeries.[1]

Randomized controlled trials have established dual antiplatelet treatment with clopidogrel and aspirin as the current standard of care for medical and interventional management of acute coronary syndromes.[3] Dual antiplatelet treatment is also recommended for patients undergoing PCI[4] with placement of stents (either bare metal or drug eluting). Randomized controlled trials support the use of clopidogrel in patients who have experienced acute cardiovascular events (e.g., stroke) and those with peripheral arterial disease.[3,5-8] For patients with atrial fibrillation and contraindications to vitamin K antagonists, the ACTIVE A (Atrial Fibrillation Clopidogrel Trial with Irbesartan for Prevention of Vascular Events) trial suggested that the combination of clopidogrel and aspirin is more effective than aspirin alone for preventing thromboembolic disease.[9]

Since the approval of clopidogrel by the U.S. Food and Drug Administration (FDA) for routine clinical use, the drug has become one of the most commonly prescribed agents in the United States. However, patient response to clopidogrel-based antiplatelet therapy is variable both between patients and across multiple measurements within a patient, with some patients showing no or minimal platelet response to clopidogrel administration (often termed clopidogrel "nonresponsiveness" or "resistance"). Alternatives to standard clopidogrel treatment include higher dose clopidogrel regimens and the use of other antiplatelet agents, such as prasugrel or ticagrelor.[10-13] Given the availability of alternative antiplatelet strategies and concern about adverse clinical outcomes in clopidogrel nonresponders, research has focused on methods to identify patients who are unlikely to benefit from clopidogrel-based treatment. The question of identifying the optimal antiplatelet therapy may also carry cost implications because generic clopidogrel products are now available in the United States.[a]

Clopidogrel Metabolism

To be biologically active, clopidogrel must be transformed to the active metabolite R-130964 by members of the CYP enzyme system, primarily the enzyme CYP2C19. R-130964 acts by binding irreversibly to the $P2Y_{12}$ receptor (the adenosine diphosphate [ADP] receptor) on the surface of platelets and inhibits platelet aggregation for the life cycle of the platelet.[14,15]

However, the relationship between genotype and clinical outcomes is not straightforward. The fact that each individual carries two CYP2C19 alleles results in combinations of alleles of varying enzymatic activity. The combined effect of the two alleles on actual enzymatic activity

---

[a]FDA release, available at www.fda.gov/NewsEvents/Newsroom/PressAnnouncements/ucm304489.htm; last accessed: October 16, 2012.

levels depends on the "true" genetic model of CYP2C19 alleles (dominant, recessive, additive, or codominant). Unfortunately, the true underlying genetic model for CYP2C19 variants is not known with certainty.[16] This is of particular concern, as the allele frequency of CYP2C19 variants is heterogeneous across populations of different ethnicities, resulting in different genotype prevalences. For example, data from the Third National Health and Nutrition Examination Survey (NHANES III) showed statistically significant heterogeneity in the prevalence of the *2 allele among non-Hispanic whites, Mexican-Americans, and non-Hispanic blacks. Non-Hispanic blacks had the highest prevalence of the *2 allele (18.3%) and of homozygotes for that allele (*2/*2; 3.8%).[17] Studies have shown that the prevalence of the rare allele is even higher in East Asian populations, with *2 allele frequencies as high as 30-40 percent.[18-20]

Furthermore, the CYP2C19 genotype is only one of many determinants of the effect of clopidogrel on platelet reactivity. For example, a genome-wide association study recently demonstrated that the *2 allele accounts for only 12 percent of the total observed variation in clopidogrel responsiveness in a selected white population.[21] Several studies have demonstrated that environmental factors and patient characteristics, such as body mass index, diabetes, and smoking habits, can influence platelet reactivity.

Predicting Response and Guiding Antiplatelet Treatment

There are currently two main approaches to determine whether a patient will have a poor response to clopidogrel: (1) genetic testing to see whether the patient has a genotype that is associated with reduced ability to metabolize clopidogrel (a "poor-metabolizer" phenotype) and (2) direct testing of the patient's blood while the patient is taking clopidogrel to see whether the platelets actually have become less prone to aggregate in response to specific agonists (phenotypic testing for platelet reactivity).

Genetic Tests for CYP2C19 Variants

Genetic testing for one or more genetic variants can be performed with various genotyping methods. For biallelic variants, these methods identify homozygotes for each variant and heterozygotes. Testing for CYP2C19 variants requires a sample of somatic genetic material, usually obtained from a blood sample or from buccal swabs. Because allelic variants at the CYP2C19 locus do not change over a person's lifetime, testing done at any time point is representative of the person's genotype.

Measurement of Platelet Reactivity

Phenotypic testing measures the reactivity of platelets while a patient is taking clopidogrel (on-clopidogrel platelet reactivity). Several assays for measuring platelet reactivity are available. These include rapid point-of-care platelet function assays (e.g., VerifyNow, Platelet Function Analyzer [PFA]-100, Plateletworks); measurements of mediators of reactivity (e.g., vasodilator-stimulated phosphoprotein [VASP] phosphorylation using flow cytometry); and functional assays (e.g., aggregometry using appropriate agonists). We refer to all these assays as "phenotypic tests" because they attempt to measure an intermediate clinical phenotype (platelet reactivity).[22]

Scope

We performed a comparative effectiveness review regarding the utility of testing for CYP2C19 variants and platelet reactivity for guiding antiplatelet treatment. We evaluated the analytic validity, predictive utility, and comparative effectiveness of genetic and phenotypic tests as biomarker tests (and of relevant test-and-treat strategies) for guiding antiplatelet therapy in patient populations who are eligible for clopidogrel treatment.

Key Questions

On the basis of the original topic nomination and an extensive process of topic development and refinement, we formulated the following Key Questions to guide the review:

Key Question 1. In patient populations who are candidates for clopidogrel therapy, does genetic testing for CYP2C19 variants predict intermediate and clinical outcomes following treatment initiation?

a. What is the analytic validity (technical test performance) of the various assays used for CYP2C19 genetic testing?
b. What is the clinical validity (predictive accuracy) of genetic testing for predicting intermediate and clinical outcomes in patients who are receiving clopidogrel therapy?
c. Do the following factors modify the association between genetic test results and clinical outcomes?
    i. Comedications
    ii. Patient-level factors (e.g., race or ethnicity, age, sex, disease severity, or comorbidities)
    iii. Test-related factors (e.g., between-assay differences)
    iv. System-level factors (e.g., settings where testing is performed)

Key Question 2. In patient populations receiving clopidogrel therapy, does phenotypic testing of platelet reactivity predict intermediate and clinical outcomes?

a. What is the analytic validity (technical test performance) of the various assays used in phenotypic testing of platelet reactivity?
b. What is the clinical validity (predictive accuracy) of phenotypic testing for predicting intermediate and clinical outcomes in patients who are receiving clopidogrel therapy?
c. Do the following factors modify the association between phenotypic test results and clinical outcomes?
    i. Comedications
    ii. Patient-level factors (e.g., race or ethnicity, age, sex, disease severity, or comorbidities)
    iii. Test-related factors (e.g., between-assay differences)
    iv. System-level factors (e.g., settings where testing is performed)

Key Question 3. What is the comparative effectiveness of alternative test-and-treat strategies (including a no-testing strategy) for therapeutic decisionmaking regarding antiplatelet therapy among patients who are candidates for clopidogrel-based treatment?

a. What is the comparative effectiveness of the following testing strategies on therapeutic decisionmaking, platelet reactivity during followup, and clinical outcomes in patients who are candidates for antiplatelet treatment?
    i. Genetic testing for CYP2C19
    ii. Genetic testing for CYP2C19 followed by phenotypic testing for platelet reactivity
    iii. Phenotypic testing for platelet reactivity
    iv. No testing
b. How do modifying factors (e.g., race or ethnicity, age, sex, comorbidities, diet, or the time between conducting the test and obtaining results) affect the association of alternative phenotypic or genetic test-and-treat strategies and patient outcomes? Alternative test-guided treatments can include nonclopidogrel antiplatelet agents or high-dose clopidogrel regimens.

Key Question 4. What are the potential adverse effects or harms from genetic or phenotypic testing per se or from test-directed treatments?

Analytic Framework

We developed an analytic framework (Figure A) that maps the Key Questions within the context of populations, interventions, comparators, and outcomes of interest, as well as the chain of logic that evidence must support to link the interventions to health outcomes. Analytic and clinical validity were straightforward to represent in the analytic framework (Key Questions 1a, 1b, 2a, and 2b). Regarding treatment decisionmaking (Key Question 3a), we conceptualized the analytic framework as a decision problem, wherein patients' disease can be managed with one of the following approaches (depicted from top to bottom in the flow diagram):

- Undergo genetic testing and then base the treatment decision on the test results.
- Undergo genetic testing and then base the treatment decision on the test results. After receiving therapy for an adequate period of time, undergo phenotypic testing for platelet reactivity and use the results to decide whether the treatment strategy should be modified.
- Receive standard treatment directly and, after an appropriate amount of time, undergo phenotypic testing for platelet reactivity and use the test results to decide whether the treatment strategy should be modified. Use of phenotypic testing (but not genetic testing) as a monitoring test can be considered a variation of this strategy in which the test is repeatedly performed.
- Receive antiplatelet therapy without undergoing any testing (the current standard of care).

The above strategies were identified as the most prevalent in published studies by preliminary searches conducted in preparation of this review. Additional variations of these strategies were uncovered by the full evidence review.

Modifiers of the effects of testing on outcomes, in terms of both predictive ability and decisionmaking, were reviewed in Key Questions 1c, 2c, and 3b. Tests and test-directed treatments may be associated with harms, investigated in Key Question 4.

Figure A. Analytic framework

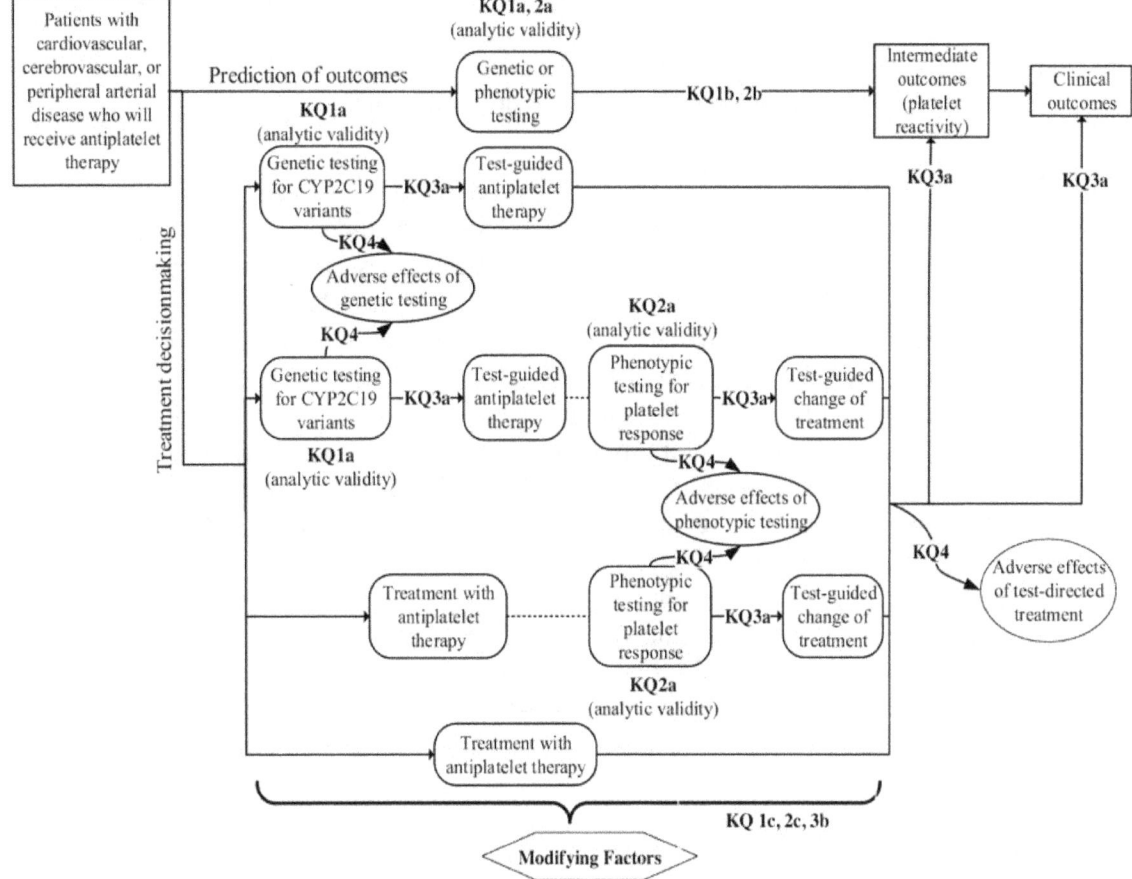

Note: KQ = Key Question.

Methods

Literature Search, Study Selection, and Data Extraction

We conducted literature searches for studies in MEDLINE®, the Cochrane Central Trials Registry, and the Cochrane Database of Systematic Reviews (from inception through July 27, 2012) without any language restriction. Our search included terms for the populations, tests, and drugs of interest. (See Appendix A of the full report for complete search strings, which were extensively validated against previous reviews on the tests of interest.) We also performed searches of the Human Genome Epidemiology Network (HuGENet) database and National Institutes of Health Genetic Association Database, using the same cutoff date (July 27, 2012). Finally, we performed a targeted search of the FDA Web site (last search performed on April 25, 2012).

We considered both comparative and noncomparative studies for Key Questions pertaining to prognostic ability but focused on comparative studies of alternative test-and-treat strategies. We did not include non–English-language studies. We excluded narrative reviews, editorials, letters to the editor, and other papers not presenting primary research data. We also excluded studies reporting exclusively on healthy individuals. Studies conducted in all relevant care settings were included. We contacted the authors of the primary studies to verify cases of suspected overlap.

A single investigator extracted data from each study; quantitative results were verified by a second reviewer. Disagreements were resolved by consensus involving a third investigator. We extracted information on the following items: patient selection criteria, population characteristics, sample size, study design, analytic details, and outcomes.

Risk-of-Bias Assessment of Individual Studies

For assessing the risk of bias, we followed recently updated guidance from the Agency for Healthcare Research and Quality "Methods Guide for Effectiveness and Comparative Effectiveness Reviews" (Methods Guide), available on the Effective Health Care Web site.[23,24] Two independent reviewers evaluated the risk of bias for each study, and disagreements were resolved by consensus including a third reviewer.

For studies of analytic validity (Key Questions 1a and 2a), we compiled a list of 11 items for assessing quality and completeness of reporting based on a recent AHRQ Methods Report.[25]

For studies of predictive ability (Key Questions 1b, 1c, 2b, and 2c), we based our assessment on the recently proposed Quality Assessment of Diagnostic Accuracy Studies (QUADAS)-2 instrument,[26] a new version of the validated QUADAS list of quality items[27-29] for systematic reviews of medical tests. We used the number of items scored as having been adequately addressed (i.e., indicative of low risk of bias) to classify studies into three categories (A, B, or C) indicating low, moderate, and high risk of bias, respectively.

Finally, for studies providing information on test-and-treatment strategies (Key Questions 3 and 4) we used a combination of items from the QUADAS-2 tool and the Cochrane risk-of-bias tool.[30]

Data Synthesis

We summarized our findings according to the order of the Key Questions. Within each Key Question, results were organized on the basis of the populations assessed and clinical indications for clopidogrel use, index tests used, and outcomes assessed.

Meta-Analysis

We performed random-effects inverse-variance meta-analysis when at least three studies were available on sufficiently similar populations using the same test and assessing the same outcomes.[31] Between-study heterogeneity was assessed on the basis of the Q statistic[32] (considered statistically significant when its p-value [P_Q] was less than 0.1). Between-study inconsistency was assessed using the I^2 index.[33] Prior to the review, we decided not to combine studies of different phenotypic tests for platelet reactivity because they are based on different principles of measurement. Similarly, we decided not to combine trials providing information about effect modification due to heterogeneous populations enrolled in trials comparing different pairs of interventions (i.e., the magnitude and direction of effect modification by the tests of interest were likely to vary among different treatment comparisons).

In the absence of consensus on the correct genetic model, we assumed a dominant model for all minor alleles because this is the model used in previous CYP2C19 meta-analyses and because it allowed fullest use of the data. We performed sensitivity analyses assuming a recessive or additive model.

We used hazard or incidence rate ratios in our meta-analyses whenever available or extractable from the reviewed studies. When such statistics were not reported and could not be calculated, we used risk (proportion) ratios because they approximate the relative incidence rate. For case-control studies, we used odds ratios because they are valid statistics for these designs and approximate the incidence rate ratio or risk ratio, depending on sampling methods.[34-36] For parsimony, we refer to all these statistics as relative risks (RRs).

Other Analyses

To assess the impact of study-level characteristics on estimates of the effect size, we used univariable random-effects metaregression.[33] Subgroup and metaregression analyses were performed for factors reported at the group level. Predefined subgroups of interest were those defined by race or ethnicity, sex, specific assay used, and clinical setting of test use (e.g., short-term administration of clopidogrel during treatment of acute cardiac events or PCI vs. chronic clopidogrel use). We also explored temporal trends in the reported effect sizes using metaregression with year of publication as the covariate. We used Egger's regression-based test[37] to assess the presence of small-study effects.[37,38]

Strength of the Body of Evidence

We graded the strength of the body of evidence for the Key Questions following the Methods Guide and recently updated recommendations for the Evidence-based Practice Center (EPC) Program.[23,39] Briefly, the strength of evidence was graded as high, moderate, low, or insufficient on the basis of four dimensions: risk of bias (described above), consistency, directness, and precision. We assessed the consistency of the data as either "no inconsistency" or "inconsistency present" (or "not applicable" if only one study). We also assessed the sparseness of the evidence. We considered evidence to be sparse if it was from only one study with a small sample size. Strength ratings were assigned on the basis of our level of confidence that the evidence reflected the true effect for the major comparisons of interest.

Assessing Applicability

We assessed applicability of the study findings on the basis of the individual study eligibility criteria and baseline characteristics of the included populations, following recommendations in the Methods Guide and recently updated recommendations for the EPC Program.[23,39] We did not assess the applicability of studies regarding the analytic validity of the tests of interest (Key Questions 1a and 2a) because technical test performance does not directly inform medical decisions, although it is a prerequisite for the clinical use of tests.[40]

Results

The literature search yielded 10,475 citations (10,374 from electronic databases, 77 from scientific information packets, and 24 from hand-searching). Of these, 1,419 articles were reviewed in full text. After full-text review, 326 were judged to have met the inclusion criteria for one or more Key Questions. We summarized the findings of the report according to the order of the Key Questions. Within each Key Question, results are organized for each appropriate subgroup on the basis of the populations assessed and clinical indications for clopidogrel use, index tests assessed, and outcomes assessed.

Key Question 1a: Analytic Validity of Tests for Genotyping CYP2C19 Variants

Eligible Studies

We identified 11 studies reporting information on the analytic validity of genotyping methods for detecting CYP2C19 variants. We also reviewed four FDA 510(k) summaries on genetic testing.

Summary of Findings

Primary studies generally indicated excellent test-retest reliability and interassay agreement. FDA 510(k) summaries did not report analyses on samples from populations and genes of interest to our review. However, the documents provided further evidence that genotyping methods have high test-retest reliability and indicated that rates of interassay agreement were high.

Primary studies reported limited information on the methods used to assess analytic validity. This probably reflects the fact that the primary focus of all included publications was not the tests' analytic validity but rather their clinical utility. Generally, studies provided adequate information on the genotyping methods used. However, they provided little information on the use of positive or negative control samples, the handling of uninterpretable results, and the test detection limits. Four studies reported information on the reproducibility of genotyping across different genotyping methods, but no study assessed reproducibility across operators. No study was conducted as part of an interlaboratory standardization project.

Key Question 1b: Predictive Value of Genetic Testing for CYP2C19 Variants

Eligible Studies

The 106 studies addressing Key Question 1b were described in 98 publications, 8 of which described 2 studies each. The vast majority of studies (100, or 94%) were of patients with ischemic heart disease. Three studies enrolled patients with different forms of vascular disease (coronary, cerebrovascular, or peripheral arterial); one enrolled patients with cerebrovascular disease; one enrolled a mixed population of patients with manifest atherothrombotic disease along with asymptomatic patients at high risk for atherothrombotic disease; and one enrolled patients with atrial fibrillation who were not candidates for vitamin K antagonist therapy.

The 106 studies had intermediate to large sample sizes: median number of enrolled individuals = 277, 25th percentile = 98, 75th percentile = 802, minimum = 30, maximum = 5,148. They were conducted recently (median year of start of enrollment, 2006, with 75% beginning enrollment after 2004), reflecting the relatively recent widespread availability of genetic testing for CYP2C19 variants. The majority of enrolled patients were men and the median age was 64 years. Across studies, the median proportions of patients with dyslipidemia and hypertension were both over 60 percent. The median proportions of patients with diabetes mellitus and patients who smoked were both greater than 25 percent. Overall, 94 percent of studies had a longitudinal (cohort) design; 11 of these were genetic substudies consisting of prospectively followed clopidogrel-treated groups from randomized trials.[b]

Overall, studies had moderate risk of bias: 12 studies were rated as quality A, 88 studies were rated as quality B, and 6 were rated as quality C. We caution that this aggregate risk-of-bias rating can be misleading, especially in the presence of poor reporting, because it assigns the same weight to all items.

Summary of Findings

The two most common genotyping methods were TaqMan genotyping (44 studies; 42%) and polymerase chain reaction with restriction fragment length polymorphism analysis (PCR-RFLP; 13 studies; 12%). In the majority of cases, analyses were conducted on genetic material isolated from blood (92 studies; 87%). Among the 56 studies that reported the genotyping success rate, the median was 100 percent (minimum = 74%; maximum = 100%). Violations of Hardy-Weinberg equilibrium (on the basis of an exact goodness-of-fit test) were not more common than would be expected by chance.

Below, findings are presented for studies providing information on the ability of genetic testing for CYP2C19 variants to predict clinical outcomes (57 studies) or platelet reactivity (74 studies) during followup.

Clinical Outcomes

Several clinical outcomes of interest were reported: all-cause mortality, cardiac mortality, acute coronary syndromes, stent thrombosis, stroke, major adverse cardiovascular events (MACE), bleeding events, and need for revascularization. Under a dominant genetic model, loss-of function CYP2C19 alleles were statistically significantly associated with stent thrombosis (RR=1.52; 95% confidence interval [CI], 1.17 to 1.97); cardiovascular mortality (RR=1.98; 95% CI, 1.13 to 3.46); and MACE (RR=1.20; 95% CI, 1.04 to 1.39). Under a dominant genetic model, gain-of-function alleles (CYP2C19*17) were statistically significantly associated with reduced risk of MACE (RR=0.82; 95% CI, 0.74 to 0.92). Studies on the predictive value of CYP2C19 variants were judged to have moderate risk of bias. There was some indication of systematic differences between larger and smaller studies (loss-of-function alleles: p<0.001, p=0.002, and p=0.049 for stent thrombosis, cardiovascular mortality, and MACE, respectively; gain-of-function alleles: p=0.046 for bleeding events). There was also substantial risk of selective outcome reporting for outcomes other than MACE.

Sensitivity analyses using alternative genetic models (recessive and additive for the variant alleles) were based on a minority of studies and possible only for the association of loss-of-function alleles with MACE and stent thrombosis. Generally, these analyses were congruent with analyses using a dominant model because they also indicated significant association between loss-of-function alleles and adverse clinical outcomes. Effect sizes using both the recessive and additive models were larger than those under the dominant model.

Intermediate Outcome: Platelet Reactivity

The intermediate outcome of platelet reactivity was reported either as a continuous variable (in 61 studies) or according to a threshold of reactivity (e.g., high vs. low; in 39 studies). The most common assays for assessing reactivity were light-transmission aggregometry (LTA), the

---

[b]When appropriate, modification of the relative treatment effect by genotype status has been considered under Key Questions 3 and 4 of this report.

VerifyNow P2Y12 assay, and the VASP assay. For platelet reactivity as a continuous outcome, the mean or median reactivity was generally higher among clopidogrel-treated patients with one or two loss-of-function alleles than those with no loss-of-function alleles. For platelet reactivity as a categorical outcome, studies generally showed that platelet reactivity above the threshold used (or in higher quantiles compared with lower quantiles of reactivity) was more common in clopidogrel-treated patients with one or two loss-of-function alleles than those with no loss-of-function alleles. Only a minority of studies reported analyses under different genetic models, and it was often impossible to reconstruct such analyses from the reported data. Because of the extensive differences among studies of either type of reactivity outcome and the often incomplete reporting of numerical information, we did not perform meta-analyses for studies using reactivity as the outcome of interest.

Key Question 1c: Factors Affecting the Predictive Value of Genetic Testing for CYP2C19 Variants

We reviewed studies to identify any evidence that patient- or system-level factors or test characteristics could modify the prognostic ability of genetic testing for CYP2C19 variants. We considered both within-study information (e.g., studies in which the predictive effect of phenotypic testing was evaluated in two or more patient subgroups) and information across studies (through metaregression analyses on study-level factors).

Effect Modification Within Studies

Twenty studies reported information on modification of the prognostic effect of the genetic test by various factors; 5 studies assessed more than two potential effect modifiers. Only two of the effects assessed were statistically significant, each in a single study: a multiplicative interaction between the *2 and *3 CYP2C19 alleles on on-clopidogrel platelet reactivity and an interaction between clinical presentation and loss-of-function CYP2C19 allele carriership (comparing a cohort of patients with myocardial infarction, ischemic stroke, or peripheral arterial disease vs. asymptomatic patients at high risk for atherothrombotic events). The following nonstatistically significant comparisons were also reported: effect modification by proton-pump inhibitors (five studies) and by ancestry (three studies), gene-gene interactions (four studies). The following modifiers were also evaluated in one study each: indication for clopidogrel use (acute coronary syndromes vs. stable angina), whether patients were clopidogrel pretreated or naïve upon study entry, whether patients required a loading dose or not (because they were on chronic clopidogrel therapy), the duration of clopidogrel therapy, smoking status (number of cigarettes per day), body-mass index (≥25 kg/m^2 vs. <25 kg/m^2), stent type (bare metal vs. drug eluting), myocardial infarction subtype (ST elevation or non–ST elevation), history of PCI (yes vs. no), interactions with a large set of clinical and procedural factors, administration of polyunsaturated fatty acids, whether patients were on calcium channel blockers or their combination with proton pump inhibitors. All results were nonsignificant. Overall, the reported findings do not provide sufficient evidence to support or exclude a differential effect of CYP2C19 variants across any of the factors assessed in the studies we reviewed. The statistically significant findings should not be overinterpreted, given the number of comparisons performed and the potential for selective reporting across studies.

Effect Modification Across Studies

Potential modifiers of the predictive effect of genetic testing for CYP2C19 that were assessed across studies using subgroup and metaregression analysis were disease subtype (acute coronary syndromes vs. mixed coronary artery disease populations), setting of care (PCI vs. other), race or ethnicity (white vs. East Asian), duration of followup (≤30 days vs. >30 days), and year when enrollment was started (continuous variable). Metaregression analyses, both for stent thrombosis and MACE, suggested that the effect of loss-of-function alleles may be more extreme among individuals of East Asian ethnicity; however, this finding needs to be interpreted with caution, given the relatively small number of publications reporting on individuals of East Asian ethnicity and the potential for confounding by other factors that differ between studies conducted in populations of different ethnicities.

Effect Modification Summary

In general, considering both analyses within studies and across studies, there is insufficient information to support or exclude the presence of substantial modification of the prognostic effect of CYP2C19 variants by any of the investigated factors because most modifiers were evaluated in a single study (in the majority of cases producing nonsignificant results) and because metaregression analyses (nonsignificant for all but one of the factors explored) may be confounded by study-level characteristics.

Key Question 2a: Analytic Validity of Tests for On-Clopidogrel Platelet Reactivity

Eligible Studies

We identified 104 studies reporting information on the analytic validity of assays for measuring platelet reactivity. We also reviewed 20 FDA 510(k) summaries on phenotypic testing assays. All published studies enrolled patients with ischemic cardiovascular disease. The six most commonly assessed assays (with some studies assessing more than one) were LTA, the VerifyNow P2Y12 assay, the VASP assay, the Multiplate analyzer, the PFA device, and thromboelastography. We summarized the reported information regarding analytic performance, interassay agreement, test reliability and assay variation, and correlations between assays applied to the same sample (by far the most common metric reported). No other aspect of analytic validity was evaluated in the studies.

Summary of Findings

Overall there appeared to be low to moderate agreement between assays. Agreement was generally greater between measurements obtained with the same assay using different agonist concentrations than between different assays.

In the 12 studies providing information on analytic performance, analytic sensitivities ranged between 0.35 and 1.00, and analytic specificities ranged between 0.42 and 0.95. In studies reporting results across multiple cutoff values, a tradeoff between sensitivity and specificity was apparent, as expected. Overall, these results indicate poor agreement in sample classification (e.g., high vs. low reactivity) when one of the two tests compared was considered a gold standard. However, the evidence suggests that no test is a gold standard (i.e., all have measurement error).

Forty studies provided information on interassay agreement. Overall, disagreements were relatively common between measurements obtained by different assays or by using different agonist concentrations within the same assays.

Forty-three studies reported information on assay variability, although more than 90 percent did not describe the methods used in their assessment. One study used the intraclass correlation coefficient for repeat measurements to assess the reliability of measurements using LTA, the VASP assay, the Multiplate analyzer, and the INNOVANCE assay. Variability or coefficient-of-variation results were less than 10 percent in all but two studies. These results need to be interpreted with caution, given the poor reporting of study methods and the fact that multiple studies were published by a limited number of investigative teams. (In most cases, we could not ascertain whether the studied populations overlapped.)

Of the 56 studies reporting correlation values, only 1 used Lin's concordance correlation coefficient (an appropriate metric), reporting a high correlation ($\rho = 0.97$) between observed and estimated platelet inhibition for the VerifyNow assay. The remaining studies used inappropriate metrics (e.g., Spearman or Pearson correlation coefficients or linear regression, which in the simple bivariate case of two measurements is equivalent to the Pearson correlation) or did not report the calculation method used.[41,42] The results indicated that the association between measurements obtained using different methods is relatively poor. However, given the inappropriateness of the methods used to assess agreement, even high correlation values would not be considered indicative of good agreement.

None of the 20 FDA 510(k) summaries on phenotypic tests of platelet reactivity reported relevant analyses that met our study selection criteria: either no data were reported or the population or agonist used in testing was not of interest, the analytic validity was not reported for clopidogrel-treated patients, or the sample size was less than 10.

Key Question 2b: Predictive Ability of Phenotypic Testing for Platelet Reactivity

Eligible Studies

Of the 128 studies addressing Key Question 2b, the vast majority (122 studies) were of patients with ischemic heart disease. Four studies enrolled patients with cerebrovascular disease; one study enrolled patients with peripheral arterial disease; and one study enrolled a mix of patients with ischemic heart disease, cerebrovascular disease, and peripheral arterial disease. Studies reported information on a variety of assays for measuring platelet reactivity. Table A summarizes information on the patient populations and outcomes assessed in the 128 studies. Detailed information on each test is presented separately under the discussion of individual assays. For parsimony, we discuss below only results for the test-outcome combinations for which the strength of the overall body of evidence was judged to be at least "low." (Please refer to the Methods section for details on our approach to rating the strength of evidence.) Complete results are available in the full report. The strength of evidence for all patient populations other than those with ischemic heart disease was judged to be insufficient owing to the very few studies and small sample sizes.

Overall, studies were considered to have a moderate risk of bias. All studies used a longitudinal design (not case control, in keeping with our inclusion criteria), and no studies had substantial loss to followup. Inappropriate exclusions were uncommon, but information on blinding was often not reported (particularly for the index test) or not used. It was often unclear whether analyses, including the definitions of increased platelet reactivity and the outcomes assessed, had been prespecified and reported in full. Using the cutoff values based on the number of adequately addressed risk-of-bias items, 36 studies were rated as quality A, 80 studies were rated as quality B, and 12 were rated as quality C. A more detailed discussion of risk of bias, focusing on the individual items assessed, is presented in the full report.

Table A. Populations, outcomes, and strength of evidence in studies for Key Question 2b, according to test used

Test Used (Total Number of Studies; Studies by Patient Population)	All-Cause Death	CV Death	ACS	ST	Stroke	Bleeding	MACE	Other Clinical Outcomes	Platelet Reactivity
LTA (total = 55; IHD = 53; PAD = 1; IHD, CVD, PAD = 1)	IHD = 13 [low]	IHD = 9 [low]	IHD = 18 [low]	IHD = 19 [low]	IHD = 12 [low]	IHD = 7 [insufficient]	IHD = 37 [low] IHD, CVD, PAD = 1 [insufficient]	IHD = 8 [insufficient]	IHD = 11 [insufficient] PAD = 1 [insufficient]
VerifyNow P2Y12 (total = 38; IHD = 35; CVD = 3)	IHD = 10 [low]	IHD = 7 [moderate]	IHD = 19 [low]	IHD = 15 [low]	IHD = 8 [insufficient]	IHD = 12 [low]	IHD = 24 [moderate]	IHD = 7 [insufficient] CVD = 3 [insufficient]	IHD = 4 [insufficient]
VASP (total = 19; IHD = 18; IHD, CVD, PAD = 1)	IHD = 4 [insufficient]	IHD = 6 [insufficient]	IHD = 6 [low]	IHD = 10 [low]	IHD = 1 [insufficient]	IHD = 1 [insufficient]	IHD = 8 [low] IHD, CVD, PAD = 1 [insufficient]	IHD = 4 [insufficient]	IHD = 7 [insufficient]
Multiplate analyzer (total = 18; IHD = 17; CVD = 1)	IHD = 6 [insufficient]	IHD = 5 [insufficient]	IHD = 9 [insufficient]	IHD = 10 [insufficient]	IHD = 3 [insufficient]	IHD = 9 [insufficient]	IHD = 13 [insufficient] CVD = 1 [insufficient]	IHD = 6 [insufficient]	IHD = 2 [insufficient]
TEG (total = 6; IHD = 6)	IHD = 2 [insufficient]	No studies	IHD = 2 [insufficient]	IHD = 1 [insufficient]	IHD = 1 [insufficient]	IHD = 3 [insufficient]	IHD = 4 [insufficient]	No studies	No studies
PFA-100 (total = 11; IHD = 10; IHD, CVD, PAD = 1)	IHD = 2 [insufficient]	IHD = 2 [insufficient]	IHD = 5 [insufficient]	IHD = 3 [insufficient]	IHD = 1 [insufficient]	IHD = 1 [insufficient]	IHD = 9 [low] IHD, CVD, PAD = 1 [insufficient]	IHD = 2 [insufficient]	IHD = 1 [insufficient]
Other (total = 9; IHD = 9)	IHD = 3 [insufficient]	No studies	IHD = 3 [insufficient]	IHD = 1 [insufficient]	IHD =1 [insufficient]	IHD = 2 [insufficient]	IHD = 6 [insufficient]	IHD = 3 [insufficient]	IHD = 3 [insufficient]

Note: Numbers indicate the number of available studies for each test-outcome combination in the population specified. Studies could have involved more than 1 combination. Text in brackets reflects our assessment of the strength of evidence for each test-outcome association.

ACS = acute coronary syndromes; CV = cardiovascular; CVD = cerebrovascular disease; IHD = ischemic heart disease; LTA = light-transmission aggregometry; MACE = major adverse cardiovascular events; PAD = peripheral arterial disease; PFA = Platelet Function Analyzer; ST = stent thrombosis; TEG = thromboelastography; VASP = vasodilator-stimulated phosphoprotein

LTA in Ischemic Heart Disease

Fifty-three studies included patients with ischemic heart disease and reported information on the predictive value of LTA for clinical outcomes (47 studies) and platelet reactivity (11 studies). Four studies reported both clinical and intermediate outcomes. Thirty-eight of the 53 studies enrolled patients with chronic stable coronary artery disease, 12 enrolled patients with acute coronary syndromes, and 3 enrolled mixed populations with chronic and acute presentations. Most studies used ADP as the agonist to assess reactivity but a few used ADP in combination with arachidonic acid (AA) to assess the response to both clopidogrel and aspirin. The strength of evidence for the prognostic effect of high platelet reactivity as measured by LTA on the following outcomes was considered low on the basis of clinical heterogeneity, variation in the metrics and cutoffs used to define reactivity, and imprecision of the study-level estimates of effect.

All-Cause Mortality (13 Studies; 12 ADP, 1 ADP + AA)

Studies did not suggest an association between increased platelet reactivity as measured by LTA and increased all-cause mortality in patients with ischemic heart disease.

Cardiovascular Mortality (9 Studies; 8 ADP, 1 ADP + AA)

Studies suggested an association between increased platelet reactivity as measured by LTA and cardiovascular mortality in patients with ischemic heart disease.

Acute Coronary Syndromes (18 Studies; 17 ADP, 1 ADP + AA)

Overall, results provided some evidence of an association between increased platelet reactivity as measured by LTA and increased risk of acute coronary syndromes in patients with ischemic heart disease.

Stent Thrombosis (19 Studies; 17 ADP, 2 ADP + AA)

Nineteen studies reported information on the ability of platelet reactivity as measured by LTA to predict stent thrombosis. Three publications reported data from the same population. Taken together, the studies suggested an association between increased platelet reactivity and increased risk of stent thrombosis in patients with ischemic heart disease.

MACE (37 Studies; 35 ADP, 2 ADP + AA)

Three of the 37 studies reported data from the same population. We evaluated data for the longest followup time available. All studies used ADP as the agonist to measure platelet reactivity; two studies used ADP in combination with AA to assess the response to both clopidogrel and aspirin. The majority of reviewed studies suggested an association between increased platelet reactivity as measured by LTA and increased risk of MACE.

Stroke (12 Studies; 11 ADP, 1 ADP + AA)

The 12 reviewed studies did not suggest an association between increased platelet reactivity as measured by LTA and increased stroke in patients with ischemic heart disease.

VerifyNow P2Y12 in Ischemic Heart Disease

Thirty-five studies included patients with ischemic heart disease and reported information on the predictive value of the VerifyNow P2Y12 assay. Of these, 33 assessed the value of the test for predicting clinical outcomes, and 3 for predicting platelet reactivity during followup. Two studies reported both clinical and platelet reactivity outcomes. Of the 35 studies, 21 enrolled patients with chronic stable coronary artery disease, 12 enrolled patients with acute coronary syndromes, and 2 enrolled a mixed population with chronic and acute presentations.

All-Cause Mortality (10 Studies; 9 ADP, 1 ADP + AA)

A meta-analysis of three studies that used ADP as the agonist and defined high platelet reactivity on the basis of platelet reactivity units found a summary RR of 1.21 (95% CI, 0.83 to 1.77; p=0.313), indicating a nonsignificant association between high platelet reactivity and all-cause mortality. There was little evidence of between-study heterogeneity (P_Q=0.902; I^2=0%). Meta-analysis was not performed for the four other studies, which either used percent platelet inhibition to define reactivity or defined reactivity using a different cutoff.

Cardiovascular Mortality (7 Studies, All ADP)

A meta-analysis of the four studies that used cutoff values based on platelet reactivity units found a summary RR of 2.50 (95% CI, 1.28 to 4.87; p=0.007), indicating a significant association between high platelet reactivity and cardiovascular mortality. There was little evidence of between-study heterogeneity (P_Q=0.527; I^2=0%). The three studies not included in the meta-analysis did not report a significant association between higher platelet reactivity and increased cardiovascular mortality.

Acute Coronary Syndromes (19 Studies; 16 ADP, 1 ADP + AA)

Nineteen studies reported information on the ability of the VerifyNow P2Y12 assay to predict myocardial infarction in patients receiving clopidogrel-based treatment. Taken together, the studies suggested an association between increased platelet reactivity as measured by VerifyNow and increased rates of both periprocedural and nonperiprocedural acute coronary syndromes in patients with ischemic heart disease. However, the strength of evidence for this association was considered low on the basis of variability in the metrics and thresholds used to define reactivity and heterogeneity of the included patient populations.

Stent Thrombosis (15 Studies; All ADP)

Fifteen studies reported information on the ability of the VerifyNow P2Y12 assay to predict stent thrombosis in patients receiving clopidogrel-based treatment. Of these, 11 did not report statistically significant results and produced relatively wide CIs, indicating substantial uncertainty around estimates of the RR; 4 studies reported statistically significant associations between high reactivity with risk of stent thrombosis. Because of heterogeneity in the metrics used to define platelet reactivity, meta-analysis was possible only for six studies that used the same metrics and cutoffs for reactivity. The summary RR was 1.67 (95% CI, 0.80 to 3.47; p=0.172). There was some evidence of between-study heterogeneity (P_Q=0.159; I^2=37%). Considering all studies, there was weak evidence to support an association between increased platelet reactivity as measured by VerifyNow and stent thrombosis in patients with ischemic heart disease.

MACE (24 Studies; 23 ADP, 1 ADP + AA)

One study that used both ADP and AA to identify a population of responders to both clopidogrel and aspirin reported significantly higher odds of MACE in those who were clopidogrel nonresponders (irrespective of aspirin response status) compared with responders. A meta-analysis was done of 13 of the 23 remaining studies that enrolled nonoverlapping patient populations and used cutoff values for platelet reactivity based on platelet reactivity units. The summary RR was 2.48 (95%, CI, 1.86 to 3.32; p<0.001) and there was evidence of moderate heterogeneity (P_Q=0.045; I^2=44%) and statistically significant small-study effects. Ten studies were not included in the meta-analysis due to differing definitions of reactivity, poor reporting, and patient overlap. Specifically, five studies used percentage of platelet inhibition to define platelet reactivity; two used a different cutoff to define reactivity; two studies did not provide adequate data for inclusion; and one overlapped with another publication that had larger sample size. Among the five studies that used percentage of platelet inhibition to define platelet reactivity, three studies reported significantly higher rates of MACE and one study reported nonsignificantly higher rates of MACE at 6 months or 1 year in those with a low response to clopidogrel. In contrast, one study reported lower rates of MACE at 30 days in those with a low response to clopidogrel.

Bleeding Events (12 Studies; All ADP)

A meta-analysis of six nonoverlapping studies with similar reactivity cutoffs found no significant difference by reactivity status for either all bleeding events (4 studies; RR=1.09; 95% CI, 0.88 to 1.37; p=0.421) with little evidence of heterogeneity (P_Q=0.738; I^2=0%) or severe bleeding events (4 studies; RR=0.85; 95% CI, 0.32 to 2.25; p=0.738) with evidence of moderate heterogeneity (P_Q=0.074; I^2=57%). Four other studies with different cutoff values reported lower but not statistically significantly different rates of major and minor bleeding for patients with a low response to clopidogrel (compared with responders), and a fifth study did not report any bleeding events.

VASP Assay With Flow Cytometry in Ischemic Heart Disease

Eighteen studies included patients with ischemic heart disease and reported information on the predictive value of the VASP assay. Of these, 13 assessed the value of the test for predicting clinical outcomes, 6 assessed the value for predicting platelet reactivity during followup, and 1 reported both clinical and platelet reactivity outcome. Eight studies enrolled patients with acute coronary syndromes, five enrolled patients with chronic stable coronary artery disease, and five enrolled mixed populations with chronic and acute presentations.

Acute Coronary Syndromes (6 Studies; All ADP)

One study reported that no events were observed regardless of platelet reactivity status and thus was not included in meta-analysis. Of the remaining five studies, two were nonoverlapping. The other three had overlapping study populations and enrollment periods, so in meta-analysis we used data from the publication reporting the largest number of events. A meta-analysis of the three studies, all of which used cutoff values based on the platelet reactivity index, found a summary RR of 1.47 (95% CI, 0.77 to 2.794; p=0.246). There was little evidence of between-study heterogeneity (P_Q=0.372; I^2=0%).

Stent Thrombosis (10 Studies; All ADP)

Two studies reported that no events were observed regardless of platelet reactivity status and thus were not included in meta-analysis. Of the remaining eight studies, three were nonoverlapping. The other five had overlapping study populations and enrollment periods, so in meta-analysis we used data from the publication reporting the largest number of events. A meta-analysis of the four studies found a summary RR of 3.37 (95% CI, 1.59 to 7.1; p=0.015), indicating a statistically significant association between high platelet reactivity and stent thrombosis. There was no evidence of between-study heterogeneity (P_Q=0.487; I^2=0%).

MACE (8 Studies; All ADP)

Two publications involved overlapping study populations; in meta-analysis we included data from the publication reporting the largest total number of cardiovascular events. A meta-analysis of the six nonoverlapping studies found a summary RR of 2.57 (95% CI, 1.21 to 5.47; p=0.015), indicating a statistically significant association between high platelet reactivity measured by the VASP assay and MACE. There was evidence of moderate between-study heterogeneity (P_Q=0.044; I^2=56%).

Multiplate Analyzer, Thromboelastography, and PFA-100 in Ischemic Heart Disease

The strength of evidence was insufficient for all outcomes for these three tests.

Comparative Studies of Test Performance Among Platelet Reactivity Assays

Twelve studies reported extractable information on clinical outcomes for at least two of the assessed tests. We focused on outcomes that were addressed by at least 3 comparative studies: major adverse cardiovascular events (composite outcome, 10 studies) and stent thrombosis (4 studies). The data could not be quantitatively synthesized because the studies involved several assays being applied to the same patient population, in which case results are likely to be correlated because the population is shared and assays done on samples of the same blood will yield correlated, if not identical, results.

MACE (Comparative Studies)

Ten studies reported comparative information regarding the ability of assays to predict MACE. The most commonly used test was LTA, which was compared with various tests (most often thromboelastography and VerifyNow P2Y12). Overall, point estimates were similar between alternative test methods within each study and CIs were overlapping, suggesting that the predictive ability of the compared tests is fairly similar.

Stent Thrombosis (Comparative Studies)

Four studies reported comparative information regarding the ability of assays to predict stent thrombosis for patients undergoing PCI with stent implantation. LTA was used in three studies, and the VerifyNow P2Y12 and PFA-100 assays were each used in two studies. Point estimates were variable within each study. However, CIs were extremely wide and overlapping, suggesting that there is substantial uncertainty regarding the relative predictive ability of the compared tests for stent thrombosis and that there is substantial uncertainty regarding comparative test performance for this outcome.

Comparative Studies of Test Performance of Genetic Testing for CYP2C19 Variants and Phenotypic Testing for Platelet Reactivity

Four studies reported information on the prognostic value of genetic and phenotypic tests for MACE and three for stent thrombosis. For each of the four studies, we plotted the points corresponding to each assay's sensitivity and specificity in the receiver operating characteristic space. Points were often close to the chance diagonal, indicating that test performance was generally poor. However, the paucity of data did not allow firm conclusions.

Key Question 2c: Factors Affecting the Predictive Value of Phenotypic Testing for Platelet Reactivity

We reviewed studies to identify any evidence that patient- or system-level factors or test characteristics could modify the predictive ability of phenotypic testing for platelet reactivity. As for Key Question 1c, we considered both within-study information (e.g., studies where the predictive effect of phenotypic testing was evaluated in two or more patient subgroups) and information across studies (through metaregression analyses on study-level factors).

Effect Modification Within Studies

In total, seven studies reported information on effect modification of the predictive effect of platelet reactivity. All studies reported information on clinical outcomes. Only a small subset of the eligible studies provided information adequate to statistically assess effect modification, and selective reporting was highly likely. Studies assessed the following factors as potential modifiers: the use of glycoprotein IIb/IIIa inhibitors as an adjunct treatment for PCI (two studies), diabetes mellitus (two studies), and chronic kidney disease (one study). Two studies used the VASP assay to assess platelet reactivity; two used the VerifyNow P2Y12 assay (one of which also used the VerifyNow ASA, which uses arachidonic acid as the agonist to measure "aspirin resistance"); and one used LTA (with ADP as the agonist). Statistically significant interaction effects were reported only in the study that assessed whether coexisting chronic kidney disease in patients with coronary artery disease modified the predictive value of the VASP assay. The study found that high on-clopidogrel platelet reactivity had statistically significantly greater effects on several clinical outcomes (all-cause mortality, cardiac death, and a composite outcome of all-cause mortality, myocardial infarction, or target-lesion revascularization) in patients with chronic kidney disease than in those without chronic kidney disease.

Effect Modification Across Studies

In analyses across studies (metaregression) the following factors did not statistically significantly modify the prognostic value of the VerifyNow P2Y12 assay on MACE (the only test-outcome combination with 10 or more available studies): disease subtype (acute coronary syndromes vs. coronary artery disease); duration of followup (≤30 days vs. >30 days); and year when enrollment was started (continuous variable).

Effect Modification Summary

In general, information on effect modification was limited, both within and across studies. Few studies reported information on the same potential effect modifiers, results were imprecise, and selective reporting was highly likely. Information across studies was also limited by the number of available studies on each test and outcome of interest. It is unclear whether the predictive effect of phenotypic testing differs across patient subgroups.

Key Question 3a: Comparative Effectiveness of Alternative Test-and-Treat Strategies

We grouped the studies we identified for this Key Question into three categories:

1. *Randomized trials of test-and-treat strategies*: These studies randomize patients to alternative management strategies, at least one of which is based on a test of interest. Patients are then followed up for intermediate or clinical outcomes.
2. *Randomized treatment trials that evaluate treatment-effect modification:* These are randomized studies in which patients in all groups undergo the test of interest at baseline. Treatment assignment is based on randomization and thus is independent of test results. Because these studies include both test-positive and test-negative patients in each treatment arm, they can be used to assess test result × treatment interactions.
3. *Randomized trials with test-based selection:* These studies select patients on the basis of baseline test results and then randomize them into non–test-based treatment groups. When properly randomized and conducted, these studies can provide unconfounded estimates of the treatment effect conditional on a particular test result.

Genetic Testing for CYP2C19 Variants

Studies of Test-and-Treat Strategies

We identified a single-center pilot study with low risk of bias that compared a strategy of testing for CYP2C19 variants versus no testing to guide treatment decisionmaking in a predominantly white population (95%). The study randomized 200 adult patients undergoing PCI for the treatment of non-ST-segment-elevation acute coronary syndrome or stable CAD to a treatment group guided by CYP2C19 genotyping or a control group with no testing.

Clinical Outcomes

The study reported information on a composite outcome of cardiovascular death, nonfatal myocardial infarction, readmission to hospital, and stent thrombosis. Twenty-three (25%) of 91 patients assigned to the rapid genotyping group were CYP2C19*2 carriers (4 were homozygotes); 23 (24%) of 96 in the standard therapy group were CYP2C19 *2 carriers (3 were homozygotes). No clinical adverse ischemic outcomes were observed in either group at 7 or 20 days of followup.

Intermediate Outcome: Platelet Reactivity During Followup

Intermediate outcomes were assessed with the VerifyNow P2Y12 assay. The primary study endpoint was the proportion of CYP2C19*2 carriers with a P2Y12 reactivity unit (PRU) value of more than 234 after 1 week of dual antiplatelet therapy. The results indicated that platelet reactivity at the last followup assessment was lower in the groups that received test-based treatment than in those that did not undergo testing.

Randomized Trials Reporting Information on Treatment-Effect Modification by CYP2C19 Genotype Status

We identified 13 publications (reporting on 12 study populations) describing randomized controlled trials that provide information on effect modification by CYP2C19 variants. Six studies provided information on clinical outcomes, five on intermediate outcomes (platelet reactivity during followup), and one on both types of outcome.

Clinical Outcomes

Six studies (reported in seven publications[c]) provided clinical outcome information. Five of the six studies were large (>1,000 participants), multicenter, randomized trials of clopidogrel-based treatment versus alternative treatments and had at least one outcome event. The sixth study, a smaller, single-center trial with a followup of 30 days, reported that no clinical outcomes of interest were observed. Studies used robust methods for randomization and allocation concealment.

The five larger studies were the CURE (Clopidogrel in Unstable Angina to Prevent Recurrent Events) trial, which included patients with non–ST-elevation acute coronary syndromes; the PLATO (Platelet inhibition and patient Outcomes) trial, which involved patients with ST-elevation or non–ST-elevation acute coronary syndromes; the TRITON-TIMI 38 (Trial to Assess Improvement in Therapeutic Outcomes by Optimizing Platelet Inhibition with Prasugrel–Thrombolysis in Myocardial Infarction 38), which included those with moderate- to high-risk acute coronary syndromes who were undergoing PCI; the CHARISMA (Clopidogrel for High Atherothrombotic Risk and Ischemic Stabilization, Management and Avoidance) trial, which included a mixed population of patients with manifest thrombotic disease (coronary, cerebrovascular, and peripheral arterial disease) along with individuals at high risk for developing atherothrombotic disease; and ACTIVE A, which enrolled patients with atrial fibrillation who were not candidates for vitamin K antagonist therapy. CURE, CHARISMA, and ACTIVE A compared aspirin plus clopidogrel (at standard doses) with aspirin monotherapy, TRITON-TIMI 38 compared aspirin plus clopidogrel versus aspirin plus prasugrel, and the PLATO trial compared aspirin plus clopidogrel versus aspirin plus ticagrelor. All trials were designed and powered to detect the main effect of antiplatelet therapy but were not specifically powered to detect heterogeneity of treatment effects and typically included only a subsample of the overall trial population.

The CURE, PLATO, CHARISMA, and ACTIVE A trials did not find statistically significant effect modification by CYP2C19 genotype for any of their efficacy outcomes. The genetic substudy of TRITON-TIMI 38 reported statistically significant treatment-effect heterogeneity among genotype groups (at least one loss-of-function allele vs. none; p=0.046), with prasugrel being superior to clopidogrel among carriers of loss-of-function CYP2C19 alleles. Overall the available studies do not suggest that CYP2C19 genotype status is a strong modifier of the treatment effects evaluated in the studies. However, these studies included only small subsets, 15 to 40 percent of the original trial populations, suggesting that selection bias may have affected their results. This was a concern particularly for the CHARISMA trial, in which differences in baseline characteristics and outcome rates were observed between the patients included and those not included in the genetic substudy. Furthermore, details were not provided regarding the timing

---

[c]Five publications reported information on a single population each and one publication reported information on two independent populations.

of obtaining samples for genetic analyses, but samples were generally not obtained at the trial baseline. In such cases, survivor bias, another form of selection bias, may also affect study results.

Because of the large differences in included populations, treatments compared, and exposure and outcome definitions among studies reporting on treatment-effect modification by CYP2C19 variants on clinical outcomes, we did not perform a meta-analysis. Given that comparators (placebo, prasugrel, or ticagrelor) differed across studies, it is plausible that interaction effects could have different magnitudes or directions. For purposes of illustration, we used the counts reported in the studies to compare the treatment effect among carriers of CYP2C19 loss-of-function alleles versus noncarriers (i.e., those with normal or gain-of-function alleles), as shown in Figure B.

Figure B. Results from large randomized trials assessing effect modification by CYP2C19 variants on MACE

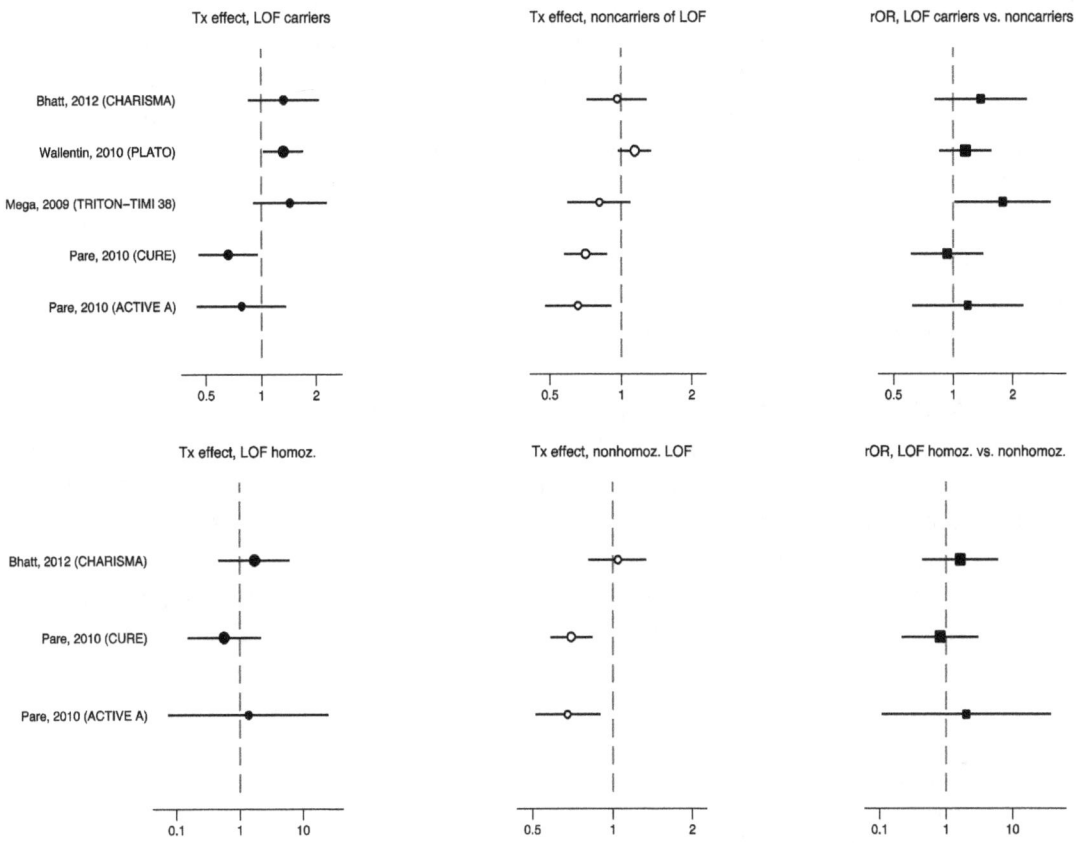

Note: The top set of panels presents forest plots of treatment effects (odds ratios) on MACE among carriers of at least 1 LOF allele (top left panel), treatment effects among noncarriers of LOF alleles (top middle panel), and relative effects (rOR) comparing the treatment effect among LOF carriers and LOF noncarriers (top right panel). The bottom set of panels presents forest plots of treatment effects on MACE among homozygotes for 2 LOF alleles (bottom left panel), treatment effects among nonhomozygotes of LOF alleles (bottom middle panel), and relative effects (rOR) comparing the treatment effect among homozygotes and nonhomozygotes of LOF alleles (bottom right panel). Two studies did not provide adequate data for the comparisons of homozygotes and nonhomozygotes. The CURE, CHARISMA, and ACTIVE A trials compared aspirin plus clopidogrel vs. aspirin monotherapy; the TRITON-TIMI 38 trial compared aspirin plus clopidogrel vs. aspirin plus prasugrel; the PLATO trial compared aspirin plus clopidogrel vs. aspirin plus ticagrelor. Point estimates for treatment effects are shown as black circles (carriers) or white circles (noncarriers); point estimates for relative treatment effects are shown as black squares. For all symbols, size is inversely proportional to the standard error of each estimate. Horizontal lines denote 95% confidence intervals for all estimates. Vertical dashed lines denote no effect. Please see Tables 18 and 19 in the full report for definitions of the genotype categories and outcomes reported by each study. References to individual studies are provided in Table 5 of the main report.

ACTIVE A = Atrial Fibrillation Clopidogrel Trial with Irbesartan for Prevention of Vascular Events A; CHARISMA = Clopidogrel for High Atherothrombotic Risk and Ischemic Stabilization, Management and Avoidance; CURE = Clopidogrel in Unstable Angina to Prevent Recurrent Events trial; homoz. = homozygotes; LOF = loss of function; MACE = major adverse cardiovascular events; nonhomoz. = nonhomozygotes; PLATO = Platelet inhibition and patient Outcomes trial; rOR = relative odds ratio; TRITON-TIMI 38 = Trial to Assess Improvement in Therapeutic Outcomes by Optimizing Platelet Inhibition with Prasugrel–Thrombolysis in Myocardial Infarction; Tx = treatment.

Intermediate Outcome: Platelet Reactivity During Followup

Seven studies assessing treatment-effect modification by CYP2C19 variants provided information on platelet reactivity during followup as an intermediate outcome. All seven were based on randomized trials comparing clopidogrel-based treatment with alternative therapies, had small to moderate sample sizes (range, 60 to 474 participants), and enrolled heterogeneous populations of patients with acute or chronic coronary artery disease. In this group of studies, 79 to 100 percent of the patients enrolled were included in the genetic substudies, suggesting that selection bias was unlikely. All had short followup periods (<7 days to 6 weeks), and they generally provided adequate descriptions of the methods used for generating the randomization sequence but did not provide sufficient information to assess methods of allocation concealment.

The studies differed in the alleles genotyped and the genotype groupings used. Platelet reactivity during followup was assessed by the VerifyNow P2Y12 assay in all seven studies, as well as by LTA in four studies and the VASP assay (based on flow cytometry) in two studies. Because of the differences in designs, populations, treatments compared, and followup durations among the included studies, we did not perform a meta-analysis. The overall results were variable and no conclusions could be drawn.

Studies With Genetic Test–Based Selection of Patients

We identified a single multicenter trial (ELEVATE-TIMI 56) that used genetic–test-based selection of patients and then randomized them to alternative antiplatelet treatments. The study enrolled 335 patients with known cardiovascular disease (57.1% with a history of myocardial infarction; 97.3% with a history of PCI) on maintenance clopidogrel therapy (75 mg daily). The trial was well conducted, with centralized randomization and blinding of both patients and outcome assessors (both for clinical and intermediate outcomes) to the treatment assessment. The sample size was based on a priori power analysis for platelet reactivity outcomes and the recruitment target was attained. There were minimal dropouts and losses to followup.

Clinical Outcomes

The study reported no deaths or cerebrovascular events. However, it was not powered to provide robust evidence on clinical outcomes and did not have adequate followup to do so. Among CYP2C19*2 noncarriers, two patients had cardiac ischemic events while taking the 75 mg dose and three with the 150 mg dose. Among carriers of a CYP2C19*2 allele, one patient experienced a cardiac ischemic event while taking the 75 mg clopidogrel dose.

Intermediate Outcome: Platelet Reactivity During Followup

Intermediate outcomes were assessed with the VASP assay (primary analysis) and the VerifyNow assay (secondary analysis). When treated with a standard clopidogrel maintenance dose of 75 mg/day, both CYP2C19*2 heterozygotes and homozygotes had significantly higher on-treatment platelet reactivity than did noncarrier patients (p<0.001 for both pairwise comparisons). Among CYP2C19*2 heterozygotes, higher clopidogrel maintenance doses up to 300 mg produced significant reductions in platelet reactivity (p<0.001 for trend). Results with the VerifyNow assay were similar to the VASP data across dose and genotype. Among CYP2C19*2 homozygotes, there was a trend toward less platelet reactivity with higher maintenance doses of clopidogrel; however, even with 300 mg daily of clopidogrel, these individuals had increased reactivity as measured by VASP and VerifyNow. In CYP2C19*2 heterozygotes, 150 mg resulted in platelet reactivity that tended to be higher than that seen in noncarrier patients treated with 75 mg daily. For CYP2C19*2 homozygotes, even 300 mg daily of clopidogrel did not result in platelet reactivity levels similar to those with standard clopidogrel dosing in noncarriers.

Phenotypic Testing for Platelet Reactivity

Studies of Test-and-Treat Strategies

We identified seven studies directly comparing alternative test-and-treat strategies. Six of the seven studies had a randomized design, and one was a nonrandomized comparative study of test-and-treat strategies. Generally, the randomized trials had moderate risk of bias, were prospectively conducted, and performed phenotypic testing immediately after sample collection, without knowledge of clinical or intermediate outcomes. However, information to judge whether outcomes were assessed without knowledge of the index-test result was often not reported. Subjects and personnel were not blinded, and reporting was incomplete regarding the methods of generating the randomization sequence and concealing allocation. The single nonrandomized comparative study had high risk of bias because the two groups being compared (test-guided treatment and non–test guided treatment) were enrolled in different research institutions, increasing the probability that results were affected by confounding or selection bias. Four studies evaluating the use of the VASP assay were of moderate size (the smallest enrolling 153 patients; the largest, 429 patients); three were multicenter studies; and 1 was a single-center investigation. One randomized controlled trial (RCT) evaluating the use of the Multiplate analyzer enrolled 192, patients and one nonrandomized comparative study evaluating the same assay enrolled 798 patients. The single study assessing VerifyNow was smaller (60 patients) and was conducted in a single research center.

The six RCTs directly comparing alternative test-and-treat strategies assessed patients undergoing PCI. Four enrolled patients with stable coronary artery disease or acute coronary syndromes, and one enrolled exclusively patients undergoing elective stenting. The experimental groups in five studies (three using the VASP assay, one using the VerifyNow assay, and one using the Multiplate analyzer) employed repeat reactivity monitoring at multiple time points with modification of the administered clopidogrel dose on the basis of test results. The other two studies performed only a single assessment of platelet reactivity, with subsequent treatment modification in patients found to have reactivity values above a predefined threshold. Control groups were given clopidogrel-based therapy at standard doses. Four studies reported a prospective power calculation and enrollment goal, which was met in all cases.

Clinical Outcomes

All seven studies comparing alternative test-and-treat strategies reported information on cardiovascular mortality. In addition, six reported on MACE (composite outcomes), five on stent thrombosis, three on acute coronary syndromes (myocardial infarction or unstable angina), three on myocardial infarction alone, two on all-cause mortality, and two on repeat revascularization. Overall, the studies had short followup durations and included moderate numbers of participants; thus, the outcome rates were low, and relative effect estimates (when possible to calculate) were often extreme (e.g., odds ratios <0.5) and had substantial uncertainty (wide CIs). Studies generally indicated that the groups with test-based monitoring had better outcomes (lower event rates) than the groups without test-based monitoring; however, the differences were often not statistically significant. Meta-analyses were not performed, owing to the differences in the populations included, interventions compared, and durations of followup used.

Intermediate Outcome: Platelet Reactivity During Followup

Four of the seven studies directly comparing alternative test-and-treat strategies reported information on platelet reactivity as an intermediate outcome. Although results generally indicated that platelet reactivity at the last followup assessment was lower in the groups that received test-based treatment than in those that received standard treatment, reporting was often incomplete and precluded statistical comparisons between groups. Furthermore, studies had short followup periods, and it was unclear whether the observed differences in reactivity affected clinical outcomes.

Studies of Treatment-Effect Modification by Baseline Platelet Reactivity

We identified three studies reporting information on effect modification by baseline platelet reactivity in patients randomized to alternative antiplatelet therapies.

Clinical Outcomes

One study, a platelet reactivity substudy of the ISAR-REACT 4 trial (Intracoronary Stenting and Antithrombotic Regimen: Rapid Early Action for Coronary Treatment-4), reported information on clinical outcomes. In the platelet sub-cohort of this trial, 205 patients (36%) had high on-clopidogrel platelet reactivity at the time of PCI (35.0% in the abciximab plus heparin group vs. 37.6% in the bivalirudin group). A significant interaction was observed between study treatment arm and platelet aggregation regarding the combined efficacy endpoint (death, myocardial infarction, or urgent target vessel revascularization; P for interaction = 0.037). This study was considered to have moderate risk of bias because the patient population was not representative of the parent trial population, suggesting the possibility of selection bias.

Intermediate Outcome: Platelet Reactivity During Followup

Two studies reported information on platelet reactivity during followup. The first study was a post hoc evaluation based on a crossover RCT comparing triple therapy (aspirin + clopidogrel + cilostazol) with double therapy (aspirin + clopidogrel + placebo) for patients with stable coronary artery disease. Based on the study results, we estimated that baseline platelet reactivity did not modify the effect of cilostazol on subsequent measurements. This study was considered to have high risk of bias because it was a post hoc assessment based on a convenience sample enrolled in a crossover trial and because the parent trial had a large withdrawal rate (23%). The second study reported the response rate among "poor responders" to the clopidogrel loading dose during prasugrel-based therapy and during clopidogrel-based therapy. Generally the response rates were higher during prasugrel therapy, regardless of the assay used to assess platelet reactivity. However, the study did not report the response status during followup for patients who were "responders" to the clopidogrel loading dose. Thus, the interaction between post–loading-dose response to clopidogrel and treatment assignment could not be assessed. This study was considered to have a high risk of bias because of incomplete outcome reporting and because information on the generation of the randomized sequence and allocation concealment was unclear.

Studies With Phenotypic Test–Based Selection of Patients

Fourteen studies met our inclusion criteria and reported information on the comparative effectiveness of treatments administered to patients selected on the basis of baseline platelet reactivity. The sample sizes ranged from 21 to more than 2,000 participants, and all 14 studies were relatively recent (published in 2008–2012). Only two trials, the GRAVITAS multicenter trial (Gauging Responsiveness with a VerifyNow Assay—Impact on Thrombosis and Safety) and the TRIGGER PCI trial (Testing Platelet Reactivity In Patients Undergoing Elective Stent Placement on Clopidogrel to Guide Alternative Therapy With Prasugrel), reported data from more than 100 randomized patients. Eleven studies were performed mainly or exclusively in the PCI setting, two studies included patients with stable coronary artery disease (noninterventional setting), and one study enrolled patients on chronic hemodialysis receiving clopidogrel treatment. On-clopidogrel platelet reactivity was used as a selection criterion in all studies; it was assessed using the VerifyNow P2Y12 assay in nine studies, LTA in three studies, the VASP assay with flow cytometry in two studies, and other assays in two studies. (One study combined measurements from three assays to define high on-treatment reactivity.) The treatment comparisons were between standard-dose clopidogrel-based therapy and high-dose clopidogrel in six studies, prasugrel in four studies, ticagrelor in two studies, and addition of a glycoprotein IIb/IIIa inhibitor in two studies.

Overall, the risk of bias varied across studies. The GRAVITAS trial had low risk of bias, both regarding aspects related to the index test of interest and regarding general aspects of randomized trial design (e.g., generation of the randomization sequence and allocation concealment). The TRIGGER-PCI trial did not provide adequate information about the randomization procedure and allocation concealment or blinding of patients to treatment assignment; however outcomes assessors were blinded to treatment assignment. Smaller studies (typically with short-term followup) were generally considered to have a higher risk of bias, owing to problems in the application of the tests of interest (e.g., an unclear rationale for the thresholds used) or incomplete reporting of outcomes. Furthermore, these studies often did not provide information sufficient to judge their risk of bias regarding general aspects of randomized trial design.

Clinical Outcomes

Clinical-outcome comparisons between the randomized treatment groups were reported in 10 of the 14 studies. Here, we discuss only the results of the two larger trials (GRAVITAS and TRIGGER-PCI). The remaining 12 studies had smaller sample sizes, ranging from 21 to 159 patients, and also had short followup durations. Information on these trials is presented in the full report.

The GRAVITAS trial (2,214 randomized patients) included patients who had undergone PCI for stable coronary artery disease or non-ST-segment-elevation acute coronary syndrome and showed increased on-clopidogrel reactivity on the VerifyNow P2Y12 assay. The patients were randomized to high-dose clopidogrel or standard-dose clopidogrel, both in combination with aspirin. After 6 months of followup, there was no statistically significant difference between the randomized groups in the rate of cardiovascular death, nonfatal myocardial infarction, stent thrombosis, all-cause mortality, or composite cardiovascular outcomes, either (1) cardiovascular death or nonfatal myocardial infarction or (2) cardiovascular death, nonfatal myocardial infarction, or stent thrombosis. The study also included followup information for a randomly selected group of patients with low platelet reactivity at baseline who were treated with standard-dose clopidogrel. (See the Results section for Key Question 1b for details.)

The TRIGGER-PCI study compared prasugrel versus standard-dose clopidogrel in 423 patients with high on-clopidogrel platelet reactivity as measured by the VerifyNow P2Y12 assay. After 236 patients had completed the planned 6-month followup, a blinded interim review identified a single primary endpoint event. Because of the very low event rate, the trial was terminated early for futility. As such, for all outcomes, event rates were very low and differences in event rates between groups were not statistically significant. Across all 10 studies reporting data on clinical outcomes, patient populations were heterogeneous, selected on the basis of different inclusion criteria, and assessed using different therapeutic regimens. For these reasons, we did not perform meta-analyses for any of the clinical outcomes reported.

Intermediate Outcome: Platelet Reactivity During Followup

Ten studies reported information on intermediate outcomes. Eight studies had a total duration of 3 months or less; five studies had a crossover design. The outcomes were assessed using different assays and were heterogeneously reported. Generally, patients on higher dose clopidogrel regimens and those receiving prasugrel showed greater responses in platelet reactivity compared with those receiving standard-dose clopidogrel regimens.

Combined Genetic Testing for CYP2C19 Variants and Phenotypic Testing To Guide Antiplatelet Treatment

We identified four studies providing information on test-based treatment strategies that also provided information on the CYP2C19 genotype of participants. All four studies reported genetic analyses based on randomized trials that had enrolled patients on the basis of baseline platelet reactivity testing. Briefly, two of the studies were conducted in the setting of small (21 and 64 patients) crossover RCTs of short duration (30 and 60 days); one was based on a short-term parallel-arm trial (2 weeks of followup); and one study (GIFT—Genotype Information and Functional Testing) was conducted in the setting of the large GRAVITAS trial with a followup of 6 months. Analyses stratified by treatment and genotype status were not reported for clinical outcomes, and all four studies reported results for the intermediate outcome of platelet reactivity. Studies did not report significant effect modification by genotype for this outcome. (All analyses assumed a dominant model for loss-of-function alleles; analyses under an alternative model were not possible.) In general, results were inconclusive because studies were small and none had been prospectively powered specifically to assess effect modification by genotype.

Key Question 3b: Factors Modifying the Comparative Effectiveness of Alternative Test-and-Treat Strategies

Only four of the studies considered relevant to Key Question 3a provided information about the use of testing for clinical decisionmaking with data stratified by patient characteristics: ancestry in two, baseline percent inhibition of on-clopidogrel reactivity in one, diabetes status in one, and history of PCI and symptomatic atherothrombosis on trial entry in one. None of the factors appeared to statistically significantly affect study results relevant to the use of testing to guide antiplatelet therapy.

Key Question 4: Harms of Testing and of Test-Directed Treatment

Harms of Test-Directed Treatment

All studies addressing Key Question 4 were also included in Key Question 3a; assessment of the risk-of-bias of individual studies is addressed in that section. We discuss studies belonging to each of three designs—studies of test-and-treat strategies, studies of treatment-effect modification, and studies with test-based selection—separately for genetic testing (for CYP2C19 variants) and for phenotypic testing (of platelet reactivity).

Genetic Testing for CYP2C19 Variants

We identified a single study comparing testing for CYP2C19 variants against a no-testing strategy to guide treatment decisionmaking. The study monitored major and minor bleeding using the thrombolysis in myocardial infarction (TIMI) classification over 30 days of followup. The frequency of minor and major bleeding was not different between the study groups.

Studies of Treatment-Effect Modification by CYP2C19 Genotype Status

Six studies (reported in five publications) provided information on treatment-effect modification of bleeding outcomes by CYP2C19 status. Five were based on large randomized trials of clopidogrel-based therapy that included more than 1,000 patients in their genetic substudies (the same studies discussed in the corresponding section of Key Question 3a). The sixth study was a small genetic substudy of 126 patients that reported no major bleeding events by TIMI criteria in either group. The five larger studies compared the effect of alternative treatment strategies, stratified by CYP2C19 genotype, on safety outcomes (in all five studies, bleeding events). The test for interaction (a test for heterogeneity of treatment effects across genotype groups) was not statistically significant for any of the reported comparisons, indicating that the impact of the compared treatments on bleeding events was not significantly different across patient groups defined by CYP2C19 genotype.

Because of the large differences in populations included, treatments compared, and exposure and outcome definitions among studies reporting on treatment-effect modification by CYP2C19 variants, we did not perform a meta-analysis. However, we used the counts reported in the studies to compare the treatment effect among carriers of CYP2C19*2 or *3 (loss-of-function alleles) versus noncarriers (i.e., carriers of CYP2C19*1 or *17 [normal and gain-of-function alleles, respectively]). The odds ratios for the treatment effect within each genotype subgroup and relative odds ratios comparing the treatment effect across genotype groups showed that treatment-effect modification was nonstatistically significant in all five studies (Figure C). Effect modification was also nonstatistically significant under a recessive genetic model; however, only three studies provided data for this analysis and CIs were wide (reflecting the low number of homozygous individuals in each study).

Figure C. Bleeding events in large randomized trials reporting information on effect modification by CYP2C19 variants

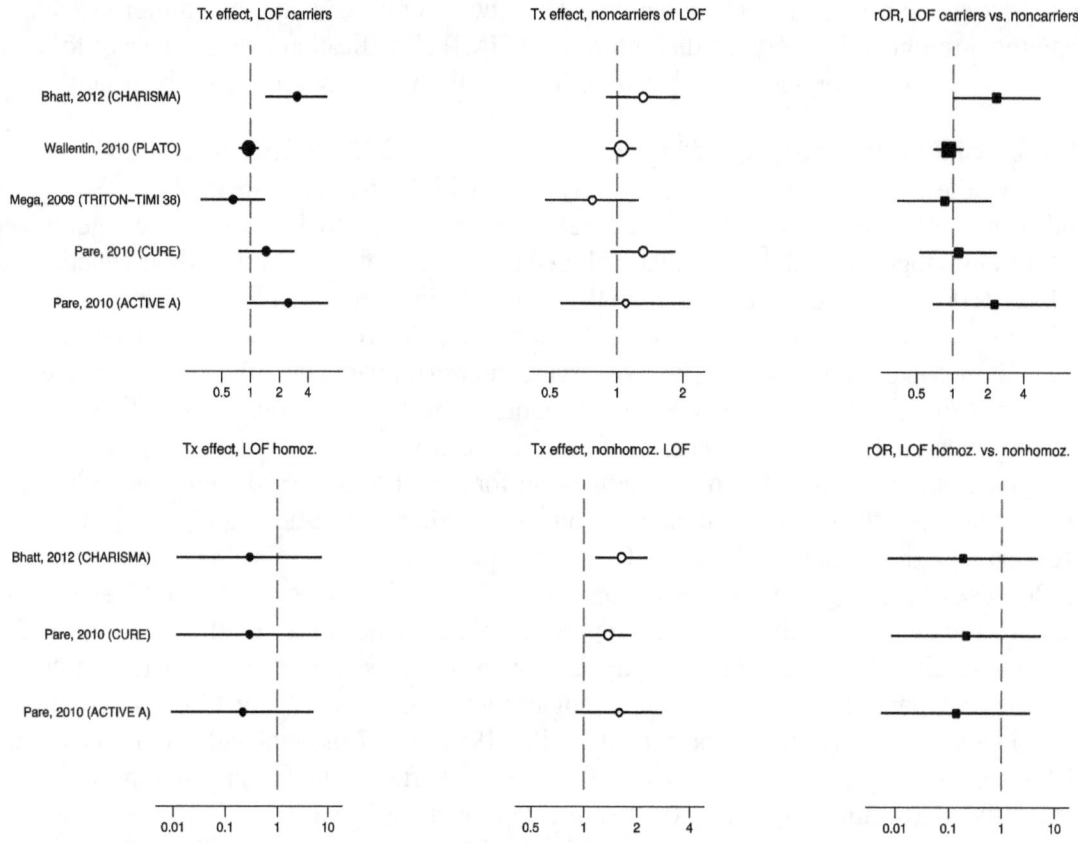

Note: The top set of panels presents forest plots for treatment effects (odds ratios) on bleeding outcomes among carriers of at least 1 LOF allele (top left panel), treatment effects among noncarriers of LOF alleles (top middle panel), and relative effects (rOR) comparing the treatment effect among LOF carriers and LOF noncarriers (top right panel). The bottom set of panels presents forest plots of treatment effects on bleeding outcomes among homozygotes for 2 LOF alleles (bottom left panel), treatment effects among nonhomozygotes of LOF alleles (bottom middle panel), and relative effects comparing the treatment effect among homozygotes and nonhomozygotes of LOF alleles (bottom right panel). Two studies did not provide adequate data for the comparisons of homozygotes and nonhomozygotes. The CURE, CHARISMA, and ACTIVE A trials compared aspirin plus clopidogrel vs. aspirin monotherapy; the TRITON-TIMI 38 trial compared aspirin plus clopidogrel vs. plus prasugrel; the PLATO trial compared aspirin plus clopidogrel vs. aspirin plus ticagrelor. Point estimates for treatment effects are shown as black circles (carriers) or white circles (noncarriers); point estimates for relative treatment effects are shown as black squares. For all symbols, size is inversely proportional to the standard error of each estimate. Horizontal extending lines denote 95% confidence intervals for all estimates. Vertical dashed lines denote no effect. Please see Table 41 in the full report for definitions of the genotype categories and outcomes reported by each study. References to individual studies are provided in Table 5 of the main report.

ACTIVE A = Atrial Fibrillation Clopidogrel Trial with Irbesartan for Prevention of Vascular Events A; CHARISMA = Clopidogrel for High Atherothrombotic Risk and Ischemic Stabilization, Management, and Avoidance; CURE = Clopidogrel in Unstable Angina to Prevent Recurrent Events trial; homoz. = homozygote; LOF = loss of function; nonhomoz. = nonhomozygote; PLATO = PLATelet inhibition and patient Outcomes trial; rOR = relative odds ratio; TRITON-TIMI 38 = Trial to Assess Improvement in Therapeutic Outcomes by Optimizing Platelet Inhibition with Prasugrel–Thrombolysis in Myocardial Infarction; Tx = treatment.

Studies With Genetic Test–Based Selection of Patients

One study, the ELEVATE-TIMI 56 trial, genotyped patients on chronic clopidogrel therapy for the presence of CYP2C19 *2 alleles, Patients with at least one *2 allele were randomized to various sequences of clopidogrel at doses of 75, 150, 225, or 300 mg daily, each for approximately 2 weeks. Noncarriers were randomized to clopidogrel 75 or 150 mg daily, each dose for two periods of approximately 2 weeks. There were no TIMI major or minor bleeding events overall, and there were no significant differences in hematologic, gastrointestinal, or musculoskeletal disorders in CYP2C19*2 carriers across different clopidogrel doses.

Phenotypic Testing for Platelet Reactivity

Studies of Test-and-Treat Strategies

Seven studies comparing alternative test-and-treat strategies provided information on harms of test-directed treatment. The studies had short followup durations (1 year in one study, 6 months in another, and 30 days in the remaining five), and few events were observed, particularly severe or major bleeding outcomes. Consequently, data were sparse and CIs around effect estimates were wide, indicating substantial uncertainty.

Studies of Treatment-Effect Modification by Baseline Platelet Reactivity

Two studies provided information on treatment-effect modification by baseline on-clopidogrel platelet reactivity. One reported no severe bleeding events and the other reported no significant effect modification.

Studies With Phenotypic Test–Based Selection of Patients

Twelve of the 14 randomized trials with phenotypic test–based patient selection reported treatment-related harms. The two larger studies (the GRAVITAS and the TRIGGER-PCI trials) found no statistically significant difference in bleeding events. The remaining 12 small studies had short followup durations (<1 month in 6 of the 12 studies) and generally reported low rates of events.

Combined Testing for CYP2C19 Variants and Phenotypic Testing To Guide Antiplatelet Treatment

Of the four studies providing information on test-based treatment strategies that also provided information on the CYP2C19 genotype of participants, none reported data on treatment-related harms stratified by treatment group and genotype status. Therefore, the interaction of genotype status and treatment could not be assessed.

Harms of Testing Per Se

We found no studies reporting on the harms of the testing process for CYP2C19 genotyping or measuring platelet reactivity in the populations of interest. However, one study comparing VASP-guided therapy with standard clopidogrel dosing in the PCI setting noted that patients in the test-guided arm had a longer time from clopidogrel loading to PCI than patients in the arm that was not test guided (p<0.001). The delay was due to the need for repeat testing and treatment modification until a predefined reactivity threshold was reached in the test-guided group. It is unclear whether this delay resulted in harm to patients.

Discussion

Clopidogrel is used extensively in the interventional management of coronary artery disease and the treatment and secondary prevention of acute coronary syndromes.[43] Furthermore, it is used for the management of patients undergoing neurointervention (with stent placement), for the prevention of stroke in patients with atrial fibrillation who are not candidates for vitamin K antagonist therapy, and for the management of selected patients with peripheral arterial disease. However, response to clopidogrel therapy—as assessed by ex vivo studies of platelet function—is variable among patients and over time. Some patients experience little suppression of platelet reactivity despite adhering to treatment, while others experience more profound suppression that may increase their risk of bleeding. Given the availability of several therapeutic options for antiplatelet treatment (e.g., increasing the loading or daily maintenance dose of clopidogrel or using adjunctive or replacement therapies such as prasugrel, ticagrelor, or cilostazol), there is interest in reliably identifying patients who are less likely to respond to standard clopidogrel treatment, as well as those who are most likely to respond to alternative treatments. This report reviewed the evidence of the effectiveness and comparative effectiveness of two types of tests that have been extensively evaluated as biomarkers for outcome prognosis for patients receiving clopidogrel therapy and as biomarkers of treatment response: genetic testing for CYP2C19 variants and phenotypic testing for on-clopidogrel platelet reactivity.

Key Findings and Assessment of the Strength of Evidence

Table B presents a summary of the report's key findings. When appropriate, results are presented separately for each of the populations and outcomes of interest. We did not assess the strength of evidence for studies of analytic validity because analytic validity is a prerequisite for the clinical use of the tests and because no framework exists for assessing the strength of evidence for analytic validity studies. We also did not assess the strength of evidence for studies exclusively assessing platelet reactivity as an outcome because platelet reactivity measurements during followup are not usually performed as part of clinical care and because platelet reactivity is not a patient-relevant outcome. Instead, we focus here on the body of evidence pertaining to predictive effects, treatment decisionmaking, and harms as related to patient-relevant clinical outcomes. Please see the Methods section for a detailed discussion of our approach to rating the strength of evidence.

Table B. Key findings from this review and assessment of strength of evidence

Key Question	Population	Test/Assay	Outcome	SOE Summary and Comments
1a: Analytic validity of tests for genotyping CYP2C19 variants	NA	Genotyping for any CYP2C19 variant	NA	SOE = NA • Few studies provided information on analytic validity specifically using samples obtained from patient populations relevant to this review. • When available, data were limited to test-retest reliability or interassay agreement. • There was limited information comparing the validity of different genetic testing assays. • However, it is generally accepted that the analytic validity of genotyping assays is robust.
1b: Predictive value of genetic testing for CYP2C19 variants	Ischemic heart disease	Genotyping for LOF CYP2C19 variants	Stent thrombosis	SOE = Moderate • Meta-analysis of 17 studies found a statistically significant association under a dominant model • RR=1.52; 95% CI, 1.17 to 1.97 • There was little evidence of heterogeneity (I^2 = 0%), but the test for small-study effects was statistically significant. • Results under additive and recessive models were consistent with a positive association and produced larger effect sizes; however, these analyses were based on a small subset of the available studies. • There was some concern about selective outcome reporting. • Studies reported few outcome events and the summary estimate was imprecise.
			MACE	SOE = Moderate • Meta-analysis of 25 studies found a statistically significant association under a dominant model • RR=1.20; 95% CI, 1.04 to 1.39 • There was some evidence of heterogeneity (I^2 = 31%). • Results under additive and recessive models were consistent with a positive association and produced larger effect sizes; however, these analyses were based on a small subset of the available studies. • The test for small-study effects was statistically significant.
			Cardiovascular mortality	SOE = Low • Meta-analysis of 7 studies found a statistically significant association under a dominant model • RR=1.98; 95% CI, 1.13 to 3.46 • There was no evidence of heterogeneity (I^2 = 0%). The summary estimate was imprecise. • The test for small-study effects was not statistically significant. • There was some concern about selective outcome reporting.

Table B. Key findings from this review and assessment of strength of evidence (continued)

Key Question	Population	Test/Assay	Outcome	SOE Summary and Comments
1b: Predictive value of genetic testing for CYP2C19 variants (continued)	Ischemic heart disease (continued)	Genotyping for LOF CYP2C19 variants (continued)	All other clinical outcomes	SOE = Insufficient • Few studies reported information for noncomposite clinical outcomes other than stent thrombosis. • There was substantial concern about selective outcome reporting. • Study-specific and meta-analysis estimates (when performed) indicated substantial uncertainty.
		Genotyping for GOF CYP2C19 variants	MACE	SOE = Low • Meta-analysis of 7 studies found a statistically significant protective effect for carriers vs. noncarriers. • RR=0.82; 95% CI, 0.74 to 0.92 • There was substantial concern about selective outcome reporting.
			All other clinical outcomes	SOE = Insufficient • Few studies provided relevant information. • There was substantial concern about selective outcome reporting. • Study-specific and meta-analysis estimates (when performed) indicated substantial uncertainty.
	Other patient groups who are candidates for clopidogrel therapy	Genotyping for any CYP2C19 variants	All clinical outcomes	SOE = Insufficient • Only few studies (often only a single study) were available for patient populations other than those with ischemic heart disease. • Some of the studies did not report information on clinical outcomes.
1c: Factors affecting the predictive value of genetic testing for CYP2C19 variants	All patient populations	Genotyping for any CYP2C19 variants	All clinical outcomes	SOE = Insufficient • 20 studies provided information on effect modification; a single study reported a statistically significant interaction effect on the prognostic performance of CYP2C19 variants for a clinical outcome. • No factor was assessed by more than 5 studies, giving rise to concerns about selective outcome reporting. • In metaregression analyses (using study-level factors as covariates) we found some evidence of effect modification by ethnicity (East Asians vs. white populations) for MACE and stent thrombosis. However, this result is based on comparisons across studies, which may be confounded by other study characteristics, and was not corroborated by within-study analyses. CIs for all interaction effects were wide for all genotype-outcome pairs assessed, and only a few studies in East Asian populations were available. • Estimates of effect modification by study-level variables are susceptible to confounding by other study-level characteristics.

Table B. Key findings from this review and assessment of strength of evidence (continued)

Key Question	Population	Test/Assay	Outcome	SOE Summary and Comments
2a: Analytic validity of tests for on-clopidogrel platelet reactivity	NA	All assays used to measure on-clopidogrel platelet reactivity	NA	SOE = NA • Few studies reported information on analytic sensitivity and specificity, possibly reflecting the research community's belief that there is no good reference standard assay for platelet reactivity. • Agreement ranged from poor to moderate and was variable between tests. • The highest agreement was observed between applications of the same assay with different concentrations of agonists rather than between different assays.
2b: Predictive ability of phenotypic testing for platelet reactivity	Ischemic heart disease	LTA	All-cause mortality	SOE = Low • 13 studies using heterogeneous methods to define increased reactivity were available. • These studies support an association between increased platelet reactivity measured by LTA and mortality. • There was some concern about selective outcome reporting.
			Cardio-vascular mortality	SOE = Low • 9 studies using heterogeneous methods to define increased reactivity were available. • Studies provided evidence of an association between increased reactivity and cardiovascular mortality; however, clinical heterogeneity precluded firm conclusions. • There was some concern about selective outcome reporting.
			Acute coronary syndromes	SOE = Low • 18 studies using heterogeneous methods to define increased reactivity were available. • Studies often found statistically significant associations between increased reactivity as measured by LTA and clinical events; however, clinical heterogeneity did not allow for stronger conclusions. • There was some concern about selective outcome reporting.
			Stent thrombosis	SOE = Low • 19 studies using heterogeneous methods to define increased reactivity were available. • Studies often found statistically significant associations between increased reactivity as measured by LTA and clinical events; however, clinical heterogeneity did not allow for stronger conclusions. • There was some concern about selective outcome reporting.
			Stroke	SOE = Low (for lack of association) • 12 studies using heterogeneous methods to define increased reactivity were available. • Studies generally did not report statistically significant associations between increased reactivity as measured by LTA and clinical events; however, clinical heterogeneity did not allow for stronger conclusions or quantitative synthesis to increase precision.

Table B. Key findings from this review and assessment of strength of evidence (continued)

Key Question	Population	Test/Assay	Outcome	SOE Summary and Comments
			MACE	SOE = Low • 37 studies using heterogeneous methods to define increased reactivity were available. • The majority of reviewed studies suggested a statistically significant association between increased platelet reactivity measured by LTA and composite cardiovascular events. • Definitions of composite outcomes were often heterogeneous.
			All other clinical outcomes	SOE = Insufficient • Clinical and population heterogeneity or small number of studies limited our ability to draw conclusions.
		VerifyNow	All-cause mortality	SOE = Low (for lack of association) • 10 studies were available. Meta-analysis of 4 studies did not find an association between increased reactivity measured by VerifyNow and all-cause mortality • RR=1.21; 95% CI, 0.83 to 1.76 • The summary estimate was imprecise and 95% CI did not rule out clinically meaningful effects.
			Cardio-vascular mortality	SOE = Moderate • 7 studies were available. Meta-analysis of 4 studies found a statistically significant association with little evidence of heterogeneity • RR=2.50; 95% CI, 1.28 to 4.87 • The CI of the summary estimate indicated substantial uncertainty. • There was some concern about selective outcome reporting.
			Acute coronary syndromes	SOE = Low • 19 studies using heterogeneous methods to define increased reactivity were available. • Studies generally suggested an association between increased reactivity as measured by VerifyNow and acute coronary syndromes, both periprocedurally and during longer followup.
			Stent thrombosis	SOE = Low (for lack of association) • 15 studies were available. Meta-analysis of 6 studies did not find an association between reactivity measured by VerifyNow and stent thrombosis • RR=1.67; 95% CI, 0.80 to 3.47 • There was some evidence of heterogeneity (I^2 = 37%) and the CI of the summary estimate indicated substantial uncertainty. • Studies not included in the meta-analysis generally produced nonsignificant results. • There was some concern about selective outcome reporting. • The test for small-study effects was statistically significant.

Table B. Key findings from this review and assessment of strength of evidence (continued)

Key Question	Population	Test/Assay	Outcome	SOE Summary and Comments
			MACE	SOE = Moderate • 24 studies were available. Meta-analysis of 13 studies identified a statistically significant association • RR=2.48; 95% CI, 1.85 to 3.32 • There was moderate statistical heterogeneity (I^2 = 44%) and studies used fairly similar definitions of increased reactivity. • The test for small-study effects was statistically significant.
			Bleeding events (major and all levels of severity combined)	SOE = Low (for lack of association) • 13 studies were available. • Meta-analysis of 4 studies with data on any bleeding event did not find an association between increased reactivity measured by VerifyNow • RR = 1.09; 95% CI, 0.88 to 1.36 • There was little evidence of heterogeneity (I^2 = 0%). • Meta-analysis of 4 studies with data on major bleeding events did not find an association between increased reactivity measured by VerifyNow • RR=0.85; 95% CI, 0.32 to 2.25 • There was evidence of moderate heterogeneity (I^2 = 57%). • For major bleeding events the summary estimate was imprecise and the 95% CI did not rule out clinically meaningful effects.
			All other clinical outcomes	SOE = Insufficient • Clinical heterogeneity or small number of studies limited our ability to draw conclusions.
		VASP assay	Cardio-vascular mortality	SOE = Insufficient • 6 studies were available. Meta-analysis of 4 studies did not identify a statistically significant association. • RR=2.42; 95% CI, 0.86 to 6.82 • Although the test for heterogeneity was nonsignificant, point estimates from individual studies ranged from protective effects to strong harmful effects. • The meta-analytic summary point estimate was far from the null and its CI was wide (imprecise). • Clinically significant effects could not be ruled out.
			Acute coronary syndromes	SOE = Low (for lack of association) • 6 studies were available. Meta-analysis of 3 studies did not identify a statistically significant association • RR=1.47; 95% CI, 0.77 to 2.79 • The test for heterogeneity was nonsignificant but point estimates from individual studies were highly variable. • The meta-analytic summary point estimate was far from the null and its CI was wide (imprecise). • Clinically significant effects could not be ruled out.

Table B. Key findings from this review and assessment of strength of evidence (continued)

Key Question	Population	Test/Assay	Outcome	SOE Summary and Comments
			Stent thrombosis	SOE = Low • 10 studies were available. Meta-analysis of 4 studies identified a statistically significant association • RR=3.37; 95% CI, 1.59 to 7.11 • There was little evidence of statistical heterogeneity and the 4 studies used fairly similar definitions of increased reactivity. • The summary estimate was imprecise but the lower bound was consistent with a 59% increase in risk in the high-reactivity group. • There was some concern about selective outcome reporting.
			MACE	SOE = Low • 8 studies were available. Meta-analysis of 6 studies identified a statistically significant association • RR=2.57; 95% CI, 1.21 to 5.47 • There was evidence of statistical heterogeneity. • The summary estimate was imprecise but the lower bound was consistent with a 21% increase in risk in the high-reactivity group. • There was some concern about selective outcome reporting.
			All other clinical outcomes	SOE = Insufficient • Few studies reported information. • Clinical heterogeneity or small number of studies limited our ability to draw conclusions.
		PFA-100	MACE	SOE = Low • 7 of the 9 studies on this assay reporting information on composite clinical outcomes produced statistically significant results indicating an association between increased reactivity and adverse outcomes. • Heterogeneity in the methods used to define increased reactivity precluded definitive conclusions; however, studies generally indicated an association between increased platelet reactivity as measured by the PFA-100 assay and composite clinical outcomes.
			All other clinical outcomes	SOE = Insufficient • Few of the available studies reported information on other outcomes. • There was concern about selective outcome reporting.
		All other assays	All clinical outcomes	SOE = Insufficient • Few studies were available. • When ≥2 studies were available for the same outcome, they used heterogeneous metrics or thresholds to define increased reactivity or used different agonists for ex vivo stimulation of platelets.

Table B. Key findings from this review and assessment of strength of evidence (continued)

Key Question	Population	Test/Assay	Outcome	SOE Summary and Comments
	Other patient groups who are candidates for clopidogrel therapy	All assays used to measure on-clopidogrel platelet reactivity	All clinical outcomes	SOE = Insufficient • Only 6 studies, using diverse assays to measure reactivity, were available in clinically heterogeneous populations. • Studies were fairly small.
2c: Factors affecting the predictive value of phenotypic testing for platelet reactivity	All patient populations	All assays used to measure on-clopidogrel platelet reactivity	All clinical outcomes	SOE = Insufficient • 7 studies provided information on effect modification; no factor was assessed by more than 3 studies. • Effect modification by study-level factors could not be assessed for most assay-outcome pairs; when such analysis was possible (for VerifyNow MACE), results indicated substantial uncertainty.
3a: Comparative effectiveness of alternative test-and-treat strategies	Ischemic heart disease	Genetic testing for CYP2C19 variants or phenotypic testing for platelet reactivity (all assays assessed)	All clinical outcomes	SOE = Insufficient • 1 RCT of testing vs. no testing was identified. The study had short duration and a small sample size; no events were observed in the 2 groups during the study period. • 3 studies provided information on treatment-effect modification for clinical outcomes and reported at least 1 outcome event. • 1 study randomized patients selected on the basis of genotype status into different clopidogrel doses. No conclusions could be drawn regarding clinical outcomes because of the short duration and small sample size of the study. • Studies compared different antiplatelet treatments and produced heterogeneous results. • Study-specific estimates were imprecise.
		Phenotypic testing for platelet reactivity	All clinical outcomes	SOE = Insufficient • The 6 RCTs of testing strategies were small, had different designs, and produced extreme results with considerable statistical uncertainty. • 1 NRCS was judged to be at high risk of bias on the basis of study design (patients in each of the 2 compared arms were enrolled at different centers). • 3 studies of effect modification were identified; studies evaluated heterogeneous interventions and used different methods to assess reactivity. • Studies of test-based patient selection assessed different treatments, enrolled heterogeneous patient populations, and did not provide robust evidence on clinical outcomes.

Table B. Key findings from this review and assessment of strength of evidence (continued)

Key Question	Population	Test/Assay	Outcome	SOE Summary and Comments
	Atrial fibrillation	Genetic testing for CYP2C19 variants or phenotypic testing for platelet reactivity (all assays assessed)	All clinical outcomes	SOE = Insufficient • Only 1 study providing information on effect modification by CYP2C19 status was identified. • The study did not find evidence of effect modification by genotype status, but there was considerable statistical uncertainty in the study estimates.
		Phenotypic testing for platelet reactivity	All clinical outcomes	SOE = Insufficient • No studies were identified.
	Other patient populations	Genetic testing for CYP2C19 variants or phenotypic testing for platelet reactivity (all assays assessed)	All clinical outcomes	SOE = Insufficient • 1 study provided information on treatment-effect modification in a mixed population of patients with atherothrombotic disease (cardiovascular, cerebrovascular, or peripheral arterial) along with asymptomatic individuals at risk for atherothrombotic disease. • The study did not provide robust evidence of effect modification.
		Phenotypic testing for platelet reactivity	All clinical outcomes	SOE = Insufficient • No studies were identified.
3b: Factors modifying the comparative effectiveness of alternative test-and-treat strategies	All patient populations	Genetic testing for CYP2C19 variants or phenotypic testing for platelet reactivity (all assays assessed)	All clinical outcomes	SOE = Insufficient • 4 studies provided information on effect modification. Each assessed different effect modifiers; no statistically significant interactions were reported.
4: Harms of testing and of test-directed treatment	All patient populations	Genetic testing for CYP2C19 variants	All clinical outcomes	SOE = Insufficient • 1 RCT of testing vs. no testing was identified. The study had short duration and a small sample size; few events were observed in the 2 groups during the study period. • 5 studies assessed treatment-effect modification by genotype status and reported at least 1 outcome event. • 1 study randomized patients selected on the basis of genotype status; it did not provide robust evidence regarding harms due to the relatively small sample size and short followup. • Studies compared different antiplatelet treatments and had heterogeneous results. • No studies provided direct information on the harms of testing per se.

Table B. Key findings from this review and assessment of strength of evidence (continued)

Key Question	Population	Test/Assay	Outcome	SOE Summary and Comments
		Phenotypic testing for platelet reactivity (all assays assessed)	All clinical outcomes	SOE = Insufficient
				• The 6 randomized studies of testing strategies were small, had different designs, produced extreme results with considerable statistical uncertainty, and in some cases did not report any outcome events.
				• 1 NRCS was judged to be at high risk of bias on the basis of study design (patients in each of the 2 compared arms were enrolled at different centers).
				• 2 studies of effect modification were identified. In 1 study safety outcomes either did not occur (regardless of reactivity status) or results were not stratified by reactivity group; the second study did not identify a significant effect but had short-term followup and reported too few outcome events to allow any robust conclusions to be drawn.
				• Studies of test-based patient selection assessed different treatments.

Note: CI = confidence interval; GOF = gain-of-function; LOF = loss-of-function; LTA = light-transmission aggregometry; MACE = major adverse cardiovascular events; NA = not applicable; NRCS = nonrandomized controlled study; PFA = Platelet Function Analyzer; RCT = randomized controlled trial; RR = relative risk; SOE = strength of evidence; VASP = vasodilator-stimulated phosphoprotein.

In summary, the analytic validity for genotyping appears well established. In contrast, the relatively poor agreement among phenotypic tests suggests that more work is needed to specify which phenotypic tests provide measurements that are usable for clinical decisionmaking. Both genetic testing for CYP2C19 variants and assays for measuring platelet reactivity appear to predict adverse cardiovascular outcomes. However, the evidence is weakened by a substantial concern about selective reporting, publication bias, and concerns about risk of bias in individual studies. Evidence of the utility of these tests to guide treatment is still inconclusive due to the small number of available studies, as well as heterogeneity in the included populations, tests used, and interventions compared. Evidence directly comparing the two testing approaches is totally lacking.

Our review has synthesized more publications than previous reviews have, with generally similar findings. Regarding the predictive effects of CYP2C19 genotype status, existing systematic reviews have reached similar conclusions to ours, both in magnitude and direction. Also consistent with our findings, previous analyses have suggested that selective outcome reporting and publication bias may have affected meta-analytic estimates.[16,44]

Compared with previous systematic reviews regarding platelet reactivity assays, our review includes a much larger number of studies and considers multiple assays assessing on-clopidogrel platelet reactivity using agonists to stimulate platelets ex vivo. In contrast to previous meta-analyses, we did not combine results across different assays (i.e., across tests using different measurement principles), different agonist concentrations, or different calculation methods or cutoff values for defining high reactivity. We believe that this choice is supported by our review of analytic validity, which found low to moderate agreement between different assays. Of note, our analyses relevant to the VerifyNow P2Y12 assay include almost double the number of studies included in a recently published meta-analysis of individual data on the same assay.[45] Despite differences in selection criteria and analysis methods, our results were similar, identifying a large effect size for the association between platelet reactivity as measured by the VerifyNow P2Y12 assay and adverse cardiovascular outcomes.

To our knowledge, this is the first review to comprehensively evaluate the use of genetic and phenotypic testing to guide clinical decisionmaking. We developed a structured approach that considered different experimental designs (randomized trials of alternative test-and-treatment strategies, randomized treatment trials assessing effect modification by biomarkers, and randomized treatment trials using the biomarkers to select patients for inclusion). Although the studies we identified were too diverse to support firm conclusions on the value of the tests of interest, we believe that our methodological approach will be helpful as the evidence base continues to grow. For example, it will be applied in our updated literature review.

Applicability

The vast majority of included studies enrolled patients with ischemic heart disease. Acute or chronic coronary disease represented almost all available studies for all Key Questions. Other populations who are potential candidates for antiplatelet therapy (e.g., patients with cerebrovascular disease, peripheral arterial disease, or atrial fibrillation) were included in a minority of studies only. This imbalance is not unexpected, given that clopidogrel's primary indications pertain to ischemic heart disease. However, it is probably not prudent to extrapolate findings from studies of ischemic heart disease to other patient populations. Given that a large number of studies included patients undergoing PCI, these findings are most applicable to interventional settings.

For CYP2C19 variants, we found limited evidence that prognostic effects were different in subgroup and metaregression analysis by ethnicity (East Asian vs. white). More evidence is needed to validate this finding and to obtain information on patient populations underrepresented in this review (e.g., blacks). Patient race or ethnicity may be an important effect modifier because the prevalence of variant alleles is substantially different among racial and ethnic groups. For example, *2 variants are much more common in East Asian populations than others.

The majority of studies were conducted in tertiary (usually academic) medical centers. Studies of treatment-effect modification by CYP2C19 genotype were based on large randomized trials, and findings may not be generalizable to everyday care settings. Because patient information on preexisting vascular disease in studies of predictive effects was generally incompletely reported, it is unclear whether patients in the included studies are representative of those seen in clinical practice. Nonetheless, the distribution of risk factors for ischemic vascular disease (male sex, hyperlipidemia, diabetes, hypertension, smoking, etc.) appeared to be representative of contemporary patient populations, and the majority of studies were conducted in recent years.

Implications for Clinical and Policy Decisionmaking

Despite the availability of a large literature on the use of genetic testing of CYP2C19 variants and phenotypic testing of platelet reactivity for predicting outcomes in patients receiving clopidogrel-based therapy, studies provided limited information on the value added by these tests over ascertainment of conventional risk factors in the populations of interest (e.g., clinical or laboratory information or disease-specific predictive scores). The data suggest that both test methods can provide prognostic information for some important clinical outcomes. However, selective outcome reporting for both types of tests, uncertainty about the underlying genetic model for CYP2C19 variants, and heterogeneity across studies in the metrics used to assess reactivity undermine certainty regarding this prognostic effect. Furthermore, there is little comparative evidence on the prognostic utility of individual tests or combinations of tests. These and other limitations of the existing literature may reduce the potential for clinical application of the tests reviewed here as prognostic markers for patients on clopidogrel-based antiplatelet therapy. The available evidence was insufficient for determining the utility of either type of testing for guiding the choice of antiplatelet therapy.

Limitations of the Evidence

On the basis of the large number of reviewed studies, we believe that the evidence regarding genetic testing for CYP2C19 variants and phenotypic testing for platelet reactivity for guiding antiplatelet treatment and predicting outcomes in patients who receive such treatment is limited in the following ways:

- Despite the large number of available studies providing information on analytic validity, most studies used inappropriate statistical methods to assess interassay agreement.
- There was a lack of comparative studies evaluating the relative predictive ability of alternative assays for measuring platelet reactivity, genetic testing of CYP2C19 variants, or combinations of these tests.
- Development ("training") and assessment ("test") samples were not separated when developing predictive markers.

- Selective outcome reporting was a concern regarding the association between test results and several clinical outcomes. Most studies reported information on composite clinical outcomes, but often they did not provide results for the component clinical events.
- There was uncertainty about the genetic model for CYP2C19 variants. Poor reporting of primary study results precluded the assessment of alternative genetic models (e.g., results were often reported only for collapsed genotype categories).
- Exposure definitions were heterogeneous because not all studies genotyped the same CYP2C19 variants and because studies used different assays, metrics, and cutoff values to define increased platelet reactivity.
- There was a paucity of studies evaluating the impact of test-guided treatment selection on the basis of CYP2C19 genotyping or reactivity measurements.
- The number of studies providing information on treatment-effect modification by CYP2C19 genotype status or baseline on-clopidogrel platelet reactivity was limited. Investigations based on completed randomized trials (repurposed RCTs) were not powered to detect treatment-effect modification and were susceptible to selection bias because included patients represented only a minority of the populations included in the parent trials.

Future Research

This review identified substantial gaps in the literature on genetic testing for CYP2C19 variants and phenotypic testing for platelet reactivity, both as biomarkers of future outcomes among patients who are receiving clopidogrel therapy and, more importantly, as tests for guiding treatment selection for patients who are candidates for antiplatelet treatment. We believe that the following evidence gaps may represent fruitful areas for future research:

- *Analytic validity of phenotypic testing:* Future studies using rigorous methods to inform the analytic validity of tests for measuring platelet reactivity are needed, particularly with regard to test-retest reliability, interassay agreement, and analytic performance.
- *Prognostic accuracy, with a focus on comparative prognostic performance:* Large-scale prospectively designed studies of the tests of interest are needed to derive reliable estimates of prognostic performance. Studies should focus on the relative performance of competing tests, prespecify "positive" and "negative" test results, and report complete data for all outcomes assessed.
- *Direct comparisons of methods for test-guided treatment selection:* Even if the predictive value of tests were established, this information is inadequate as a basis for treatment decisionmaking. The most promising tests could be prioritized for assessment in directly comparative studies of testing versus no testing for guiding treatment choice. Such studies could provide unconfounded estimates of the relative benefits and harms of the compared strategies.[46] However, randomized comparisons of alternative testing strategies are costly and time consuming. Furthermore, recruitment may be challenging or impossible if one of the treatment groups is standard clopidogrel-based therapy, in view of the current FDA-approved labeling and recent results from studies using pharmacodynamic endpoints. Still, such designs may be appropriate when comparing antiplatelet therapies other than standard clopidogrel dosing (including high-dose clopidogrel treatment). When experimental studies are not considered logistically or ethically feasible, observational data may be useful, especially given that CYP2C19 testing is not universally implemented.

- *"Repurposing" completed randomized trials to assess effect modification:* An alternative to direct comparative studies of testing strategies is to assess effect modification by genotype status by repurposing already completed randomized trials, in which the drugs of interest were tested against a suitable comparator, by genotyping samples from enrollees. Results of genetic analyses could be associated with the prospectively recorded clinical outcomes.[47,48] Although this approach did not provide definitive answers in this review due to limitations of the existing studies, future repurposed trials could yield more informative results if they were properly planned. Such planning must include a strategy for obtaining samples from all participants (or a random sample thereof), acquiring specimens prior to treatment, and using appropriate methods to control for multiple testing. When randomized trials are not available for repurposing, a similar approach can be implemented in the setting of registries linking DNA information to electronic health records. Patients receiving different antiplatelet therapies whose choice of treatment was not based on CYP2C19 status, but for whom material for genotyping is available, are candidates for such research.
- *Monitoring of platelet reactivity to guide treatment:* Strategies of monitoring platelet reactivity can be conceptualized as "dynamic treatment regimes"[49-51] (i.e., rules for sequential decisionmaking based on the evolution of reactivity measurements over time). With these methods, the impact of alternative monitoring strategies on clinical outcomes can be evaluated using observational data. The most promising monitoring strategies can then be evaluated in randomized comparative studies.

Conclusions

In summary, we found limited evidence on the analytic validity of genetic testing for platelet reactivity. However, using evidence from other populations and genetic variants, we believe that the available assays for CYP2C19 genotyping have adequate technical test performance. In contrast, we found a large body of evidence on the analytic validity of assays for measuring platelet reactivity suggesting that interassay agreement is only poor to moderate. No phenotypic assays can be considered a "gold standard" test.

We found some evidence supporting a significant association between loss-of-function CYP2C19 variants and increased risk of stent thrombosis, cardiovascular mortality, and MACE. We also found a significant association between gain-of-function alleles and reduced risk of MACE. The interpretation of these associations should be cautious, given the potential for selective reporting and small-study effects to have affected study results. Furthermore, the applicability of findings to patient populations other than those with ischemic coronary artery disease, particularly those undergoing revascularization procedures, was limited. We also found evidence supporting an association between high on-clopidogrel platelet reactivity as measured by various assays (particularly LTA, VerifyNow P2Y12, and the VASP assay) and adverse cardiovascular events. Our confidence in these findings is limited by the relatively small number of studies available for each test-outcome combination, the potential for selective outcome reporting, and the common lack of separation between the populations used to derive test thresholds of optimal predictive value and those used to assess predictive value at these thresholds.

The evidence on the use of testing to guide treatment choice was insufficient. A single randomized trial of CYP2C19 testing versus no testing provided limited evidence on clinical outcomes. Subanalyses of five well-conducted randomized controlled trials generally did not find strong evidence of effect modification by CYP2C19 status. However, concern regarding selection bias in the genetic substudies and the heterogeneity of patient populations and treatments rendered the evidence inconclusive. Similarly, the short followup periods and low numbers of outcome events in trials of platelet reactivity–guided treatment versus standard antiplatelet therapy did not offer a firm base for conclusions. No studies comparing genetic and phenotypic testing strategies were identified.

Additional research is needed to better establish the prognostic value and clinical utility for treatment decisionmaking of both genetic testing for CYP2C19 variants and phenotypic testing for platelet reactivity, focusing on standardizing testing methods and assessing the relative impact of testing strategies on patient-relevant clinical outcomes in large well-conducted clinical trials.

References

1. Writing Group Members, Roger VL, Go AS, et al. Executive Summary: Heart Disease and Stroke Statistics—2012 Update. Circulation. 2012 Jan 3;125(1):188-97.

2. Keenan NL, Shaw KM. Coronary heart disease and stroke deaths - United States, 2006. MMWR Surveill Summ. 2011 Jan 14;60(Suppl):62-6.

3. Squizzato A, Keller T, Romualdi E, et al. Clopidogrel plus aspirin versus aspirin alone for preventing cardiovascular disease. Cochrane Database Syst Rev. 2011 Jan;(1):CD005158.

4. Writing Committee, Levine GN, Bates ER, et al. 2011 ACCF/AHA/SCAI Guideline for Percutaneous Coronary Intervention. Circulation. 2011 Dec 6;124(23):e574-e651.

5. Bowry AD, Brookhart MA, Choudhry NK. Meta-analysis of the efficacy and safety of clopidogrel plus aspirin as compared to antiplatelet monotherapy for the prevention of vascular events. Am J Cardiol. 2008 Apr 1;101(7):960-6.

6. Sabatine MS, Hamdalla HN, Mehta SR, et al. Efficacy and safety of clopidogrel pretreatment before percutaneous coronary intervention with and without glycoprotein IIb/IIIa inhibitor use. Am Heart J. 2008 May;155(5):910-7.

7. Sudlow CL, Mason G, Maurice JB, et al. Thienopyridine derivatives versus aspirin for preventing stroke and other serious vascular events in high vascular risk patients. Cochrane Database Syst Rev. 2009 Oct 7;(4):CD001246.

8. Antithrombotic Trialists' Collaboration. Collaborative meta-analysis of randomised trials of antiplatelet therapy for prevention of death, myocardial infarction, and stroke in high risk patients. BMJ. 2002 Jan 12;324(7329):71-86.

9. ACTIVE Investigators, Connolly SJ, Pogue J, et al. Effect of clopidogrel added to aspirin in patients with atrial fibrillation. N Engl J Med. 2009 May 14;360(20):2066-78.

10. Bellemain-Appaix A, Brieger D, Beygui F, et al. New P2Y12 inhibitors versus clopidogrel in percutaneous coronary intervention: a meta-analysis. J Am Coll Cardiol. 2010 Nov 2;56(19):1542-51.

11. Wallentin L, Becker RC, Budaj A, et al. Ticagrelor versus clopidogrel in patients with acute coronary syndromes. N Engl J Med. 2009 Sep 10;361(11):1045-57.

12. Wiviott SD, Braunwald E, McCabe CH, et al. Prasugrel versus clopidogrel in patients with acute coronary syndromes. N Engl J Med. 2007 Nov 15;357(20):2001-15.

13. Navarese EP, Verdoia M, Schaffer A, et al. Ischaemic and bleeding complications with new, compared to standard, ADP-antagonist regimens in acute coronary syndromes: a meta-analysis of randomized trials. QJM. 2011 Jul 1;104(7):561-9.

14. Geiger J, Brich J, Honig-Liedl P, et al. Specific impairment of human platelet P2Y(AC) ADP receptor-mediated signaling by the antiplatelet drug clopidogrel. Arterioscler Thromb Vasc Biol. 1999 Aug;19(8):2007-11.

15. Kazui M, Nishiya Y, Ishizuka T, et al. Identification of the human cytochrome P450 enzymes involved in the two oxidative steps in the bioactivation of clopidogrel to its pharmacologically active metabolite. Drug Metab Dispos. 2010 Jan;38(1):92-9.

16. Bauer T, Bouman HJ, van Werkum JW, et al. Impact of CYP2C19 variant genotypes on clinical efficacy of antiplatelet treatment with clopidogrel: systematic review and meta-analysis. BMJ. 2011;343:d4588.

17. Chang MH, Lindegren ML, Butler MA, et al. Prevalence in the United States of selected candidate gene variants: Third National Health and Nutrition Examination Survey, 1991-1994. Am J Epidemiol. 2009 Jan 1;169(1):54-66.

18. Chan MY, Tan K, Tan HC, et al. CYP2C19 and PON1 polymorphisms regulating clopidogrel bioactivation in Chinese, Malay and Indian subjects. Pharmacogenomics. 2012 Apr;13(5):533-42.

19. Yin SJ, Ni YB, Wang SM, et al. Differences in genotype and allele frequency distributions of polymorphic drug metabolizing enzymes CYP2C19 and CYP2D6 in mainland Chinese Mongolian, Hui and Han populations. J Clin Pharm Ther. 2012 Jun;37(3):364-9.

20. Veiga MI, Asimus S, Ferreira PE, et al. Pharmacogenomics of CYP2A6, CYP2B6, CYP2C19, CYP2D6, CYP3A4, CYP3A5 and MDR1 in Vietnam. Eur J Clin Pharmacol. 2009 Apr;65(4):355-63.

21. Shuldiner AR, O'Connell JR, Bliden KP, et al. Association of cytochrome P450 2C19 genotype with the antiplatelet effect and clinical efficacy of clopidogrel therapy. JAMA. 2009 Aug 26;302(8):849-57.

22. Bonello L, Tantry US, Marcucci R, et al. Consensus and future directions on the definition of high on-treatment platelet reactivity to adenosine diphosphate. J Am Coll Cardiol. 2010 Sep 14;56(12):919-33.

23. Agency for Healthcare Research and Quality. Methods Guide for Effectiveness and Comparative Effectiveness Reviews. AHRQ Publication No. 10(11)-EHC063-EF. Rockville (MD): Agency for Healthcare Research and Quality; March 2011. Chapters available at www.effectivehealthcare.ahrq.gov.

24. Viswanathan M, Ansari MT, Berkman ND, et al. Assessing the risk of bias of individual studies in systematic reviews of health care interventions. In: Methods Guide for Effectiveness and Comparative Effectiveness Reviews. AHRQ Publication No. 10(11)-EHC063-EF. Rockville (MD): Agency for Healthcare Research and Quality; March 2011. Chapters available at www.effectivehealthcare.ahrq.gov.

25. Agency for Healthcare Research and Quality. Methods Guide for Medical Test Reviews. AHRQ Publication No. 12-EC017. Rockville, MD: Agency for Healthcare Research and Quality; June 2012.

26. Whiting PF, Rutjes AWS, Westwood ME, et al. QUADAS-2: a revised tool for the quality assessment of diagnostic accuracy studies. Ann Intern Med. 2011 Oct 18;155(8):529-36.

27. Whiting P, Rutjes AW, Reitsma JB, et al. The development of QUADAS: a tool for the quality assessment of studies of diagnostic accuracy included in systematic reviews. BMC Med Res Methodol. 2003 Nov 10;3:25.

28. Whiting P, Rutjes AW, Dinnes J, et al. Development and validation of methods for assessing the quality of diagnostic accuracy studies. Health Technol Assess. 2004 Jun;8(25):iii, 1-iii234.

29. Whiting PF, Weswood ME, Rutjes AWS, et al. Evaluation of QUADAS, a tool for the quality assessment of diagnostic accuracy studies. BMC Med Res Methodol. 2006;6:9.

30. Higgins JPT, Douglas GA, Peter CG, et al. The Cochrane Collaboration's tool for assessing risk of bias in randomised trials. BMJ. 2011 Oct 18;343.

31. DerSimonian R, Laird N. Meta-analysis in clinical trials. Control Clin Trials. 1986 Sep;7(3):177-88.

32. Cochran WG. The combination of estimates from different experiments. Biometrics. 1954 Mar;10(1):101-29.

33. Higgins JPT, Thompson SG. Quantifying heterogeneity in a meta-analysis. Statist Med. 2002;21(11):1539-58.

34. Pearce N. What does the odds ratio estimate in a case-control study? Int J Epidemiol. 1993 Dec;22(6):1189-92.

35. Knol MJ, Vandenbroucke JP, Scott P, et al. What do case-control studies estimate? Survey of methods and assumptions in published case-control research. Am J Epidemiol. 2008 Nov 1;168(9):1073-81.

36. Miettinen OS. Theoretical Epidemiology: Principles of Occurrence Research in Medicine. New York: Wiley; 1985.

37. Egger M, Davey SG, Schneider M, et al. Bias in meta-analysis detected by a simple, graphical test. BMJ. 1997 Sep 13;315(7109):629-34.

38. Lau J, Ioannidis JP, Terrin N, et al. The case of the misleading funnel plot. BMJ. 2006 Sep 16;333(7568):597-600.

39. Owens DK, Lohr KN, Atkins D, et al. AHRQ series paper 5: grading the strength of a body of evidence when comparing medical interventions--Agency for Healthcare Research and Quality and the effective health-care program. J Clin Epidemiol. 2010 May;63(5):513-23.

40. Atkins D, Chang SM, Gartlehner G, et al. Assessing applicability when comparing medical interventions: AHRQ and the Effective Health Care Program. J Clin Epidemiol. 2011;64:1198-207.

41. Bland JM, Altman DG. Statistical methods for assessing agreement between two methods of clinical measurement. Lancet. 1986 Feb. 8;1(8476):307-10.

42. Lin LI. A concordance correlation coefficient to evaluate reproducibility. Biometrics. 1989;45(1):255-68. PMID: 2720055.

43. Holmes DR Jr, Dehmer GJ, Kaul S, et al. ACCF/AHA clopidogrel clinical alert: approaches to the FDA "boxed warning": a report of the American College of Cardiology Foundation Task Force on clinical expert consensus documents and the American Heart Association endorsed by the Society for Cardiovascular Angiography and Interventions and the Society of Thoracic Surgeons. J Am Coll Cardiol. 2010 Jul;56(4):321-41.

44. Holmes MV, Perel P, Shah T, et al. CYP2C19 genotype, clopidogrel metabolism, platelet function, and cardiovascular events. JAMA. 2011 Dec 28;306(24):2704-14.

45. Brar SS, ten Berg J, Marcucci R, et al. Impact of platelet reactivity on clinical outcomes after percutaneous coronary intervention: a collaborative meta-analysis of individual participant data. J Amer Coll Cardiol. 2011 Nov 1;58(19):1945-54.

46. Lord SJ, Irwig L, Simes RJ. When is measuring sensitivity and specificity sufficient to evaluate a diagnostic test, and when do we need randomized trials? Ann Intern Med. 2006;144(11):850-5.

47. Dahabreh IJ, Terasawa T, Castaldi PJ, et al. Systematic review: anti-epidermal growth factor receptor treatment effect modification by KRAS mutations in advanced colorectal cancer. Ann Intern Med. 2011 Jan 4;154(1):37-49.

48. Simon RM, Paik S, Hayes DF. Use of archived specimens in evaluation of prognostic and predictive biomarkers. J Natl Cancer Inst. 2009 Nov 4;101(21):1446-52.

49. Cain LE, Robins JM, Lanoy E, et al. When to start treatment? A systematic approach to the comparison of dynamic regimes using observational data. Int J Biostat. 2010;6(2):18.

50. Hernan MA, Lanoy E, Costagliola D, et al. Comparison of dynamic treatment regimes via inverse probability weighting. Basic Clin Pharmacol Toxicol. 2006;98(3):237-42.

51. Orellana L, Rotnitzky A, Robins JM. Dynamic regime marginal structural mean models for estimation of optimal dynamic treatment regimes, Part I: main content. Int J Biostat. 2010;6(2):8.

Introduction

Platelets play a role in the development of atherosclerotic vascular diseases such as acute and chronic coronary artery disease, ischemic cerebrovascular disease (i.e., ischemic stroke or transient ischemic attack), and peripheral arterial disease. Specifically, platelet activation and aggregation, and the interaction of platelets with blood cells and the endothelium, contribute to the pathophysiology of these diseases. Furthermore, platelets participate in thrombus formation in the setting of atrial fibrillation.[1] Because of the importance of platelets in disease processes that often culminate in major adverse clinical events (e.g., myocardial infarction, ischemic stroke, or cardiovascular death), there is a strong rationale for the development of therapies specifically targeting platelet function for the primary and secondary prevention of cardiovascular disease. Because patient response to antiplatelet treatments is variable, there is also great interest in developing biomarkers to predict treatment response and guide treatment selection.

Burden of Disease and Clinical Setting

Approximately 82 million Americans currently suffer from some form of cardiovascular disease.[2] Coronary heart disease alone is the cause of 1 of every 6 deaths in the United States; and stroke, 1 of every 18 deaths.[3] In spite of widespread prevention efforts, it is estimated that every year more than a million Americans have a myocardial infarction and approximately 795,000 Americans experience a first or recurrent stroke.[2] There were approximately seven million inpatient cardiovascular operations and procedures in the United States in 2007, of which one million were either percutaneous coronary intervention (PCI) or coronary artery bypass graft (CABG) surgeries.[2]

Randomized controlled trials have established dual antiplatelet treatment with clopidogrel and aspirin as the current standard of care for medical and interventional management of acute coronary syndromes.[4] Dual antiplatelet treatment is also recommended for patients undergoing PCI[5] with placement of stents (either bare metal or drug eluting). Randomized controlled trials support the use of clopidogrel in patients who have experienced acute cardiovascular events (e.g., stroke) and those with peripheral arterial disease.[4,6-9] In patients with atrial fibrillation and contraindications to vitamin K antagonists, the ACTIVE-A trial suggested that the combination of clopidogrel and aspirin is more effective than aspirin alone for preventing thromboembolic disease.[10]

Since the approval of clopidogrel by the Food and Drug Administration (FDA) for routine clinical use, the drug has become one of the most commonly prescribed agents in the United States. However, patient response to clopidogrel-based antiplatelet therapy is variable (both between patients and across multiple measurements within a patient), with some patients showing no or minimal platelet response to clopidogrel administration (often termed clopidogrel "nonresponsiveness" or "resistance"). Alternatives to standard clopidogrel treatment include higher-dose clopidogrel regimens and the use of other antiplatelet agents, such as prasugrel or ticagrelor.[11-14] Given the availability of alternative antiplatelet strategies and concern about adverse clinical outcomes in clopidogrel nonresponders, research has focused on methods to identify patients who are unlikely to benefit from clopidogrel-based treatment. The question of identifying the optimal antiplatelet therapy may also carry cost implications because generic clopidogrel products are now available in the United States.[a]

Clopidogrel Metabolism

To be biologically active, clopidogrel must be transformed to the active metabolite R-130964 by members of CYP enzyme system, primarily the enzyme CYP2C19. R-130964 acts by binding irreversibly to the $P2Y_{12}$ receptor (the adenosine diphosphate [ADP] receptor) on the surface of platelets and inhibits platelet aggregation for the life cycle of the platelet.[15,16] Platelet aggregation in a patient returns to pretreatment levels approximately 5 days after clopidogrel is stopped, owing to the production of new (noninhibited) platelets by the hematopoietic system.[17,18]

The CYP2C19 gene is highly polymorphic, with more than 35 identified variants. Following the recommendations of the Human Cytochrome P450 Allele Nomenclature Database,[b] each of these variants is designated by a number (e.g., "*1," "*2," and so on). CYP2C19*1 alleles lead to normal enzymatic activity (i.e., a normal metabolizer phenotype). Some alleles, including the relatively common CYP2C19*2, *3, and *4 alleles, are all known to be "loss-of-function" alleles that lead to complete elimination of enzymatic activity (i.e., a poor metabolizer phenotype). The relatively common CYP2C19*17 alleles are known to be "gain-of-function" alleles that lead to increased enzymatic activity (i.e., an enhanced metabolizer phenotype).[19]

However, the relationship between genotype and clinical outcomes is not straightforward. The fact that each individual carries two CYP2C19 alleles results in combinations of alleles of varying enzymatic activity. The combined effect of the two alleles on actual enzymatic activity levels depends on the "true" genetic model of CYP2C19 alleles (dominant, recessive, additive, or co-dominant). For example, if the inheritance model of a loss of function allele is dominant, then a patient with only one loss of function allele would have very low levels of enzymatic activity. If, however, the inheritance model is recessive then a patient could have one loss of function allele but still have normal levels of enzymatic activity. Because different combinations of alleles have different metabolic activity—potentially leading to variability in platelet reactivity and clinical outcomes—analyses of the prognostic effect of CYP2C19 genotype need to consider the underlying genetic model. To complicate matters further, the genetic model for different outcomes is not necessarily the same. Unfortunately, the "true" underlying genetic model for CYP2C19 variants is not known with certainty.[20-24] This is of particular concern as the allele frequency of CYP2C19 variants is heterogeneous across populations of different ethnicity, resulting in different genotype prevalences. For example, data from the Third National Health and Nutrition Examination Survey (NHANES III) showed statistically significant heterogeneity in the prevalence of the *2 allele among non-Hispanic whites, Mexican-Americans, and non-Hispanic blacks. The latter group had the highest prevalence of the *2 allele (18.3%) and of homozygotes for that allele (*2/*2; 3.8%).[25] Studies have shown that the prevalence of the rare allele is even higher in East-Asian populations (with *2 allele frequencies as high as 30-40%); in these populations an increased number of individuals will be susceptible to the effects of reduced clopidogrel metabolism.[26-28]

Furthermore, the CYP2C19 genotype is only one of many determinants of the effect of clopidogrel on platelet reactivity. For example, a genome-wide association study recently

---

[a]FDA release, available at: www.fda.gov/NewsEvents/Newsroom/PressAnnouncements/ucm304489.htm; last accessed October 16, 2012.

[b]Available at: www.cypalleles.ki.se; last accessed April 18, 2012.

demonstrated that the *2 allele accounts for only 12 percent of the total observed variation in clopidogrel responsiveness in a selected white population.[29] Several studies have demonstrated that environmental factors and patient characteristics, such as body mass index, diabetes, and smoking habits, can influence platelet reactivity.

Predicting Response and Guiding Antiplatelet Treatment

There are currently two main approaches to determine whether a patient will have a poor response to clopidogrel: (1) genetic testing to see whether the patient has a genotype that is associated with reduced ability to metabolize clopidogrel (a poor-metabolizer phenotype), and (2) direct testing of the patient's blood while the patient is taking clopidogrel to see whether the platelets actually have become less prone to aggregate in response to specific agonists (phenotypic testing for platelet reactivity).

Genetic Tests for CYP2C19 Variants

Genetic testing for one or more genetic variants can be performed with various genotyping methods, such as restriction-fragment-length polymorphism analysis, other polymerase chain reaction (PCR)–based methods, or single nucleotide polymorphism (SNP) microarray methods. Testing for CYP2C19 variants requires a sample of somatic genetic material, usually obtained from a blood sample or from buccal swabs. Because allelic variants at the CYP2C19 locus do not change over a person's lifetime, testing done at any time point is representative of the person's genotype. Several studies have evaluated associations between loss-of-function CYP2C19 alleles and major adverse cardiovascular events as well as intermediate endpoints (e.g., platelet reactivity). Research has also focused on whether CYP2C19 genotypes can be used to predict the phenotype of on-clopidogrel platelet reactivity and whether the association of genotype and phenotype can be modified by alternative treatment strategies (e.g., higher clopidogrel dosing or use other antiplatelet agents).

Measurement of Platelet Reactivity

Phenotypic testing measures the reactivity of platelets while a patient is taking clopidogrel (on-clopidogrel platelet reactivity). Several assays for measuring platelet reactivity are available. These include rapid (point-of-care) platelet function assays (e.g., VerifyNow, Platelet Function Analyzer [PFA]-100, Plateletworks), measurements of mediators of reactivity (e.g., vasodilator-stimulated phosphoprotein [VASP] phosphorylation using flow cytometry), and functional assays (e.g., turbidimetric, impedance, and conductance aggregometry using appropriate agonists). The technical characteristics and principles of measurement of these tests have been described in recent reviews.[30-37] We refer to all these assays as "phenotypic tests," because they attempt to measure an intermediate clinical phenotype (platelet reactivity).[38] A potential advantage of phenotypic tests is that some assays can be easily used during routine care (point-of-care testing). In addition, because platelet reactivity reflects the combined impact of an individual's entire genetic makeup (not limited to CYP2C19) along with environmental exposures on clopidogrel pharmacodynamics, phenotypic testing may better predict clinical outcomes among clopidogrel treated patients. However a number of different assays using diverse measurement techniques are available and the prognostic value and potential clinical utility of platelet reactivity testing are still unclear.

Modifiers of the Prognostic Ability and Clinical Utility of Tests

Proton-pump inhibitors (PPIs) are often prescribed along with antiplatelet therapy to limit the potential for gastrointestinal bleeding complications. Because CYP2C19 is the key enzyme in the metabolism of several PPIs, it has been hypothesized that coadministration of these drugs could inhibit the activation of clopidogrel.[39] A recent systematic review that examined studies investigating the association between PPI use and adverse cardiovascular events among patients receiving clopidogrel concluded that PPI use was associated with an approximately 40 percent increase in the risk of major adverse cardiovascular outcomes and an 18 percent increase in mortality.[40] However, no systematic review has assessed the interaction of PPIs with the clopidogrel treatment effect within categories defined by CYP2C19 status or platelet reactivity.

Other potential modifiers of the utility of genetic and phenotypic test results include the specific indication for clopidogrel use (because the prognostic ability of testing may vary among patient populations), race or ethnicity (because of the varying prevalence of CYP2C19 alleles among different groups), comorbid conditions (that may affect the baseline event rate or serve as markers for the coadministration of drugs metabolized by CYP2C19), baseline disease severity, sex, and age.

Current Uncertainties Regarding Genetic and Phenotypic Testing

There are several areas of uncertainty regarding the use of both genetic tests for CYP2C19 variants and phenotypic tests to assess on-clopidogrel platelet reactivity. First, there is controversy regarding the prognostic ability of these tests for clinical outcomes in patients who are receiving clopidogrel: several studies have reported significant associations between CYP2C19 status or high on-clopidogrel platelet reactivity and clinical outcomes; however concerns have been raised regarding the potential for selective outcome reporting and publication bias to have affected study results.[20,41,42,42] The relative prognostic value of genetic and phenotypic testing is also unclear.

Second, there are conflicting views on whether the results of these tests can be used to guide therapeutic decisionmaking for antiplatelet therapy. Although clinicians and patients may find it helpful to know the probability of future outcomes under clopidogrel therapy, medical tests are most valuable when they can be used to guide treatment decisions. Thus, beyond prognostic ability, there is interest in evaluating whether genetic or phenotypic testing can improve patient outcomes by identifying patients who would benefit more (or experience less harm) by using treatment strategies other than standard clopidogrel-based treatment (e.g., using alternative clopidogrel dosing schemes or other antiplatelet agents). The observation that specific CYP2C19 variants or levels of on-treatment platelet reactivity above a threshold predict worse outcomes does not necessarily mean that changing treatment on the basis of these tests will improve outcomes. It is possible that the genotype or phenotype is simply a marker for poor outcome regardless of the treatment strategy used.[41] Therefore the evidence of the test's impact on treatment decisions and subsequent patient outcomes must be considered separately from outcome prediction. Some investigators advocate clinical use,[43,44] while others suggest that the tests are not ready for clinical application because the evidence on their clinical utility is limited.[41,42,45] The best evidence on the use of testing for guiding treatment decisionmaking can be obtained from comparative studies of alternative testing strategies (including no-testing). As discussed above, prognostic value is not enough to establish the utility of testing for guiding treatment choice; it is also important to demonstrate that the prognostic effect is modified by the treatment received. Third, the modifiers of these tests' effects, both in terms of prognostic ability and therapeutic decisionmaking, also have not been fully evaluated.

Scope of the Review

The purpose of this review was to systematically evaluate the analytic validity, prognostic utility, and comparative effectiveness of two types of biomarker tests (and relevant test-and-treat strategies) for guiding antiplatelet therapy in patient populations who are eligible for clopidogrel treatment. The impact of biomarkers such as genotype or phenotype on patient-relevant outcomes is indirect; any effects of testing are mediated through the impact of test results on clinical thinking and therapeutic decisionmaking. In the case of antiplatelet therapy, the effects of treatment on clinical outcomes are believed to be mediated through platelet reactivity (a surrogate outcome). We aimed to assess the impact of testing on both intermediate and patient-relevant clinical outcomes.

Key Questions

On the basis of the original topic nomination and an extensive process of topic development and refinement, we formulated the following Key Questions to guide the review. These questions broadly follow the "ACCE framework," covering Analytic validity, Clinical validity, Clinical utility, and test-related harms, as proposed by the Evaluation of Genomic Applications in Practice and Prevention Working Group of the Centers for Disease Control and Prevention.

Key Question 1. In patient populations who are candidates for clopidogrel therapy, does genetic testing for CYP2C19 variants predict intermediate and clinical outcomes following treatment initiation?

a. What is the analytic validity (technical test performance) of the various assays used for CYP2C19 genetic testing?
b. What is the clinical validity (predictive accuracy) of genetic testing for predicting intermediate and clinical outcomes in patients who are receiving clopidogrel therapy?
c. Do the following factors modify the association between genetic test results and clinical outcomes?
    i. Co-medications
    ii. Patient-level factors (e.g., race or ethnicity, age, sex, disease severity, or comorbidities)
    iii. Test-related factors (e.g., between-assay differences)
    iv. System-level factors (e.g., settings where testing is performed)

Key Question 2. In patient populations receiving clopidogrel therapy, does phenotypic testing of platelet reactivity predict intermediate and clinical outcomes?

a. What is the analytic validity (technical test performance) of the various assays used in phenotypic testing of platelet reactivity?
b. What is the clinical validity (predictive accuracy) of phenotypic testing for predicting intermediate and clinical outcomes in patients who are receiving clopidogrel therapy?

Do the following factors modify the association between phenotypic test results and clinical outcomes?

    i. Comedications
    ii. Patient-level factors (e.g., race or ethnicity, age, sex, disease severity, or comorbidities)
    iii. Test-related factors (e.g., between-assay differences)
    iv. System-level factors (e.g., settings where testing is performed)

Key Question 3. What is the comparative effectiveness of alternative test-and-treat strategies (including a no-testing strategy) for therapeutic decisionmaking regarding antiplatelet therapy among patients who are candidates for clopidogrel-based treatment?

a. What is the comparative effectiveness of the following testing strategies on therapeutic decisionmaking, platelet reactivity during followup, and clinical outcomes in patients who are candidates for antiplatelet treatment?
    i. Genetic testing for CYP2C19
    ii. Genetic testing for CYP2C19 followed by phenotypic testing for platelet reactivity
    iii. Phenotypic testing for platelet reactivity
    iv. No testing
b. How do modifying factors (e.g., race or ethnicity, age, sex, comorbidities, diet, or the time between conducting the test and obtaining results) affect the association of alternative phenotypic or genetic test-and-treat strategies and patient outcomes? Alternative test-guided treatments can include nonclopidogrel antiplatelet agents or high-dose clopidogrel regimens.

Key Question 4. What are the potential adverse effects or harms from genetic or phenotypic testing per se or from test-directed treatments?

Methods

This comparative effectiveness review evaluated the analytic validity, prognostic value, and comparative effectiveness of two types of medical tests (genetic testing for CYP2C19 variants and phenotypic testing to measure platelet reactivity) for patients who are candidates for or are already receiving antiplatelet therapy. A primary focus was the evaluation of test-guided therapeutic decisionmaking on patient-relevant clinical outcomes.

We performed a systematic review of the published literature using established methodologies as outlined in the Agency for Healthcare Research and Quality (AHRQ) "Methods Guide for Effectiveness and Comparative Effectiveness Reviews" (hereafter referred to as the Methods Guide; available at www.effectivehealthcare.ahrq.gov/methodsguide.cfm). The main sections in this chapter reflect the elements of the protocol established for the comparative effectiveness review; certain methods map to the Preferred Reporting Items for Systematic Reviews and Meta-Analyses (PRISMA) checklist.[46] All methods and analyses were determined a priori. The protocol was developed with input from external clinical and methodological experts and in consultation with officers from AHRQ; it was posted online to solicit additional public comments.

AHRQ Task Order Officer

The AHRQ Task Order Officer (TOO) assigned to this project was responsible for overseeing all aspects of this report. The TOO facilitated a common understanding among all parties involved in the project, resolved ambiguities, and fielded all queries from the Evidence-based Practice Center (EPC) regarding the scope and processes of the project. The TOO and other staff at AHRQ reviewed the report for consistency, clarity, and to ensure that it conforms to AHRQ standards.

External Stakeholder Input

An initial set of questions for evidence review were nominated to the Effective Healthcare Program by a Federal agency. During a topic refinement phase, the initial questions that had previously been nominated for this report were refined with input from a panel of Key Informants. The Key Informants included a general internist, a cardiologist, a representative from the FDA, a representative from the Evaluation of Genomic Applications in Practice and Prevention (EGAPP) Working Group, health care payers (one public and one private), and a patient representative. After a public review of the proposed Key Questions, a group of experts was convened to form the Technical Expert Panel (TEP), which served in an advisory capacity to help refine the Key Questions, identify important issues, and define parameters for the review of evidence. TEP members included a representative of the EGAPP Working Group (who also nominated the topic and participated in Topic Refinement), experts in cardiovascular disease (including an interventional cardiologist), experts on the tests of interest, and a methodologist with expertise in health technology assessment. Discussions among the EPC, TOO, Key Informants, and, subsequently, the TEP occurred during a series of teleconferences and via email. In addition, input from the TEP was sought during compilation of the report when questions arose about the scope of the review.

Key Questions

Four Key Questions were posed. Key Questions 1 and 2 pertains to the analytic validity and prognostic validity of the index tests of interest. Key Question 3 pertains to the comparative effectiveness of alternative test-and-treatment strategies (including a no-testing strategy). Finally, Key Question 4 pertains to the harms of test-directed treatment and testing per se. The complete Key Questions are presented at the end of the Introduction section.

Analytic Framework

We developed an analytic framework (Figure 1) that maps the Key Questions within the context of populations, interventions, comparators, and outcomes of interest, as well as the chain of logic that evidence must support to link the interventions to health outcomes. Analytic and clinical validity were straightforward to represent in the analytic framework (Key Questions 1a, 1b, 2a, and 2b). Regarding treatment decisionmaking (Key Question 3a), we conceptualized the analytic framework as a decision problem, wherein patients' disease can be managed with one of the following approaches (depicted from top to bottom in the flow diagram):

1. Undergo genetic testing and then base the treatment decision on the test results.
2. Undergo genetic testing and then base the treatment decision on the test results. After receiving therapy for an adequate period of time, undergo phenotypic testing for platelet reactivity and use the results to decide whether the treatment strategy should be modified.
3. Receive standard treatment directly and, after an appropriate amount of time, undergo phenotypic testing for platelet reactivity and use the test results to decide whether the treatment strategy should be modified. Use of phenotypic testing (but not genetic testing) as a monitoring test can be considered a variation of this strategy in which the test is repeatedly performed.
4. Receive antiplatelet therapy without undergoing any testing (the current standard of care).

The above strategies were identified as the most prevalent in published studies by preliminary searches conducted in preparation of this review. Additional variations of these strategies were uncovered by the full evidence review.

Modifiers of the effects of testing on outcomes (both in terms of predictive ability and decisionmaking) were reviewed in Key Questions 1c, 2c, and 3b. Tests and test-directed treatments may be associated with harms; this was investigated in Key Question 4.

Figure 1. Analytic framework

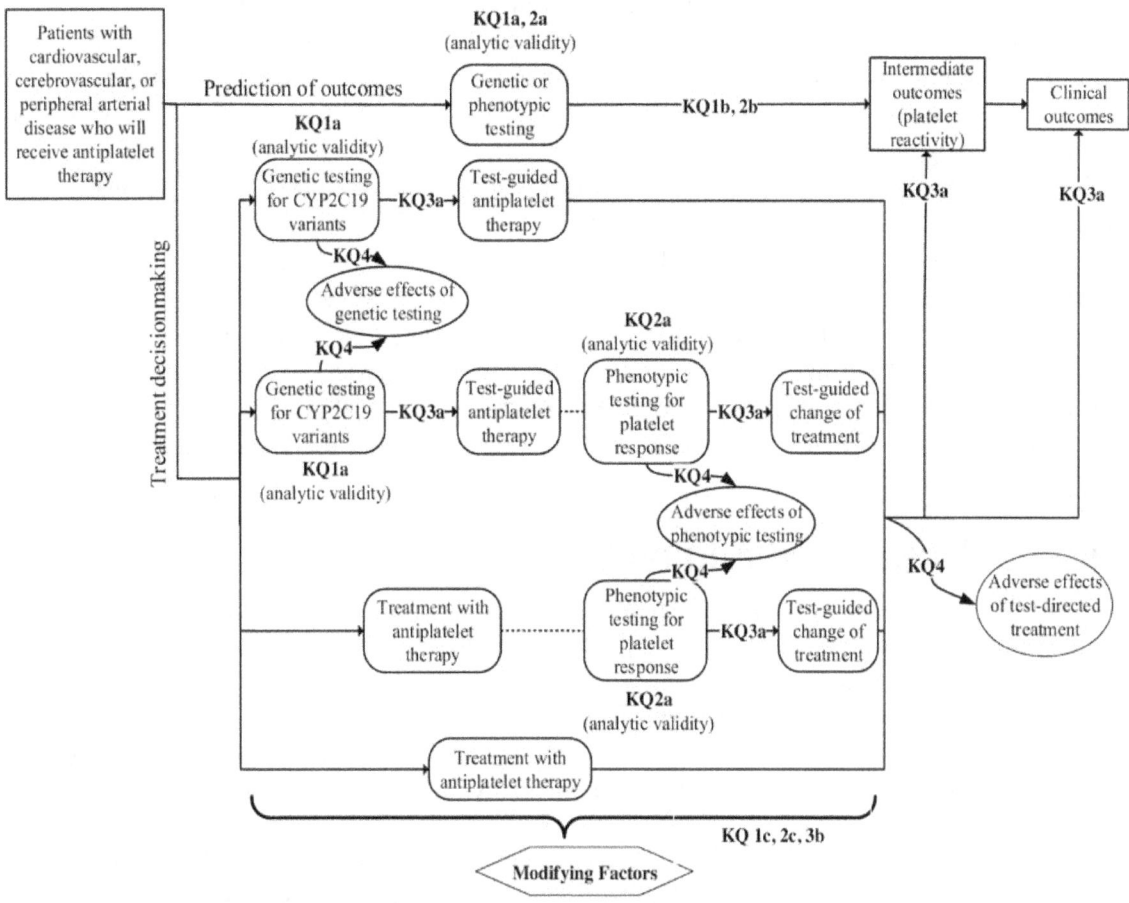

Abbreviation: KQ = Key Question.

Literature Search and Abstract Screening

We conducted literature searches for studies in MEDLINE®, the Cochrane Central Trials Registry®, and the Cochrane Database of Systematic Reviews (from inception through July 27, 2012) without any language restriction. Our search included terms for the populations, tests, and drugs of interest (see Appendix A for complete search strings, which were extensively validated against previous reviews on the tests of interest). We also performed searches of the Human Genome Epidemiology Network (HuGENet) database and National Institutes of Health Genetic Association Database, using the same cutoff date (July 27, 2012). Finally, we performed a targeted search of the FDA Web site (last search performed on April 25, 2012).

A common set of 200 abstracts was first screened by four investigators and discrepancies were discussed in order to standardize screening practices and ensure understanding of the criteria by all team members. Two hundred additional abstracts were screened by all investigators to ensure that selection criteria were standardized. The remaining citations were split into nonoverlapping sets, each screened by a single reviewer. Abstracts were manually screened, using *Abstrackr*.[47] Reviewers were specifically instructed to be inclusive in order to increase the sensitivity of abstract screening. Abstracts considered not relevant by a reviewer were rereviewed by a second team member. We retrieved the full text of articles for citations considered potentially relevant by at least one investigator.

We asked technical experts to provide additional citations of potentially relevant articles. Additional studies were identified through the perusal of reference lists of eligible studies, published clinical practice guidelines, and relevant narrative and systematic reviews. We also performed a targeted search of the FDA Web site (with the last search performed on April 25, 2012). On the basis of preliminary searches conducted during topic refinement, we provided the Scientific Resource Center (SRC, an entity within the Effective Health Care Program independent of the EPC) with a list of relevant technologies and manufacturers. The SRC solicited information from the manufacturers and organized all obtained material into scientific information packets (SIPs), which were then forwarded to the EPC for review. All articles identified through sources other than electronic database searches were reviewed for eligibility in full text, using the same criteria as for articles identified through our database searches.

Finally, we searched the ClinicalTrials.gov Web site (with the last search performed on May 3, 2012) to identify ongoing comparative trials of test-and-treat strategies for guiding antiplatelet treatment. We did not consider unpublished data other than that included in FDA documents or ClinicalTrials.gov.

Study Selection and Eligibility Criteria

Full-text articles were reviewed independently by two investigators to determine eligibility. Disagreements regarding inclusion or relevance to a specific question were resolved by consensus including at least one additional senior investigator.

We considered both comparative and noncomparative studies for Key Questions pertaining to prognostic ability but focused on comparative studies of alternative test-and-treat strategies. Below we detail the study selection criteria for each Key Question. The criteria are also summarized in Table 1.

We did not include non–English language studies but we recorded the number of studies that were excluded on the grounds of language for each Key Question. We excluded narrative reviews, editorials, letters to the editor, and other papers not presenting primary research data. We also excluded studies reporting exclusively on healthy individuals. Appendix B lists all the studies excluded after full-text screening and the reason for exclusion.

Populations and Conditions of Interest

For all Key Questions, the populations of interest consisted of adult patients with cardiovascular, cerebrovascular, or peripheral arterial disease who were candidates for or were receiving clopidogrel. Specifically, we included studies enrolling: (1) patients with acute coronary syndromes, including those who had experienced a myocardial infarction (ST-elevation or non–ST-elevation), or patients who had unstable angina; (2) patients who were undergoing PCI for acute coronary syndromes, those who had undergone PCI with stent implantation (of either bare-metal or drug-eluting stents), or those who had undergone CABG (and had a contraindication to acetylsalicylic acid); (3) patients with a previous ischemic stroke or transient ischemic attack; (4) patients with established peripheral arterial disease; and (5) patients with atrial fibrillation for whom vitamin K antagonist therapy was not suitable. We also reviewed studies evaluating the use of clopidogrel for the prevention of vascular events in high-risk populations (e.g., patients on hemodialysis).

Interventions

For Key Questions 1 and 2 we reviewed studies of genetic testing (for CYP2C19 variants) or phenotypic testing. Genetic variants of interest were all variants of the CYP2C19 locus, including loss- and gain-of-function alleles. Phenotypic tests of interest were those assessing on-clopidogrel platelet reactivity (the degree to which platelets are able to be activated by an agonist). After consultation with the TEP and the TOO, it was decided that tests of platelet activation (where an agonist is not used) would not be reviewed, because they are not in wide clinical use and are less standardized than tests of reactivity.

For Key Questions 3 (comparative effectiveness of test-and-treat strategies) and 4 (harms) we reviewed studies of management strategies involving genetic testing for CYP2C19 variants or phenotypic testing for platelet reactivity, followed by therapeutic management decisions based on test results. Potential test-and-treat strategies included testing for CYP2C19 genetic variants, testing for platelet reactivity, or both, to guide the choice among alternative antiplatelet treatment strategies (including standard clopidogrel dosing, increased clopidogrel dosing, and use of non–clopidogrel-based antiplatelet therapies such as ticagrelor or prasugrel).

Comparators

For Key Questions 1 and 2 (prognostic effects), a common implicit comparator is not performing any testing; in studies where information was reported on the prognostic effect of testing without comparisons against alternative tests, we considered the comparison to be testing versus no testing (implicit). However, we included studies comparing the prognostic accuracy of more than one genetic or phenotypic test applied to the same patient population.

For Key Questions 3 (comparative effectiveness of test-and-treat strategies) and 4 (harms), we considered as comparators either a no-testing strategy or alternative test-and-treat strategies.

Outcomes

For Key Questions 1a and 2a (analytic validity) we considered the following outcomes: analytic accuracy (e.g., analytic sensitivity and specificity), analytic precision, test detection limits, dilution linearity, test–retest reliability (e.g., intra-assay agreement, measurement reproducibility), interassay agreement, interlaboratory comparisons (e.g., interlaboratory agreement, measurement reproducibility), and the proportion of nonevaluable samples.

For Key Questions 1b–c and 2b–c we considered both intermediate outcomes (platelet reactivity, when used as a biomarker of outcome status) and clinical outcomes: overall mortality, myocardial infarction (fatal or nonfatal), ischemic stroke (fatal or nonfatal), cardiovascular mortality, stent thrombosis (for patients with implanted stents), combinations of the above (composite clinical outcomes), bleeding events (categorized by severity and by the organ system affected), and health-related and overall quality of life. Following discussions with Key Informants, it was decided that the review would not cover pharmacokinetic outcomes because they do not directly translate into clinical outcomes and because pharmacokinetic assessments are not routinely performed in patients receiving antiplatelet treatment.

For Key Question 3 we considered intermediate outcomes (platelet reactivity, when used as a biomarker of outcome status, and impact on therapeutic decisionmaking [i.e., change in clinical decisions on the basis of test results) and clinical outcomes (see previous paragraph).

Finally, for Key Question 4, we considered adverse effects of test-directed treatment (including bleeding events and others such as gastrointestinal events and liver toxic effects) and adverse effects of testing per se (such as test-related anxiety and adverse events secondary to venipuncture).

Study Designs

Key Questions 1 and 2

For Key Questions 1a and 2a, we reviewed studies of analytic validity (single laboratory studies or interlaboratory comparisons) reporting on metrics of intra-assay variability, reliability, analytic sensitivity against a reference standard, or agreement between methods.

For Key Questions 1b–c and 2b–c, we included prospective or retrospective cohort studies using the index tests of interest to predict outcomes. For Key Question 1b we also considered case–control studies. We excluded case–control studies from Key Question 2b because platelet reactivity is modified by coronary events, is variable over time, and is affected by treatments that are bound to be systematically different between cases and controls [i.e., platelet reactivity in the cases is modified by post-event exposures (e.g., treatment instituted after an ischemic event) and may be nonrepresentative of reactivity levels preceding the event of interest]. For analyses of prognostic ability, we also included clopidogrel-treated arms of comparative studies (of clopidogrel versus alternative strategies). We included studies assessing a single index test as well as those assessing more than one test (directly comparative studies). For Key Questions pertaining to effect modification (1c, 2c, and 3c) we required that studies reported formal interaction tests or allowed for the calculation of statistics that compare the test effect among strata of the modifier of interest.

Key Questions 3 and 4

For Key Questions 3 and 4 we included randomized and nonrandomized comparative studies of test-and-treat strategies in unselected populations. Because such studies are rare we also considered "repurposed" randomized controlled trials.[c,48-50] These studies are randomized investigations comparing alternative therapeutic interventions (e.g., clopidogrel-based vs. non–clopidogrel-based management). Biological samples are collected from all patients (all comparison groups) and are analyzed for one or more biomarker of interest. Because for each patient there is information on biomarker status, treatment assignment, and outcomes, the studies can provide information on effect modification (i.e., the presence of a differential treatment effect in biomarker-"positive" vs. biomarker-"negative" patients). This effect modification provides information about whether the biomarker can be used to guide therapeutic decisionmaking. In addition, we included studies where patients were selected on the basis of tests of interest (e.g., platelet reactivity above some threshold) and then randomly assigned to one of at least two alternative treatment strategies. For this study design we only considered randomized comparative studies (parallel arm or cross-over) because they can provide information on the unconfounded effect of treatment conditional on the test result. For Key Question 4 we planned to include noncomparative studies reporting on the harms of testing per se, but none of these studies were identified.

---

[c]These studies are also referred to as "prospective–retrospective" studies in the oncology literature, which is where the design has been applied mostly (presumably because of the availability of archived tissue samples in randomized trials of cancer therapeutics).[48]

Sample Size and Timing

For Key Questions relevant to analytic validity, we used a minimum sample size of 50 patients (or data points, depending on the design and analysis of the primary studies). This minimum sample size is often recommended for statistical comparisons of analytic validity (e.g., test–retest reliability or Bland–Altman test for agreement between continuous measurements). The precision of estimates of analytic validity depends on the specific statistic used; generally, a sample size of 50 excludes studies that are too small to be informative without being otherwise restrictive. For all other Key Questions (1b–c, 2b–c, 3, and 4), we included studies reporting on at least 10 patients (in total or, when there were ≥ 2 study groups, per group), because smaller studies produce very imprecise estimates.

We included studies of any duration of followup, including those that did not report this information. We considered short-term and long-term outcomes separately (using a cutoff time of 30 days, wherever appropriate). For patients undergoing invasive or interventional procedures (e.g., PCI or CABG), we also considered periprocedural events separately.

Settings

Studies conducted in all relevant care settings (e.g., primary and secondary care or rural and urban clinics) were included. Study selection was not based on cointerventions.

Data Extraction

A single investigator extracted data from each study; quantitative results were verified by a second reviewer. Disagreements were resolved by consensus involving a third investigator. Data were extracted into standard forms; separate forms were generated for each Key Question. Extraction forms were piloted on three to five articles for each Key Question and revisions were made as needed. We extracted information on the following items: patient selection criteria, population characteristics, sample size, study design, analytic details, and outcomes.

Table 1. Summary of the selection criteria used

Key Question	Population*	Intervention	Comparator	Outcomes	Study Design	Sample Size
KQ1a	Adult patients with vascular disease who were candidates for or were receiving clopidogrel	Genetic testing of CYP2C19 variants	Alternative genotyping assays or repeat testing	Analytic accuracy, analytic precision, test detection limits, dilution linearity, test–retest reliability, interassay agreement; interlaboratory comparison, and proportion of nonevaluable samples for genetic test	Laboratory studies reporting on assay variability, reliability, accuracy, or agreement	≥50 data points
KQ1b	Same as above	Phenotypic testing of on-clopidogrel platelet reactivity	No testing or other predictive tests	Intermediate outcomes (e.g., platelet reactivity as a biomarker of outcome status) Clinical outcomes: overall or cardiovascular mortality, fatal or nonfatal MI or ischemic stroke, stent thrombosis, bleeding, and health-related and overall quality of life	Prospective or retrospective cohort or case–control studies using genetic test to predict outcomes, comparative studies (of clopidogrel vs. alternative treatment), or clopidogrel-based treatment groups from RCTs	≥10 patients
KQ1c	Same as above	Genetic testing of CYP2C19 variants	No testing or other predictive tests	Same as for KQ1b	Same as for KQ1b but in addition, formal interaction tests or statistics comparing the test effect among strata of the modifier of interest must have been reported or calculation permitted	≥10 patients
KQ2a	Same as above	Phenotypic testing of on-clopidogrel platelet reactivity	Alternative phenotypic test assays or repeat testing	Analytic accuracy, analytic precision, test detection limits, dilution linearity, test–retest reliability, interassay agreement; interlaboratory comparison, and proportion of nonevaluable samples for phenotypic test	Laboratory studies reporting on assay variability, reliability, accuracy, or agreement	≥50 data points

14

Table 1. Summary of the selection criteria used (continued)

Key Question	Population*	Intervention	Comparator	Outcomes	Study Design	Sample Size
KQ2b	Same as above	Genetic testing of CYP2C19 variants	No testing or other predictive tests	Intermediate outcomes (e.g., platelet reactivity as a biomarker of outcome status) Clinical outcomes: overall or cardiovascular mortality, fatal or nonfatal MI or ischemic stroke, stent thrombosis, bleeding, and health-related and overall quality of life	Prospective or retrospective cohort studies using phenotypic test to predict outcomes, comparative studies (of clopidogrel vs. alternative treatment), or clopidogrel-based treatment groups from RCTs	≥10 patients
KQ2c	Same as above	Phenotypic testing of on-clopidogrel platelet reactivity	No testing or other predictive tests	Same as for KQ2b	Same as for KQ2b but fin addition, normal interaction tests or statistics comparing the test effect among strata of the modifier of interest must have been reported or calculation permitted	≥10 patients
KQ3a	Same as above	Management strategies involving CYP2C19 testing, followed by treatment decision on basis of test result†	No-testing strategy or alternative test-and-treat strategy	Intermediate outcomes (e.g., platelet reactivity as a biomarker of outcome status) Impact on therapeutic decisionmaking Clinical outcomes: overall or cardiovascular mortality, fatal or nonfatal MI or ischemic stroke, stent thrombosis, bleeding, and health-related and overall quality of life	Randomized and nonrandomized comparative studies of test-and-treat strategies in unselected populations or "repurposed" RCTs (e.g., clopidogrel-based vs. non-clopidogrel-based management; see text for more information)	≥10 patients per group

15

Table 1. Summary of the selection criteria used (continued)

Key Question	Population*	Intervention	Comparator	Outcomes	Study Design	Sample Size
KQ3b	Same as above	Management strategies involving phenotypic testing of on-clopidogrel platelet reactivity, followed by treatment decision on basis of test result†	No-testing strategy or alternative test-and-treat strategy	Same as for KQ 3a	Same as for KQ3a	≥10 patients per group
KQ4	Same as above	Same as for KQ3a and 3b	Same as for KQ3a and 3b	Adverse effects of test-directed treatment (e.g., bleeding, gastrointestinal event, liver toxic effect) and of testing (e.g., test-related anxiety, events secondary to venipuncture)	Same as for KQ3a; also noncomparative studies reporting harms of testing	≥10 patients (per group, for comparative studies)

Abbreviations: KQ = Key Question; MI = myocardial infarction; RCT = randomized controlled trial.

*The population of interest was the same for all the Key Questions and included cardiovascular, cerebrovascular, or peripheral arterial disease (acute coronary syndromes; percutaneous coronary intervention or coronary artery bypass grafting with a contraindication to acetylsalicylic acid; previous ischemic stroke or transient ischemic attack; established peripheral arterial disease; and atrial fibrillation with contraindications to vitamin K antagonist treatment).

†Potential test-and-treat strategies included testing for CYP2C19 genetic variants, testing for platelet reactivity, or both, to guide selection among alternative antiplatelet treatment strategies (including standard clopidogrel dosing, increased clopidogrel dosing, and non–clopidogrel-based antiplatelet therapies such as ticagrelor or prasugrel).

16

Data Synthesis

Qualitative Synthesis

We summarized the findings of the report according to the order of the Key Questions. Within each Key Question, results were organized for each appropriate subgroup on the basis of the populations assessed and clinical indications for clopidogrel use (e.g., acute coronary syndromes, stroke, atrial fibrillation not suitable for vitamin K antagonists, etc.), index tests used, and outcomes assessed. Data are presented in evidence tables and are summarized narratively in the full text. We use tables and graphs (histograms, weighted scatterplots, and others) to synthesize information across studies.

Predefined subgroups of interest were those defined by race or ethnicity, sex, specific assay used, and clinical setting of test use (e.g., short-term administration of clopidogrel during treatment of acute cardiac events or PCI vs. chronic clopidogrel use).

Quantitative Synthesis

Meta-Analysis

We performed meta-analysis when at least three studies were available on sufficiently similar populations, using the same test, and assessing the same outcomes. Sufficient similarity was judged on the basis of the clinical heterogeneity of patient populations, interventions, and testing strategies, as well as the methodological heterogeneity of study designs and outcomes reported. The determination on the appropriateness of meta-analysis was made before any statistical analysis was conducted; we did not base the decision to perform meta-analysis on statistical criteria for heterogeneity. Such criteria are often inadequate (e.g., low power when the number of studies is small) and do not account for the ability to explore and explain heterogeneity by examining study-level characteristics. We provide our rationale for performing (or not performing) meta-analysis on a case-by-case basis in the Results section. Of particular note was our decision not to combine studies of different phenotypic tests for platelet reactivity. This decision was based on the different principles of measurement implemented in different assays and our own findings on interassay agreement (presented under Key Question 2a), which indicated that agreement for identifying lack of response may be limited. Similarly, we decided not to combine randomized treatment trials providing information about effect modification because they had enrolled heterogeneous patient populations and compared different pairs of interventions (i.e., the magnitude and direction of effect modification by the tests of interest was likely to vary among different treatment comparisons).

Meta-analyses of relative risk (RR) estimates from individual studies were performed using random effects inverse-variance models that account for unexplained heterogeneity between studies. Fixed effects models were evaluated in sensitivity analyses. We estimated between-study heterogeneity using the DerSimonian–Laird method.[51] Between-study heterogeneity was assessed on the basis of Cochran's chi-square–based Q statistic.[52] Heterogeneity was considered statistically significant when the p-value of the Q statistic (P_Q) was less than 0.1, to account for the low power of the test when the number of studies is relatively low (as was the case in our review). Between-study inconsistency was assessed using the I^2 index.[53] I^2 values higher than 50 percent were considered to indicate moderate inconsistency; values above 75 percent, severe inconsistency. These cutoff values are arbitrary and I^2 estimates are typically associated with

17

substantial uncertainty.[54] In these analyses, for studies where no events were observed in a single arm we used a continuity correction of 0.5. Studies in which no events were observed in both arms ("zero total event" studies) were excluded from meta-analyses.

For meta-analyses of studies of prognostic effects, we also estimated summary prognostic sensitivity and specificity, using bivariate random effects models with the exact binomial likelihood to model within study variability.[55,56] Analyses using the exact binomial likelihood do not require continuity corrections when zero events are observed. Although analyses of prognostic sensitivity and specificity can supplement the information from meta-analyses of RRs, we note that they are unadjusted for other patient level covariates and do not account for the time-to-event nature of the outcomes of interest (the necessary information is never reported in individual published studies).

Genetic Model for Studies of CYP2C19 Variants

In the case of biallelic loci dominant, recessive, additive, or co-dominant genetic models of inheritance are possible. Inferences under a misspecified model can lead to misleading conclusions regarding the magnitude and direction of genotype-phenotype associations. The "true" genetic model for the effect of CYP2C19 polymorphisms on pharmacodynamic and clinical outcomes is not known. Some evidence suggests that the loss-of-function trait for the CYP2C19 gene has a dominant mode of inheritance, whereas others support an additive or recessive model.[21-23] Similar data exist for the gain-of-function (*17) allele. Following previous meta-analyses on the same variants, in our primary analyses we used a *dominant model* for all minor alleles (i.e., a model that assumes carriers of one and carriers of two minor alleles have the same phenotype).[20,41] In addition to having been used by other investigators, the dominant genetic model allows the inclusion of data from the maximum possible number of studies (because data in relevant publications were often inadequate to perform analyses under an additive model). However, to assess the robustness of our findings under different genetic models we repeated meta-analyses using a *recessive genetic model* (i.e., a model that assumes carriers of one minor allele and non-carriers have the same phenotype) and an *additive (per-allele) genetic model* (i.e., a model that quantifies the effect of each additional variant allele on the phenotype). Although a model-free approach for meta-analysis of genetic associations is particularly appealing in the presence of uncertainty about the underlying mode of inheritance, available methods are impractical unless the number of studies is fairly large. For this reason they were not implemented for this review.[24]

Measures of Association for Prognostic Studies

Because the majority of studies reporting on clinical outcomes included in this report had longitudinal designs, the most appropriate statistical analyses take into account the time to occurrence of events (e.g., by using survival analysis methods). For this reason, we used hazard or incidence rate ratios in our meta-analyses whenever available or extractable from the reviewed studies. When such statistics were not reported (and could not be calculated), we used risk (proportion) ratios because they approximate the relative incidence rate. For case–control studies we used odds ratios (reported or calculated) because they are valid statistics for these designs and approximate the risk ratio or incidence rate ratio (depending on sampling methods).[57-59] For parsimony, we refer to all these statistics as "relative risks" (RRs).

Subgroup and Meta-Regression Analysis

To assess the impact of study-level characteristics on estimates of the effect size, we performed univariable (one study-level characteristic used as a predictor at a time) random effects meta-regression.[53] We did not perform analyses using averages of patient-level measurements as predictors (e.g., mean age or percent smokers) because these are prone to ecological bias.[60] Subgroup and meta-regression analyses were performed for prespecified factors if reported at the group level (i.e., race or ethnicity, sex, specific assay used, and clinical setting of test use) and for quality items included in our quality assessment. We also explored temporal trends in the reported effect sizes using meta-regression with year of publication as the covariate.

Small-Study Effects

We used Egger's regression-based test[61] to assess the presence of "small-study effects"[62]—that is, differences between larger (more precise) and smaller (less precise) studies. Although this test is often referred to as a test for "publication bias,"[61] theoretical and empirical studies show that the test, and related visualization methods ("funnel plots"), cannot differentiate publication bias from "true" heterogeneity between smaller and larger studies.[63,64] Furthermore, selective outcome reporting, other biases, or chance can also lead to significant results. Because of these reasons, we interpreted the results of tests for small-study effects with caution[65] and did not display funnel plots.

Sensitivity Analyses

When meta-analyses were conducted, we performed the following sensitivity analyses, as appropriate: leave-one-out meta-analysis, analysis under a fixed effects model, and analysis after excluding the first study of a specific association (to assess "first-study effects"[66,67]).

Population Overlap Across Publications

We took particular care to avoid double counting (both in qualitative and quantitative analyses) when published papers reported on potentially (fully or partially) overlapping patient populations. Potential overlap was assessed on the basis of the sampling population of each study, the enrollment period for each publication, the patient selection criteria, and information on overlap provided by the authors in the published papers. We used a conservative approach of considering as potentially overlapping the populations of studies conducted by the same investigators when overlap could not be ruled out on the basis of the above criteria. In the presence of suspected overlap we based our analysis on the study reporting the largest number of outcome events (typically, the study reporting on the longest followup for longitudinal studies). In all cases of suspected overlap we contacted the corresponding authors of each paper using a standardized protocol with a primary contact email and 2 reminders over a period of 6 weeks. Only two authors (corresponding to 6 publications that we considered as overlapping) replied; in all cases they confirmed our suspicions.

Software

All analyses were performed using Stata IC, version 12.1 (Stata Corp., College Station, TX). All tests were two-sided (except those for heterogeneity) and statistical significance was defined as a p-value of less than 0.05. We did not perform any adjustments for multiple comparisons.

Risk of Bias and Completeness of Reporting of Individual Studies

For assessing the risk of bias, we followed recently updated guidance from the Methods Guide.[68,69] We used different criteria for assessing the risk of bias (and when appropriate, the completeness of reporting) for each Key Question.

For studies of analytic validity (Key Questions 1a and 2a), we compiled a list of 11 items for assessing quality and completeness of reporting based on a recent AHRQ Methods Report.[70] The list of criteria is provided in Appendixes D (for Key Question 1a) and E (for Key Question 2a). Each item was rated as "Yes," "No," "Unclear/Not reported," or "Not applicable."

For studies of predictive ability (Key Questions 1b–c and 2b–c), we based our assessment on the recently proposed Quality Assessment of Diagnostic Accuracy Studies (QUADAS)–2 instrument,[71] a new version of the validated QUADAS list of quality items[72-74] for systematic reviews of medical tests. Briefly, the tool assesses four domains for risk of bias: patient selection, index test, reference standard test (outcome), and flow and timing. Each domain is evaluated according to a set of relevant "signaling" questions answered as "Yes," "No," or "Unclear/Not reported. The complete tool and the operational definitions we used for each item are presented in Appendix D (for Key Question 1b) and Appendix E (for Key Question 2b). After scoring each item, a summary risk-of-bias assessment is performed for each of the four domains and then an overall determination (across the four domains) is made. We used arbitrary thresholds based on the number of items scored as having been adequately addressed (i.e., indicative of low risk of bias) to classify studies into three categories (A, B, or C) indicating low, moderate, and high risk of bias, respectively. This approach was used as a shorthand description of the available evidence; throughout the report we emphasize the component items that contributed to the summary rate.

Finally, for studies providing information on test-and-treatment strategies (Key Questions 3 and 4) we used a combination of items from the QUADAS-2 tool and the Cochrane risk of bias tool.[75] The complete list of items assessed is provided in Appendix F. Each item was labeled as "Yes," "No," or "Unclear/Not reported." Two independent reviewers evaluated the risk of bias for each study and disagreements were resolved by consensus including a third reviewer.

Grading the Body of Evidence

We graded the strength of the body of evidence for the Key Questions following the Methods Guide and recently updated recommendations for the EPC program.[68,76] Briefly, the grading of the strength of evidence was based on four dimensions: risk of bias, consistency, directness, and precision. The risk of bias assessment of individual studies was performed as described in the preceding section.

We assessed consistency of the data as either "no inconsistency" or "inconsistency present" (or "not applicable" if only one study). We did not use rigid counts of studies as standards of evaluation (e.g., four of five studies agree, therefore the data are consistent); instead, we assessed the direction, magnitude, and statistical significance of all studies, and our meta-analysis results (when performed), to reach conclusions. We describe our logic when studies were not unanimous. We assessed the directness of the evidence ("direct" vs. "indirect") on the basis of the use of surrogate outcomes (e.g., platelet reactivity vs. clinical events as the outcomes of interest) or the need for indirect comparisons (e.g., when tests had not been directly compared in terms of predictive ability or utility for treatment decisionmaking and inference was based on observations across studies). We assessed the precision of the evidence as "precise" or "imprecise" on the basis of the degree of certainty surrounding each effect estimate. A precise estimate is one that allows for a clinically useful conclusion. An imprecise estimate is one for which the CI is wide enough to include clinically distinct conclusions (e.g., situations in which the direction of effect is unknown and CIs are consistent with both clinically important superiority and inferiority; or situations were a statistically significant result is produced but CIs are consistent with a broad range of effect sizes) and that therefore precludes a conclusion. As a component of precision, the sparseness of the evidence was also assessed. We considered evidence to be sparse if it was from only one study with a small sample size. Because this review assessed many outcomes, the evaluation of overall strength of evidence was based on patient-relevant clinical outcomes, which we broadly defined as any outcomes that affect the patient's well-being.

We focused our assessment of the strength of evidence on studies reporting patient-relevant clinical outcomes (for Key Questions 1b–c, 2b–c, 3, and 4); we did not assess the strength of evidence for intermediate outcomes because they were ascertained using diverse methods (platelet reactivity measured with different assays) and their clinical importance is unclear at present. We also did not assess the strength of evidence of studies of analytic validity (Key Questions 1a and 2a) because technical test performance does not directly inform medical decisions (even though it is a prerequisite for the clinical use of tests).

We rated the strength of evidence for each comparison and outcome of interest according to four levels: high, moderate, low, and insufficient. Ratings reflect the investigators' level of confidence that the evidence reflects the true effect for the major comparisons of interest, and are defined as follows:

- *High:* There is high confidence that the evidence reflects the true effect. Further research is very unlikely to change our confidence in the estimate of effect. No important scientific disagreement exists across studies.
- *Moderate:* There is moderate confidence that the evidence reflects the true effect. Further research may change our confidence in the estimate of effect and may change the estimate. Little disagreement exists across studies.
- *Low:* There is low confidence that the evidence reflects the true effect. Further research is likely to change the confidence in the estimate of effect and is likely to change the estimate. Underlying studies may report conflicting results.
- *Insufficient:* Evidence is either unavailable or does not permit a conclusion. There are sparse or no data. In general, when only one study has been published the evidence is considered insufficient, unless the study was particularly large, robust, and of good quality. We emphasize that when a body of evidence is deemed "insufficient," the absence of conclusive evidence should not be interpreted as evidence of absence of an association.

These ratings provide a shorthand description of the strength of evidence supporting the major questions we addressed. However, they by necessity may oversimplify the many complex issues involved in the appraisal of a body of evidence. It is important to remember that the individual studies evaluated in formulating the composite rating differed in their design, reporting, and quality. The strengths and weaknesses of the individual reports, as described in detail in the text and tables, should also be taken into consideration.

Assessing Applicability

We assessed applicability of the study findings on the basis of the individual study eligibility criteria and baseline characteristics of the included populations, following recommendations in the AHRQ Methods Guide and recently updated recommendations for the EPC program.[68,76] We did not assess the applicability of studies on the analytic validity of the tests of interest (Key Questions 1a and 2a) because technical test performance does not directly inform medical decisions (it is, however, a prerequisite for the clinical use of tests).[77]

For studies of predictive ability (Key Questions 1b–c and 2b–c), we judged applicability on the basis of study eligibility criteria (e.g., narrow vs. broad range of demographics [men only vs. men and women]), the use of tests that are not widely available (tests developed "in-house" ["home-brew" assays]), and the assessment of outcomes that required laboratory measurement of platelet reactivity (rather than patient-relevant outcomes). We took a similar approach for studies considered relevant to test-and-treatment strategies (Key Questions 3 and 4). We address applicability along with other key issues relevant to the body of evidence pertaining to each Key Question and also provide comments on specific issues that, according to our best judgment, affected applicability.

Results

The literature search yielded 10,475 citations (10,374 from electronic databases; 77 from submission information packages; and 24 from hand-searching; Figure 2). Of these, 1419 articles were reviewed in full text. After full text review, 326 were judged to have met the inclusion criteria for one or more Key Questions. The most common reason for exclusion of articles was that the results of the genetic or phenotypic tests studied were not used for prediction of intermediate or clinical outcomes or physician/patient decisionmaking. Other common reasons for exclusion were that the tests, populations, or outcomes studied were not of interest to this review; that the sample size was too small to yield useful estimates (n<50 for Key Question 1a or 2a about analytic validity or n<10 for Key Question 1b, 2b, or 3 about clinical utility or decisionmaking); that no primary data were reported; or that the full text was written in a language other than English. See Appendix B for a list of the excluded studies with the reason for exclusion. Appendix C contains a list of FDA documents that we reviewed. The summary tables for the 325 accepted studies are in Appendixes D through F.

Figure 2. Literature flow diagram

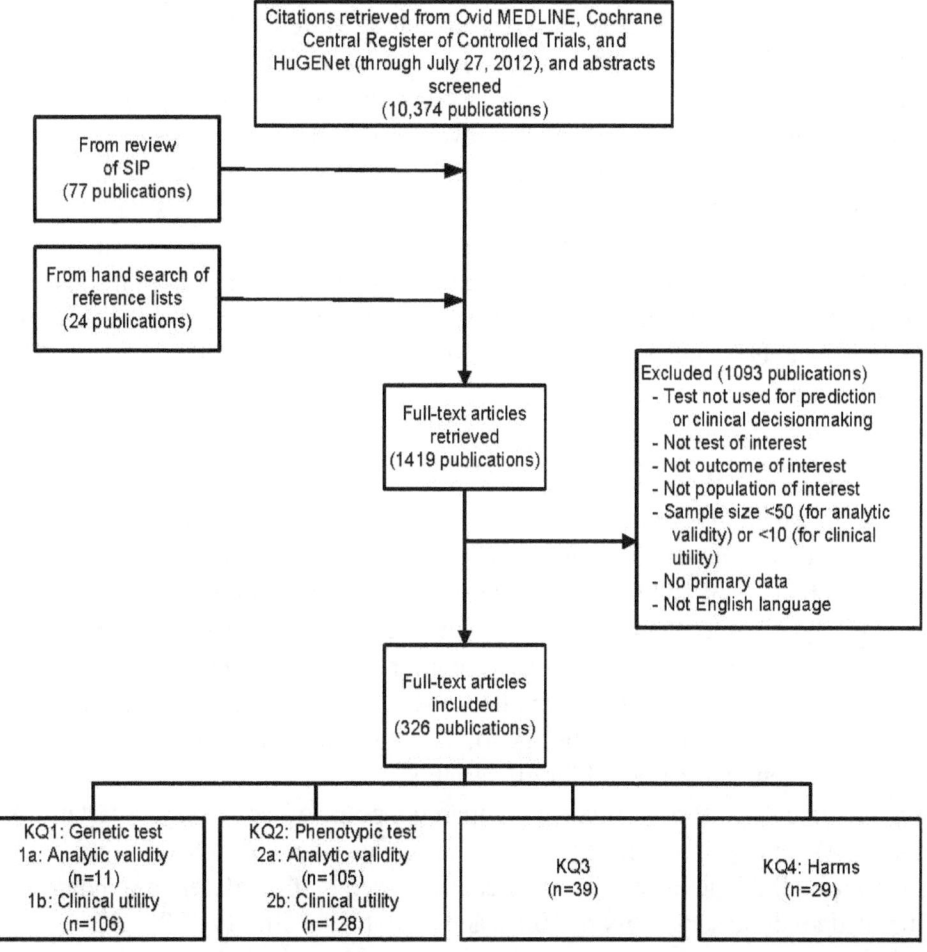

Abbreviations: KQ = Key Question; SIP = scientific information packet. A single article may report information on more than one study. Detailed reasons for exclusion of studies reviewed in full text but not considered further are presented in Appendix B.

Key Question 1a. What is the analytic validity (technical test performance) of the various assays used for CYP2C19 genetic testing?

Eligible Studies for Key Question 1a

We identified 11 studies[29,78-87] reporting information on the analytic validity of genotyping methods for detecting CYP2C19 variants. Information on the patient populations, assays evaluated, test timing, and study designs used is presented in Appendix D. Studies reported limited information regarding the methods used to assess technical test performance, possibly reflecting their focus on clinical (rather than analytic) validity. Three of the studies were conducted by the same team of investigators and reported laboratory and clinical findings on patients identified at a single center in Germany (typically, these were participants in ongoing clinical trials); thus, at least partial overlap is likely. We also reviewed four FDA 510(k) summaries on genetic testing assays (see Appendix C).

Eight studies included patients undergoing PCI for coronary artery disease;[29,78-83,86] one included a mixed population of patients with MI or undergoing PCI;[84] one included patients with chronic cardiovascular disease;[87] and one included a mixed population of vascular patients (coronary, cerebrovascular or peripheral artery disease) along with patients at high risk for the development of vascular disase.[85] Seven studies assessed test–retest reliability (repeat testing of samples for the detection of CYP2C19 polymorphisms); three assessed agreement between alternative genotyping methods;[82,83,87] and one study assessed the analytic sensitivity and specificity against a reference standard.[86] Among the seven studies assessing test-retest reliability four reported the proportion of retested samples (20% in three cases; 11% in the fourth study), corresponding to 305 samples (in each of two studies), 497 samples (in the third study), and 535 samples in the fourth study. In the remaining two studies, the proportion of retested samples was not reported (and could not be calculated). Among the three studies assessing agreement between alternative genotyping methods, one reported the number of tested samples (333 samples). The study assessing analytic test performance against a reference standard reported results on 187 samples.

Summary of Findings on Analytic Validity

Among the seven clinical studies providing information on analytic validity for CYP2C19 genotyping presenting results on test–retest reliability six reported that the concordance rate on repeat genotyping was 100 percent; and two reported that the rate was "higher than 98%." Four of the seven studies genotyped more than one variant; however, it was unclear whether agreement was assessed for all variants, and results were not reported for each variant separately.

All three studies assessing agreement between alternative genotyping methods reported perfect agreement.[82,83,87] Two of the three studies genotyped more than one variant; however, it was unclear whether agreement was assessed for all variants.

The study assessing analytic test performance compared a point-of-care assay (Spartan RX CYP2C19; the index test) versus direct sequencing (the reference standard). One sample identified as a *2 carrier by the index test was a non-carrier based on the reference standard, resulting in an estimated analytic sensitivity of 100% and analytic specificity of 99.3%.[86] This comparison of analytic performance is noteworthy because it was conducted in the setting of randomized trial of testing versus no-testing (results on intermediate and clinical endpoints from this trial have been summarized under Key Questions 2-4).

FDA 510(k) summaries did not report analyses on samples from populations and gene of interest in our review. However, the documents provided evidence that genotyping methods have high test–retest reliability and indicated that rates of interassay agreement were high (based on fairly extensive studies of test-retest reliability and inter-assay agreement).

Risk of Bias and Completeness of Reporting for Studies Reviewed for Key Question 1a

We evaluated risk of bias and completeness of reporting based on 11 predefined questions. Studies reported limited information on the methods they used to assess analytic validity. This probably reflects the fact that the primary focus of all included publications was not the tests' analytic validity (but rather their clinical utility). Generally, studies provided adequate information on the genotyping methods used. However, they provided little information on the use of positive or negative control samples, the handling of uninterpretable results, and the test detection limits. Four studies reported information on the reproducibility of genotyping across different genotyping methods, but no study assessed reproducibility across operators. No study was conducted as part of an interlaboratory standardization project. Appendix D summarizes our assessment of risk of bias and completeness of reporting for studies of genetic testing for CYP2C19 variants.

Key Question 1b. What is the clinical validity (predictive accuracy) of genetic testing for predicting intermediate and clinical outcomes in patients who are receiving clopidogrel therapy?

Eligible Studies for Key Question 1b

The studies included for this Key Question enrolled patients on clopidogrel-based antiplatelet therapy. Of the 106 studies addressing Key Question 1b (in 98 publications; 8 publications described 2 studies each), the vast majority (100 [94 percent]) were of patients with ischemic heart disease; three studies enrolled patients with different forms of vascular disease (coronary, cerebrovascular, or peripheral arterial); one enrolled patients with cerebrovascular disease; one enrolled a mixed population of patients with manifest atherothrombotic disease along with patients at high risk for atherothrombotic disease; and one enrolled patients with atrial fibrillation who were not candidates for vitamin K antagonist therapy. In 81 studies (76 percent), 80 percent or more patients were undergoing PCI; 4 studies (4 percent) included patients undergoing angiography; and 21 (20 percent) included populations in which less than 80 percent of patients were undergoing a procedure or did not provide information on the proportion of patients undergoing revascularization. The majority of studies were of patients receiving dual antiplatelet therapy with clopidogrel in combination with aspirin. Detailed information on the selection criteria, settings, and treatment strategies (including adjunctive treatments) is presented in Appendix D.

The 106 studies had intermediate to large sample sizes (median number of enrolled individuals=277; 25th percentile=98; 75th percentile=802; minimum=30; maximum=5148). They were conducted recently (median year of start of enrollment was 2006, with 75 percent beginning enrollment after 2004), reflecting the relatively recent widespread availability of genetic testing for CYP2C19 variants. Across studies, men represented the majority of enrolled patients (median proportion across studies was 75 percent; men were the majority sex in 95 of the 97 studies noting the sex of participants). In 98 studies providing information on patient age, the median of the average age reported in each study was 64 years; average age was equal to or older than 65 years in 37 of the studies. Patients had a relatively high burden of risk factors for coronary artery disease (which are associated with adverse cardiovascular outcomes): the median proportion of patients with dyslipidemia was 61 percent (in the 74 studies with data; 25th percentile=49 percent; 75th percentile=76 percent); hypertension, 68 percent (in 86 studies; 25th percentile=56 percent; 75th percentile=81 percent); diabetes mellitus, 28 percent (in 95 studies; 25th percentile=21 percent; 75th percentile=35 percent); and tobacco use, 32 percent (in 88 studies; 25th percentile=16 percent; 75th percentile=42 percent). Detailed information about patient characteristics and preexisting vascular disease is summarized in Appendix D.

A total of 100 of the 106 studies (94 percent) had a longitudinal (cohort) design; 5 were case–control studies; and 1 was a case-cohort study. Of the longitudinal studies, 11 were genetic substudies consisting of prospectively followed clopidogrel-treated groups from randomized trials. (When appropriate, possible modification of the relative treatment effect by genotype status has been considered under Key Questions 3 and 4 of this report.)

Overall studies had moderate risk of bias (12 studies were rated as quality "A;" 88 studies were rated as quality "B;" and 6 were rated as quality "C"). We caution that this aggregate risk-of-bias rating can be misleading, especially in the presence of poor reporting. A more detailed discussion of risk of bias, focusing on the individual items assessed is presented later in this chapter.

Genotyping Methods, Hardy–Weinberg Equilibrium, Variant Allele Frequencies

The 106 studies addressing Key Question 1b used a variety of genotyping methods for identifying CYP2C19 variants. The two most common were TaqMan genotyping (44 studies; 42 percent) and PCR-RFLP (13 studies; 12 percent). In the majority of cases analyses were conducted on genetic material isolated from blood (92 studies; 87 percent). Among the 56 studies that reported the genotyping success rate, the median was 100 percent (minimum=74 percent; maximum=100 percent). The vast majority of studies genotyped samples for the CYP2C19 *2 allele; additional alleles were genotyped in a minority of studies and were rare in the sampled population. Detailed information on the genotyping methods used and the distribution of observed genotypes for each study are presented in Appendix D.

Seventy-five of the eligible studies provided information adequate to calculate goodness-of-fit p-values for Hardy–Weinberg equilibrium (using an exact test); some studies reported information on more than one patient group and more than one genetic variant. Table 2 shows summary results across studies, and Figure 3 shows a quantile–quantile plot of p-values for deviations from Hardy–Weinberg equilibrium against the uniform distribution, for the *2 allele.

Table 2. P-values for deviation from Hardy–Weinberg equilibrium

CYP2C19	No. of Studies Reporting Genotype Distributions	Median P-Value [25th, 75th percentile]	No. of Studies With p<0.05 (%)
*2	77	0.50 [0.25, 0.81]	5 (6%)
*3	28	1.00 [0.70, 1.00]	0 (0%)
*17	29	0.64 [0.19, 0.84]	2 (7%)
Other	14	1.00 [1.00,1.00]	0 (0%)
Total	148	0.69 [0.30, 1.00]	7 (5%)

Studies not reporting the complete genotype distribution (n=12) have not been included in the table. The 44 studies included could have reported genotype distributions for more than one allele. For the two case–control studies and the one case-cohort study, we assessed violations for Hardy–Weinberg equilibrium (HWE) for the control group only. Variants other than *2, *3, and *17 were fairly uncommon, leading to p-values for HWE violation equal to 1 in many cases.

Figure 3. Quantile–quantile plot (observed vs. uniform distribution) of p-values for deviation from Hardy–Weinberg violation in studies reporting the genotype distribution for the CYP2C19*2 allele

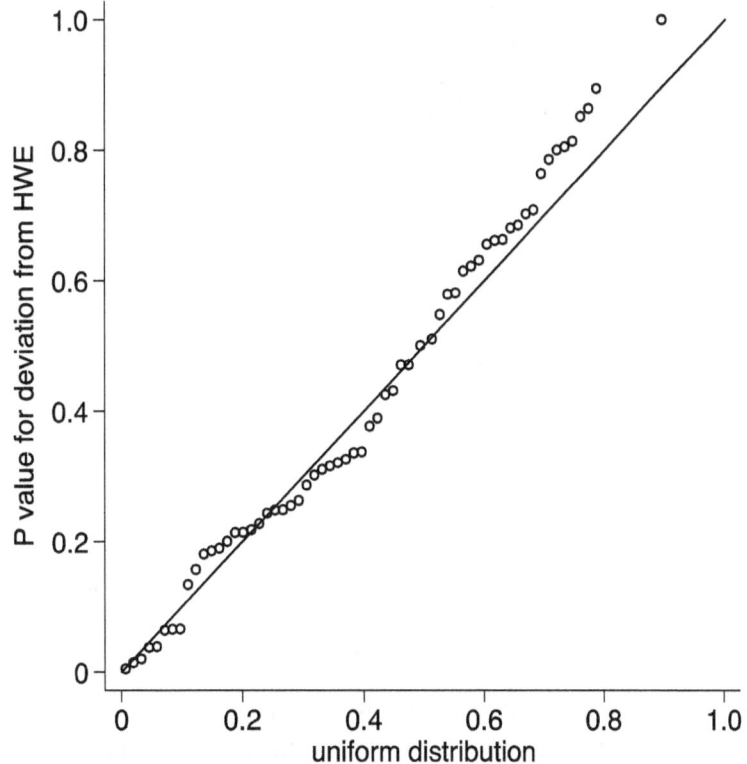

Abbreviations: HWE=Hardy–Weinberg equilibrium. P-values are from an exact test.

Figure 4 presents forest plots of the CYP2C19*2 allele frequency (number of *2 alleles over total number of alleles in the population) and the prevalence of homozygotes for the rare variant (*2/*2 individuals over total number of study participants) from eligible studies. The graph highlights that the allele frequency and the prevalence of *2/*2 homozygotes is higher among East Asian populations (white circles) as compared to populations of European ancestry (black circles). Less information was available for black populations (black squares) and populations of mixed (or not reported) ancestry (white squares).

Figure 4. *2 Allele frequency and *2/*2 genotype prevalence in eligible studies

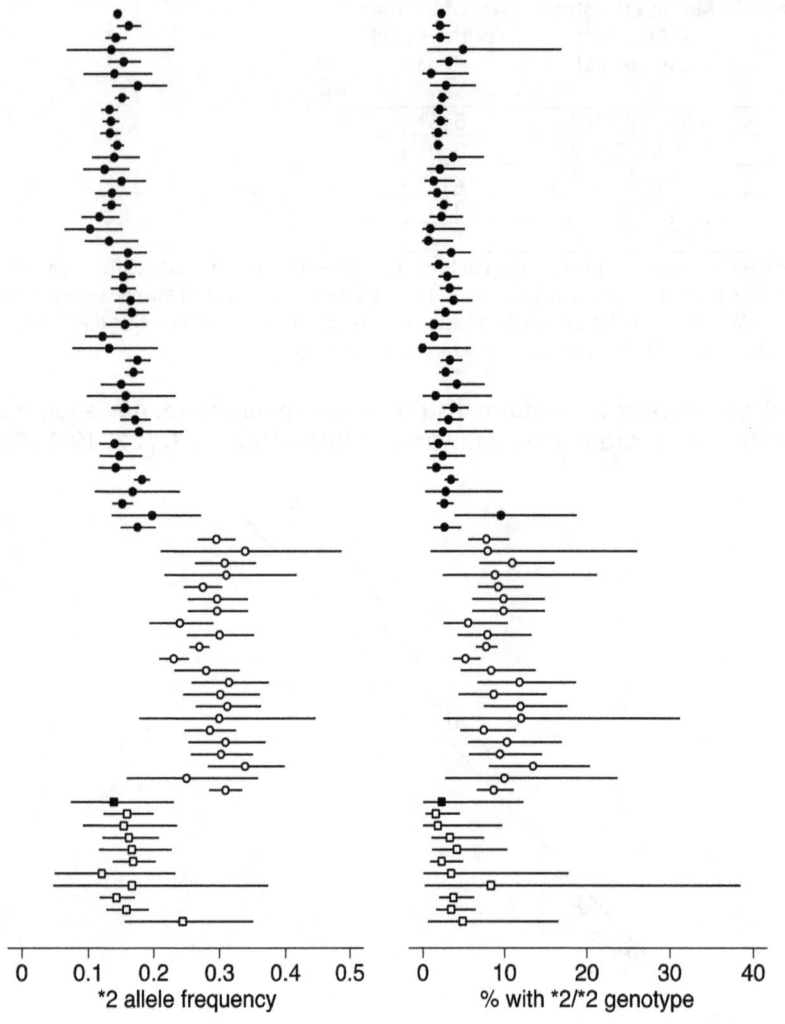

*2 allele frequency (left panel) and *2/*2 genotype prevalence (right panel) in eligible studies providing relevant information. Black circles = European ancestry; white circles = East Asian populations; black squares = black populations; white squares = population of other/mixed ancestry or not reported. Extending lines denote exact (binomial) 95% confidence intervals.

Overall, statistically significant deviations were uncommon (n=7 across all genotyped alleles), and at the 0.05 alpha level, roughly seven significant results would be expected by chance alone (= 0.05 × 148). In addition, these results need to be interpreted with caution given that patients were selected for inclusion in the studies on the basis of the presence of ischemic heart disease (or other atherosclerotic vascular disease).

Of the 106 eligible studies, 57 provided information on the predictive value of genetic testing for CYP2C19 variants for predicting clinical outcomes, and 74 reported data appropriate for predicting on-clopidogrel platelet reactivity. In the following section we discuss studies according to the outcomes reported for each population of interest. Because the study designs and outcome definitions used across studies of ischemic coronary artery disease were considered sufficiently similar, we performed meta-analyses if at least three studies provided information for an outcome of interest. We synthesized findings across studies, on the assumption that their patient populations were nonoverlapping. (Please see the Methods section for additional details on how we assessed potential population overlap.) Subgroup and effect modification analyses for the same set of studies are presented in the next section (results for Key Question 1c).

Summary of Findings on the Predictive Value of CYP2C19 Variants for Patients on Clopidogrel-Based Antiplatelet Therapy

Table 3 summarizes our findings on the predictive value of CYP2C19 variants for clinical outcomes across studies reporting on nonoverlapping of clopidogrel-treated patient populations included in meta-analyses or synthesized quantitatively in patient populations with ischemic heart disease. We performed meta-analyses when at least three studies reported on the comparison of interest and the occurrence of at least one outcome event. Three studies enrolled mixed patient populations with different forms of vascular disease (coronary, cerebrovascular, or peripheral arterial); one enrolled patients with cerebrovascular disease; one enrolled a mixed population of patients with manifest atherothrombotic disease along with patients at high risk for atherothrombotic disease; and one enrolled patients with atrial fibrillation. Results from these studies are summarized separately below. As we discuss in subsequent sections, results regarding platelet reactivity (when used as an outcome) were not amenable to quantitative synthesis.

Table 3. Summary of results on the predictive value of CYP2C19 variants for clinical outcomes among clopidogrel-treated patients with ischemic heart disease

Exposure	Outcome	No. of Studies with Nonoverlapping Populations	Summary of Findings	P-Value for Small-Study Effects
LOF vs. no LOF	All-cause mortality	7	RR=1.00 (95% CI, 0.64 to 1.55) P_Q=0.403; I^2=3%	0.163
	Cardiovascular mortality	7	RR=1.98 (95% CI, 1.13 to 3.46) P_Q=0.936; I^2=0%	0.719
	ACS	9	RR=1.35 (95% CI, 0.91 to 2.00) P_Q=0.828; I^2=0%	0.092
	Stent thrombosis	17	RR=1.52 (95% CI, 1.17 to 1.97) P_Q=0.772; I^2=0%	**<0.001**
	Stroke	7	RR=2.07 (95% CI, 0.68 to 6.33) P_Q=0.374; I^2=7%	0.950
	MACE	25	RR=1.20 (95% CI, 1.04 to 1.39) P_Q=0.076; I^2=31%	**0.002**
	Bleeding events	6	RR=1.02 (95% CI, 0.86 to 1.21) P_Q=0.701; I^2=0%	**0.049**
	Other clinical outcomes	4 studies (5 outcomes)	Studies suggested that revascularization outcomes and "net clinical" benefit are more common among carriers of loss-of-function alleles.	NA
GOF vs. no GOF	All-cause mortality	3	RR=1.28 (95% CI, 0.81 to 2.02) P_Q=0.505; I^2=0%	0.351
	Cardiovascular mortality	0	NA	
	ACS	2	Both studies reported non–statistically significant results. Confidence intervals were wide; the two point estimates for the RR differed by >0.3.	NA
	Stent thrombosis	5	RR=0.83 (95% CI, 0.52 to 1.32) P_Q=0.754; I^2=0%	0.399
	Stroke	1	The study did not find a statistically significant association.	NA
	MACE	7	RR=0.82 (95% CI, 0.74 to 0.92) P_Q=0.966; I^2=0%	0.882
	Bleeding events	6	RR=1.51 (95% CI, 1.08 to 2.11) P_Q=0.088; I^2=48%	**0.046**
	Revascularization	0	NA	NA

Abbreviations: ACS = acute coronary syndromes; CI = confidence interval; GOF = gain-of-function alleles; LOF = loss-of-function alleles; MACE = major adverse cardiovascular events; NA = not applicable; RR = relative risk.
Significant p-values are in bold type.

Studies of Patients With Ischemic Heart Disease

Clinical Outcomes

Fifty-seven of the 106 studies eligible for Key Question 1b reported information on the predictive value of CYP2C19 genotyping for predicting clinical outcomes in patients with ischemic heart disease. Eligible studies were fairly large (median number of genotyped individuals=428) and recent (median year enrollment started=2005).

All-Cause Mortality

Seven studies with nonoverlapping populations of patients with ischemic heart disease reported information on the predictive value of loss-of-function alleles for all-cause mortality (and reported the occurrence of at least one outcome event).[78,84,88-93] The studies were large

30

(minimum sample size=160) but represented a minority of all 57 studies reporting clinical outcomes. The summary RR for all-cause mortality comparing carriers of any loss-of-function allele with noncarriers was 1.00 (95% CI, 0.64 to 1.55; p=0.988). Overall, there was little between-study heterogeneity ($P_Q = 0.403$; $I^2 = 3$ percent). Figure 5 presents the meta-analysis results, along with study-specific event rates.

Figure 5. Meta-analysis of all-cause mortality comparing carriers and noncarriers of loss-of-function CYP2C19 alleles

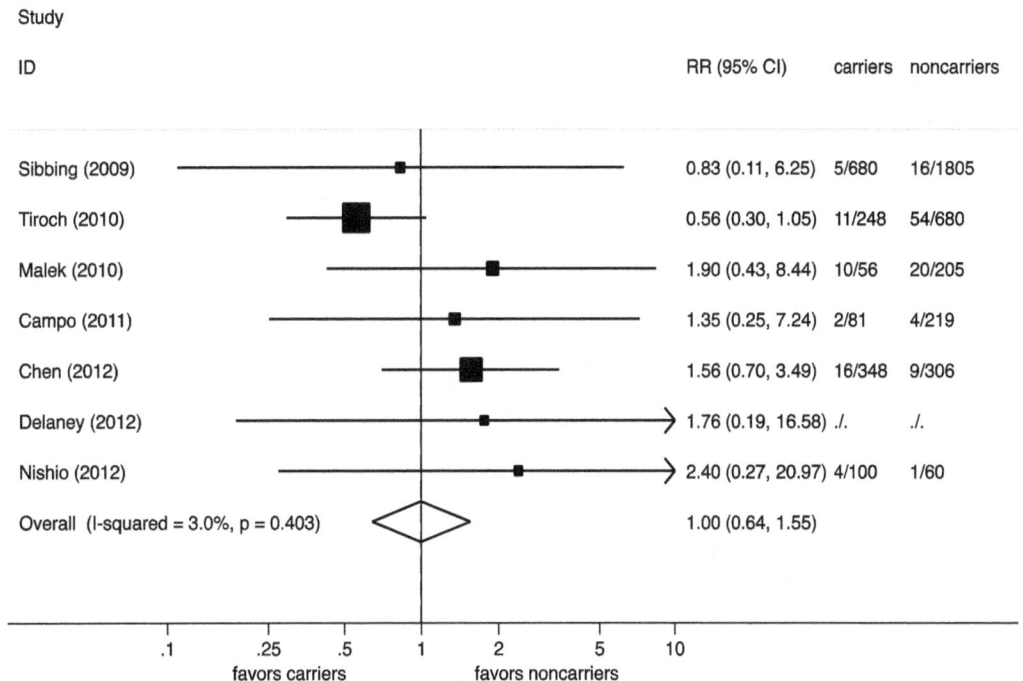

Abbreviations: CI = confidence interval; LOF = loss-of-function; RR = relative risk.
The solid squares (and horizontal lines) indicate the RR of all-cause mortality (and the corresponding 95% CI) for individual studies. The affected numbers of carriers or noncarriers are shown to the right of the plot. The size of the squares is proportional to the weight of each study in the meta-analysis. The dashed vertical line represents the summary RR, with the open diamond showing the corresponding CI. The solid line indicates an RR of 1.

The summary RR for all-cause mortality comparing carriers of any gain-of-function allele versus noncarriers (based on only three studies reporting relevant data[79,88,91]) was 1.28 (95% CI, 0.81 to 2.02; p=0.288). Overall, there was little between-study heterogeneity ($P_Q = 0.505$; $I^2 = 0$ percent). Figure 6 presents the meta-analysis results, along with study-specific event rates.

Figure 6. Meta-analysis of all-cause mortality comparing carriers and noncarriers of gain-of-function CYP2C19 alleles

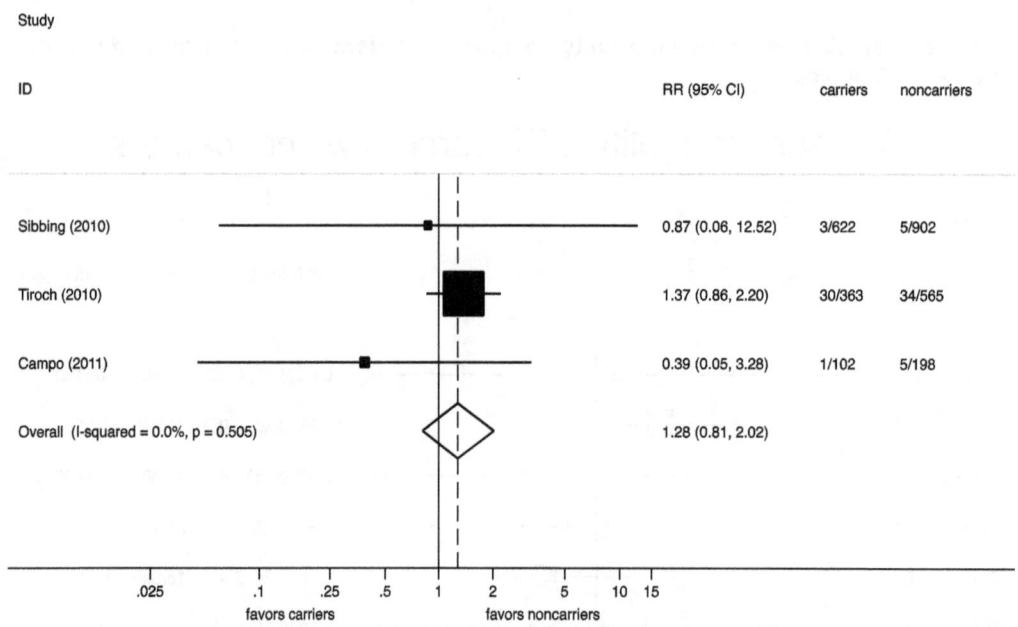

Abbreviations: CI = confidence interval; GOF = gain-of-function; RR = relative risk.
The solid squares (and horizontal lines) indicate the RR of all-cause mortality (and the corresponding 95% CI) for individual studies. The affected numbers of carriers or noncarriers are shown to the right of the plot. The size of the squares is proportional to the weight of each study in the meta-analysis. The dashed vertical line represents the summary RR, with the open diamond showing the corresponding CI. The solid line indicates an RR of 1.

Cardiovascular Mortality

Information on the predictive value of genetic testing for mortality due to cardiovascular causes was reported in seven studies with nonoverlapping populations of patients with ischemic heart disease (in which at least one event was observed).[92-98] Studies were fairly large (minimum sample size=105) but represented a minority of the 57 studies reporting clinical outcomes. The summary RR for cardiovascular mortality comparing carriers of any loss-of-function allele and noncarriers was 1.98 (95% CI, 1.13 to 3.46; p=0.017). Overall, there was little between-study heterogeneity (P_Q = 0.936; I^2 = 0 percent). Figure 7 presents the meta-analysis results, along with study-specific event rates.

No studies provided information on the impact of gain-of-function alleles on risk of cardiovascular mortality.

Figure 7. Meta-analysis of cardiovascular mortality comparing carriers and noncarriers of loss-of-function CYP2C19 alleles

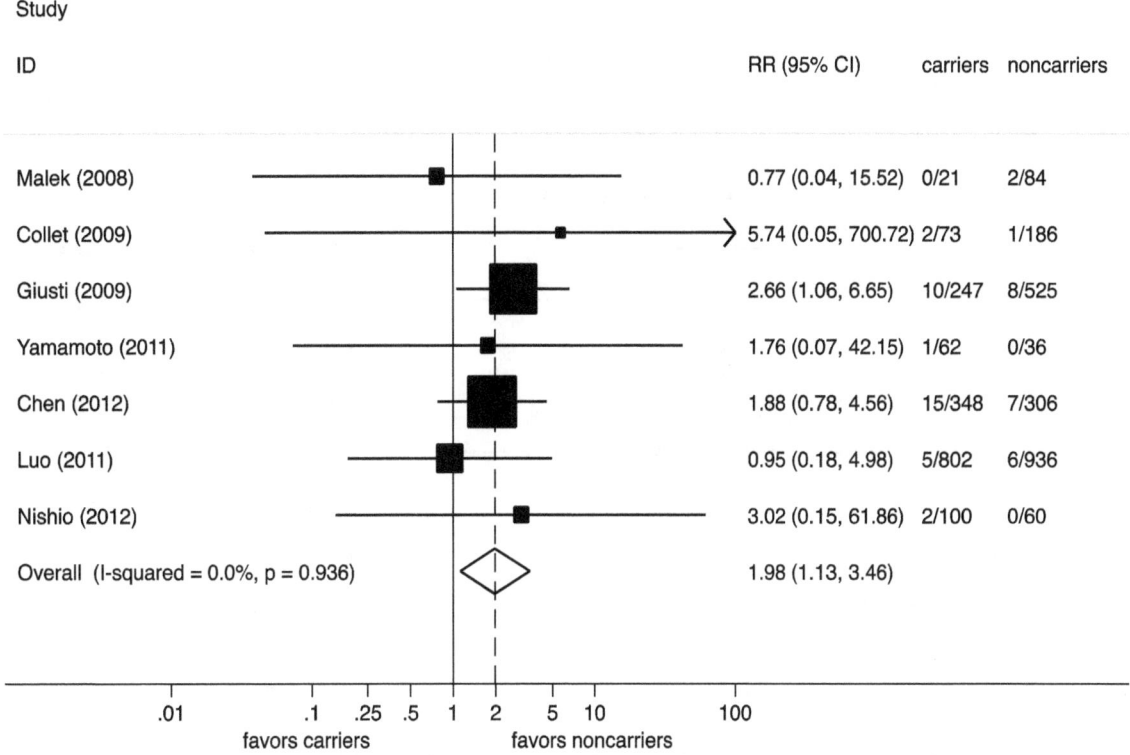

Abbreviations: CI = confidence interval; LOF = loss-of-function; RR = relative risk.
The solid squares (and horizontal lines) indicate the RR of cardiovascular mortality (and the corresponding 95% CI) for individual studies. The affected numbers of carriers or noncarriers are shown to the right of the plot. The size of the squares is proportional to the weight of each study in the meta-analysis. The dashed vertical line represents the summary RR, with the open diamond showing the corresponding CI. The solid line indicates an RR of 1.

Acute Coronary Syndromes

Information on the predictive value of genetic testing for acute coronary syndromes (including myocardial infarction) was reported in nine studies with nonoverlapping populations of patients with ischemic heart disease.[78,84,91,93,94,96,97,97-99] Studies were large (minimum sample size=105) but represented a minority of the 57 studies reporting clinical outcomes in patients with ischemic heart disease. The summary RR for acute coronary syndromes comparing carriers of any loss-of-function allele versus noncarriers was 1.35 (95% CI, 0.91 to 2.00; p=0.136). Overall, there was little between-study heterogeneity ($P_Q = 0.828$; $I^2 = 0$ percent). Figure 8 presents the meta-analysis results, along with study-specific event rates.

Figure 8. Meta-analysis of acute coronary syndromes comparing carriers and noncarriers of loss-of-function CYP2C19 alleles

-

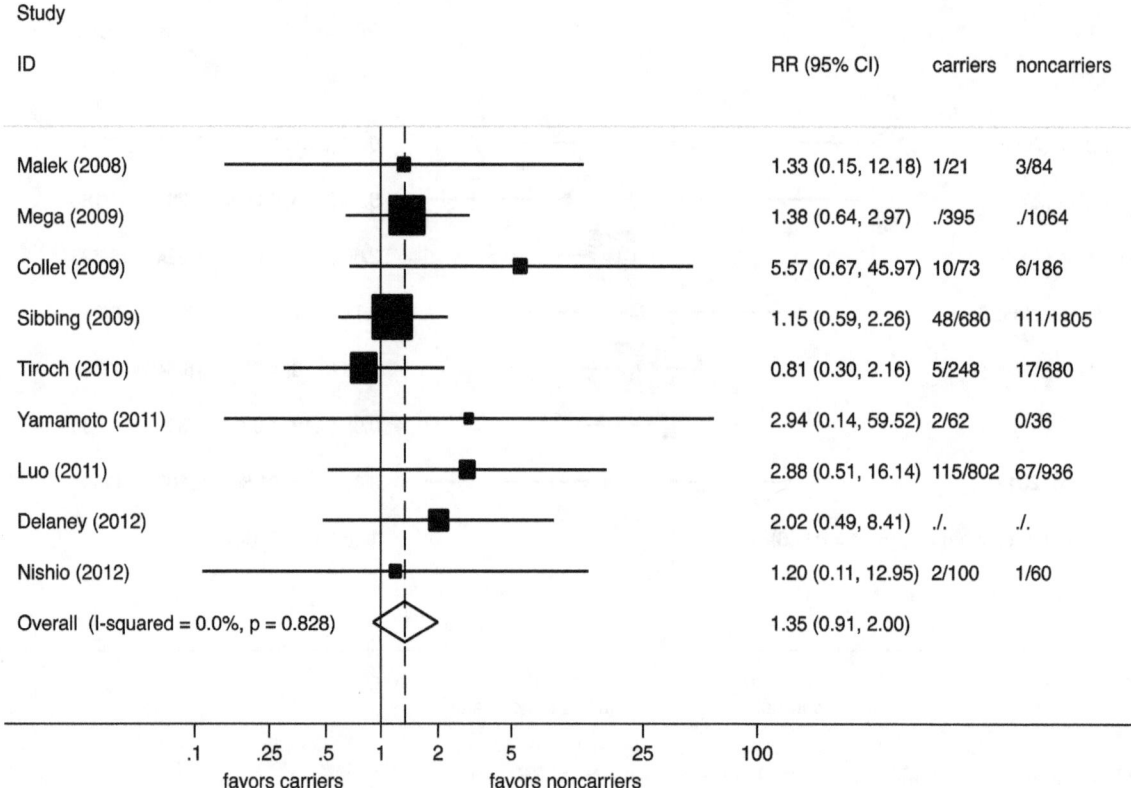

Acute coronary syndromes, LOF carriers vs. noncarriers

Study ID		RR (95% CI)	carriers	noncarriers
Malek (2008)		1.33 (0.15, 12.18)	1/21	3/84
Mega (2009)		1.38 (0.64, 2.97)	./395	./1064
Collet (2009)		5.57 (0.67, 45.97)	10/73	6/186
Sibbing (2009)		1.15 (0.59, 2.26)	48/680	111/1805
Tiroch (2010)		0.81 (0.30, 2.16)	5/248	17/680
Yamamoto (2011)		2.94 (0.14, 59.52)	2/62	0/36
Luo (2011)		2.88 (0.51, 16.14)	115/802	67/936
Delaney (2012)		2.02 (0.49, 8.41)	./.	./.
Nishio (2012)		1.20 (0.11, 12.95)	2/100	1/60
Overall (I-squared = 0.0%, p = 0.828)		1.35 (0.91, 2.00)		

.1   .25   .5   1   2   5   25   100
favors carriers   favors noncarriers

Abbreviations: CI = confidence interval; LOF = loss-of-function; RR = relative risk.
One study (Mega et al. 2009[99]) did not report the number of observed events.
The solid squares (and horizontal lines) indicate the RR of acute coronary syndromes (and the corresponding 95% CI) for individual studies. The affected numbers of carriers or noncarriers are shown to the right of the plot. The size of the squares is proportional to the weight of each study in the meta-analysis. The dashed vertical line represents the summary RR, with the open diamond showing the corresponding CI. The solid line indicates an RR of 1.

Only two studies[78,91] reported information on the impact of gain-of-function alleles on the risk of acute coronary syndromes. Both studies did not find a statistically significant association between carriage of gain-of-function alleles and acute coronary syndromes, but the CIs were wide (RR=1.05; 95% CI, 0.34 to 3.29 and RR=0.73; 95% CI 0.30 to 1.76, respectivelly), indicating substantial uncertainty in the estimates.

Stent Thrombosis

Information on the predictive value of loss-of-function alleles for stent thrombosis (definite or probable, based on study-specific definitions when available) was reported in 17 studies with nonoverlapping populations of patients with ischemic heart disease (in which at least one outcome event was observed).[78,82,84,88,90-92,94-96,98-106] Studies were large (minimum sample size=60; median sample size=596). The summary RR for stent thrombosis comparing carriers of any loss-of-function allele versus noncarriers was 1.52 (95% CI, 1.17 to 1.97; p=0.002). Overall, there was little between-study heterogeneity ($P_Q = 0.772$; $I^2 = 0$ percent). Figure 9 presents the meta-analysis results, along with study-specific event rates.

Figure 9. Meta-analysis of stent thrombosis comparing carriers and noncarriers of loss-of-function CYP2C19 alleles

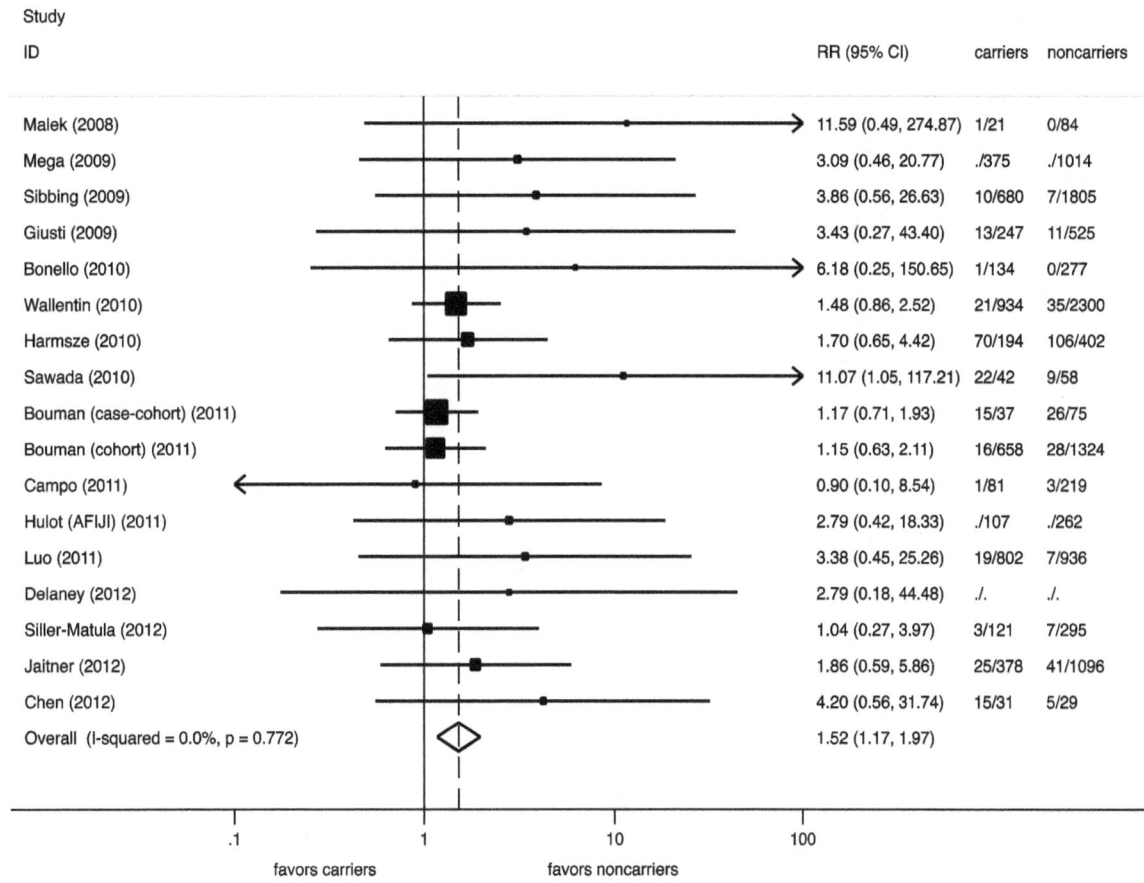

Abbreviations: CI = confidence interval; LOF = loss-of-function; RR = relative risk.
One study (Mega et al. 2009[99]) did not report the number of observed events; one study (Delaney et al. 2012[84]) reported only an effect size.
The solid squares (and horizontal lines) indicate the RR of stent thrombosis (and the corresponding 95% CI) for individual studies. The affected numbers of carriers or noncarriers are shown to the right of the plot. The size of the squares is proportional to the weight of each study in the meta-analysis. The dashed vertical line represents the summary RR, with the open diamond showing the corresponding CI. The solid line indicates an RR of 1.

Figure 10 presents an analysis of predictive accuracy for the same group of studies (14 of 17 studies provided the needed data) under a dominant genetic model. The summary sensitivity was 0.47 (95% CI, 0.39 to 0.56) and the average specificity was 0.69 (95% CI, 0.66 to 0.72) using a random effects model.

Figure 10. Prognostic performance of CYP2C19 genetic testing for stent thrombosis

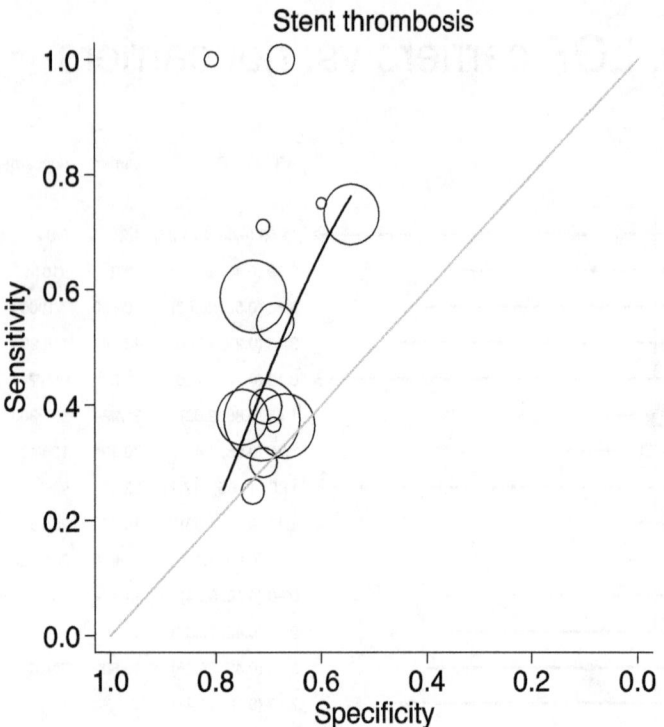

Bivariate meta-analysis of sensitivity and specificity for predicting stent thrombosis. The black solid line shows the fitted summary receiver operating characteristic curve; the gray solid line is the chance diagonal. Individual studies are shown as bubbles with size proportional to study size.

Information on the predictive value of gain-of-function alleles for stent thrombosis (definite or probable) was reported in five studies with nonoverlapping populations of patients with ischemic heart disease.[78,88,91,101,107] Studies were large (minimum sample size=300); however, they represented a minority of the 17 studies reporting stent thrombosis. The summary RR for stent thrombosis comparing carriers of any gain-of-function allele versus noncarriers was 0.83 (95% CI, 0.52 to 1.32; p=0.425). Overall, there was little between-study heterogeneity (P_Q = 0.754; I^2 = 0.0 percent). Figure 11 presents the meta-analysis results, along with study-specific event rates.

Figure 11. Meta-analysis of stent thrombosis comparing carriers and noncarriers of gain-of-function CYP2C19 alleles

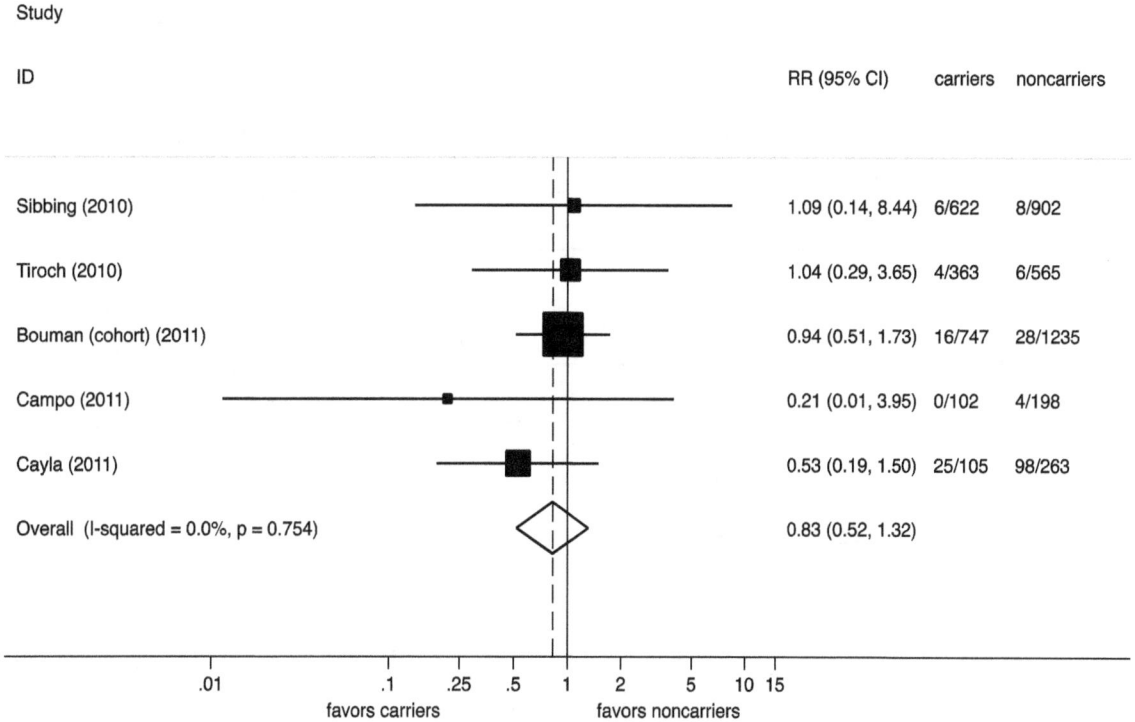

Stent thrombosis, GOF carriers vs. noncarriers

Study ID		RR (95% CI)	carriers	noncarriers
Sibbing (2010)		1.09 (0.14, 8.44)	6/622	8/902
Tiroch (2010)		1.04 (0.29, 3.65)	4/363	6/565
Bouman (cohort) (2011)		0.94 (0.51, 1.73)	16/747	28/1235
Campo (2011)		0.21 (0.01, 3.95)	0/102	4/198
Cayla (2011)		0.53 (0.19, 1.50)	25/105	98/263
Overall (I-squared = 0.0%, p = 0.754)		0.83 (0.52, 1.32)		

.01 .1 .25 .5 1 2 5 10 15
favors carriers   favors noncarriers

Abbreviations: CI = confidence interval; GOF = gain-of-function; RR = relative risk.
The solid squares (and horizontal lines) indicate the RR of stent thrombosis (and the corresponding 95% CI) for individual studies. The affected numbers of carriers or noncarriers are shown to the right of the plot. The size of the squares is proportional to the weight of each study in the meta-analysis. The dashed vertical line represents the summary RR, with the open diamond showing the corresponding CI. The solid line indicates an RR of 1.

Stroke

Information on the predictive value of loss-of-function alleles for stroke was reported in seven studies with nonoverlapping populations of patients with ischemic heart disease.[78,91,97-100,108] Studies had heterogeneous sample sizes (minimum sample size = 201; maximum = 2,485) and represented a minority of the 57 studies reporting clinical outcomes. The summary RR for stent thrombosis comparing carriers of any loss-of-function allele versus noncarriers was 2.07 (95% CI 0.68, 6.33); p=0.201. Overall, there was limited evidence of between-study heterogeneity ($P_Q = 0.374$; $I^2 = 7$ percent). Figure 12 presents the meta-analysis results, along with study-specific event rates.

Figure 12. Meta-analysis of stroke comparing carriers and noncarriers of loss-of-function CYP2C19 alleles

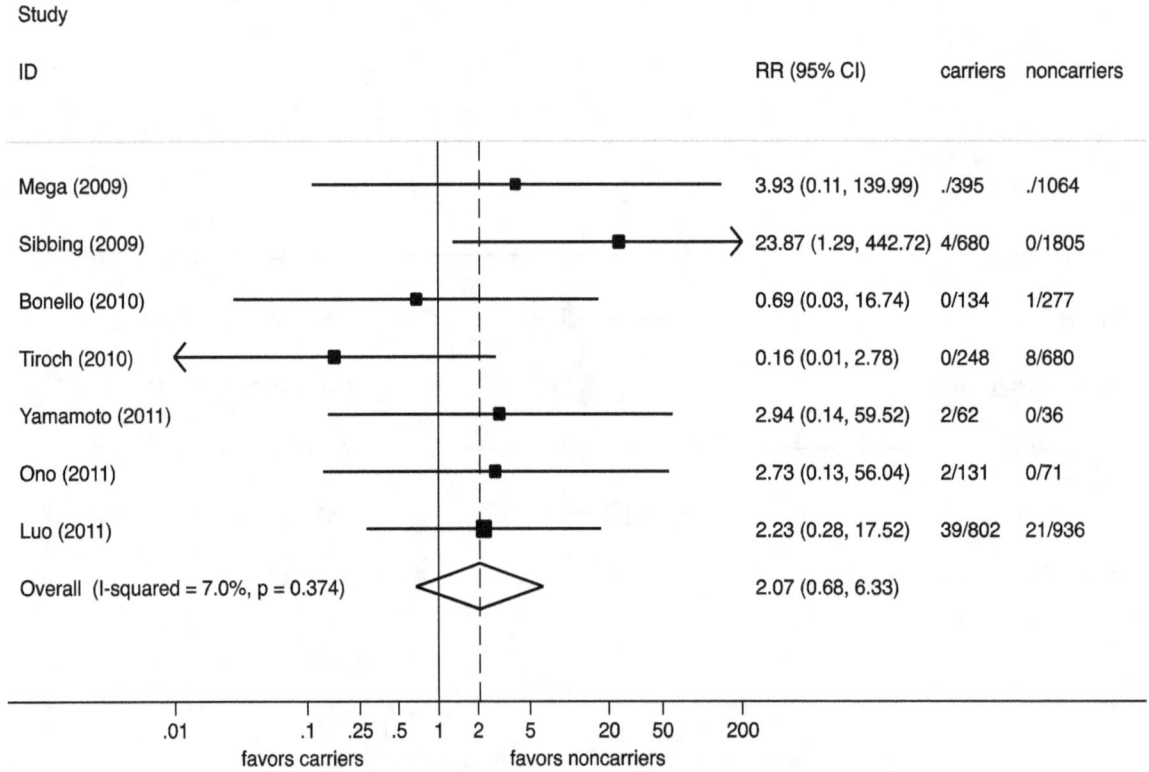

Stroke, LOF carriers vs. noncarriers

Study ID	RR (95% CI)	carriers	noncarriers
Mega (2009)	3.93 (0.11, 139.99)	./395	./1064
Sibbing (2009)	23.87 (1.29, 442.72)	4/680	0/1805
Bonello (2010)	0.69 (0.03, 16.74)	0/134	1/277
Tiroch (2010)	0.16 (0.01, 2.78)	0/248	8/680
Yamamoto (2011)	2.94 (0.14, 59.52)	2/62	0/36
Ono (2011)	2.73 (0.13, 56.04)	2/131	0/71
Luo (2011)	2.23 (0.28, 17.52)	39/802	21/936
Overall (I-squared = 7.0%, p = 0.374)	2.07 (0.68, 6.33)		

favors carriers   favors noncarriers

Abbreviations: CI = confidence interval; LOF = loss-of-function; RR = relative risk.
One study (Mega et al. 2009[99]) did not report the number of observed events.
The solid squares (and horizontal lines) indicate the RR of stroke (and the corresponding 95% CI) for individual studies. The affected numbers of carriers or noncarriers are shown to the right of the plot. The size of the squares is proportional to the weight of each study in the meta-analysis. The dashed vertical line represents the summary RR, with the open diamond showing the corresponding CI. The solid line indicates an RR of 1.

Only a single study[91] reported information on the association between gain-of-function alleles (*17) and stroke risk. The study reported a non-statistically significant RR of 0.93 (95% CI, 0.23 to 3.88), suggesting that there is substantial uncertainty regarding the effect of gain-of-function alleles on stroke risk.

MACE

Composite clinical outcomes, often called MACE, were the most commonly reported clinical outcome across the eligible studies. Although definitions of these composite outcomes were somewhat variable, we reasoned that the most inclusive definition used by each study (i.e., the one including as many events as possible) would provide an estimate of the cardiovascular morbidity experienced by individuals in each study. (This is also common practice in meta-analyses in cardiovascular disease topics.) Details about the exposure and outcome definitions used in the eligible studies are presented in Appendix D.

Of the studies reporting on MACE, 25 were considered to have included nonoverlapping patient populations and compared event rates among patients with at least one loss-of-function allele versus those with no loss-of function alleles.[29,79,82,84,88,91-93,95-97,99,100,104,105,108-117] Studies were fairly large (minimum sample size=86; median sample size=428). The summary RR comparing carriers of any loss-of-function allele versus noncarriers was 1.20 (95% CI 1.04, 1.39; p=0.015). Overall, there was moderate between-study heterogeneity ($P_Q = 0.076$; $I^2 = 31$ percent). Figure 13 presents the meta-analysis results, along with study-specific event rates.

Figure 13. Meta-analysis of MACE comparing carriers and noncarriers of loss-of-function CYP2C19 alleles

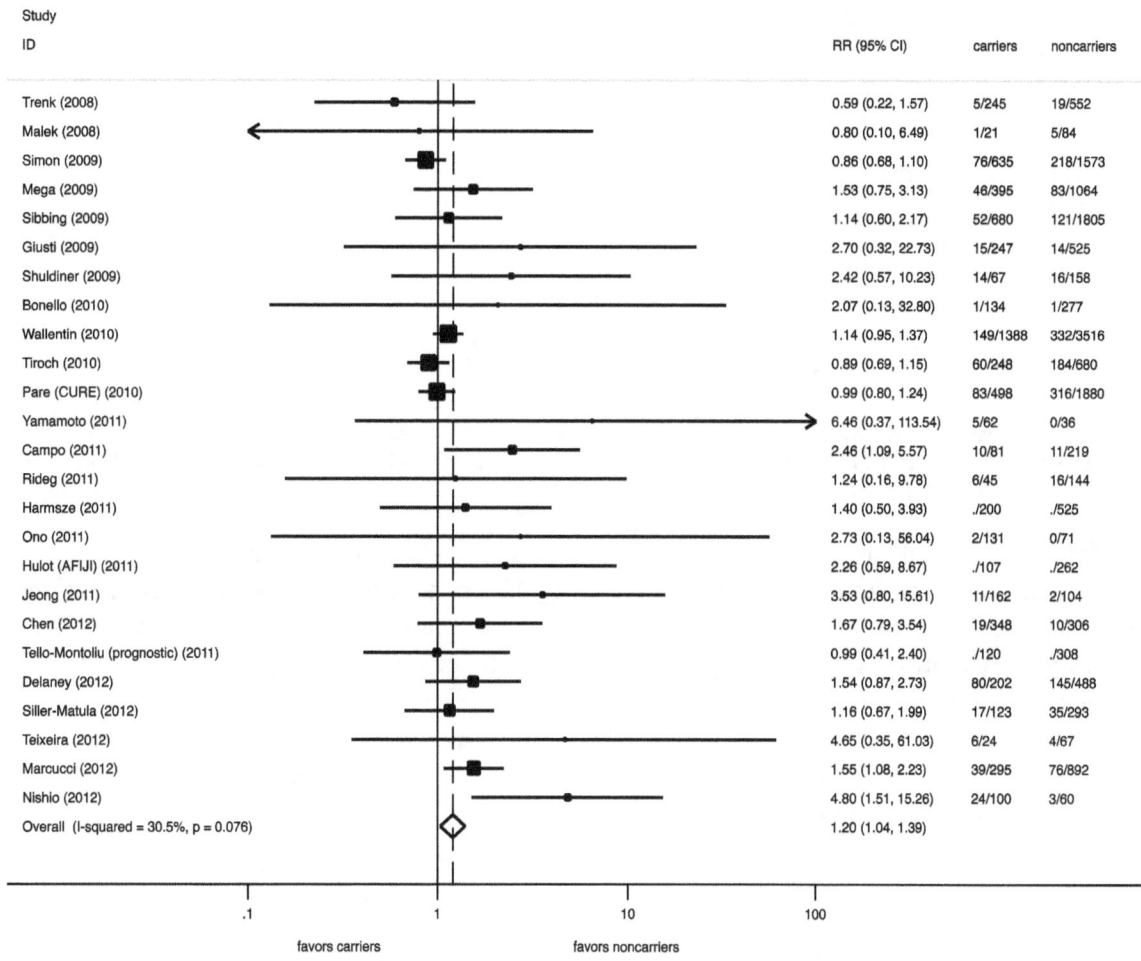

Abbreviations: CI = confidence interval; LOF = loss-of-function; MACE = major adverse cardiovascular events; RR = relative risk.

The solid squares (and horizontal lines) indicate the RR of MACE (and the corresponding 95% CI) for individual studies. The affected numbers of carriers or noncarriers are shown to the right of the plot. The size of the squares is proportional to the weight of each study in the meta-analysis. The dashed vertical line represents the summary RR, with the open diamond showing the corresponding CI. The solid line indicates an RR of 1.

Figure 14 presents an analysis of predictive accuracy for the same group of studies (22 of 25 studies provided the necessary data) under a dominant genetic model. The summary sensitivity was 0.44 (95% CI 0.33, 0.56) and the average specificity was 0.67 (95% CI 0.61, 0.72) using a random effects model.

Figure 14. Prognostic performance of CYP2C19 genetic testing for MACE

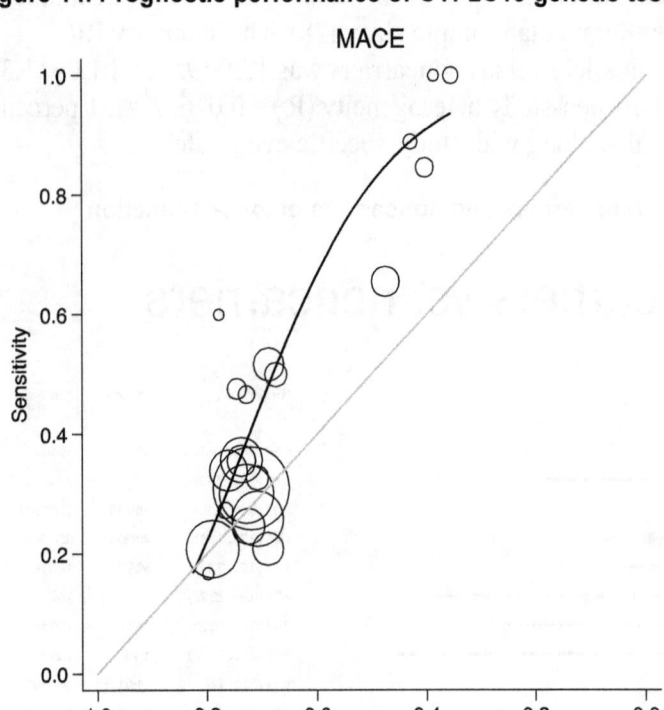

Bivariate meta-analysis of sensitivity and specificity for predicting MACE. The black solid line shows the fitted summary receiver operating characteristic curve; the gray solid line is the chance diagonal. Individual studies are shown as bubbles with size proportional to study size. MACE = major adverse cardiovascular events.

Information on the predictive value of gain-of-function alleles for major adverse cardiovascular events was reported in seven studies with nonoverlapping populations of patients with ischemic heart disease.[79,84,91,109,110,113,115] Studies were large (minimum sample size=428); however, they represented a minority of the 25 studies reporting on MACE outcomes. The summary RR for all-cause mortality comparing carriers of any gain-of-function allele versus noncarriers was 0.82 (95% CI 0.74, 0.92; p<0.001). Overall, there was little between-study heterogeneity (P_Q = 0.966; I^2 = 0 percent). Figure 15 presents the meta-analysis results, along with study-specific event rates.

Figure 15. Meta-analysis of MACE comparing carriers and noncarriers of gain-of-function CYP2C19 alleles

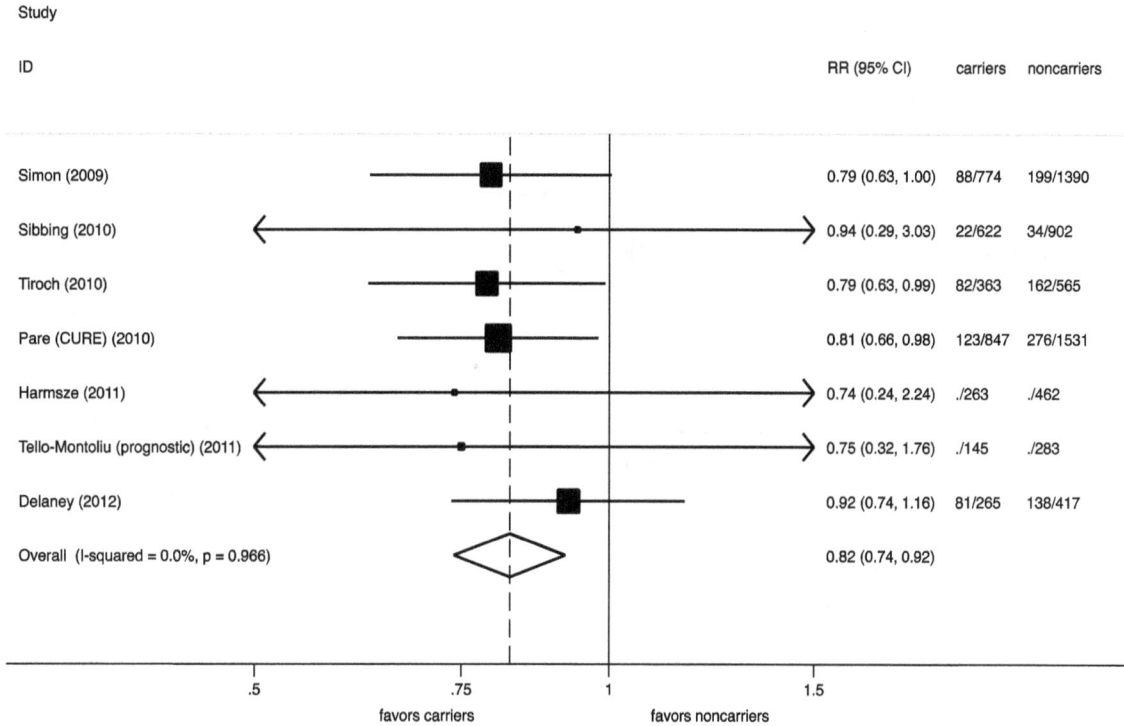

MACE, GOF carriers vs. noncarriers

Study ID	RR (95% CI)	carriers	noncarriers
Simon (2009)	0.79 (0.63, 1.00)	88/774	199/1390
Sibbing (2010)	0.94 (0.29, 3.03)	22/622	34/902
Tiroch (2010)	0.79 (0.63, 0.99)	82/363	162/565
Pare (CURE) (2010)	0.81 (0.66, 0.98)	123/847	276/1531
Harmsze (2011)	0.74 (0.24, 2.24)	./263	./462
Tello-Montoliu (prognostic) (2011)	0.75 (0.32, 1.76)	./145	./283
Delaney (2012)	0.92 (0.74, 1.16)	81/265	138/417
Overall (I-squared = 0.0%, p = 0.966)	0.82 (0.74, 0.92)		

.5   .75   1   1.5

favors carriers   favors noncarriers

Abbreviations: CI = confidence interval; CURE = Clopidogrel in Unstable Angina to Prevent Recurrent Events trial; GOF = gain-of-function; MACE = major adverse cardiovascular events; RR = relative risk.
The solid squares (and horizontal lines) indicate the RR of MACE (and the corresponding 95% CI) for individual studies. The affected numbers of carriers or noncarriers are shown to the right of the plot. The size of the squares is proportional to the weight of each study in the meta-analysis. The dashed vertical line represents the summary RR, with the open diamond showing the corresponding CI. The solid line indicates an RR of 1.

Bleeding Events

Of the studies reporting on bleeding events, six were considered to have included nonoverlapping patient populations and compared event rates among patients with at least one loss-of-function allele versus those with no loss-of function alleles.[88,98,100,104,109,114] Studies were large (minimum sample size=266). The summary RR comparing carriers of any loss-of-function allele versus noncarriers was 1.02 (95% CI 0.86, 1.21; p=0.81). Overall, there was little between-study heterogeneity (P_Q = 0.701; I^2 = 0 percent). Figure 16 presents the meta-analysis results, along with study-specific event rates.

Figure 16. Meta-analysis of bleeding events comparing carriers and noncarriers of loss-of-function CYP2C19 alleles

Bleeding events, LOF carriers vs. noncarriers

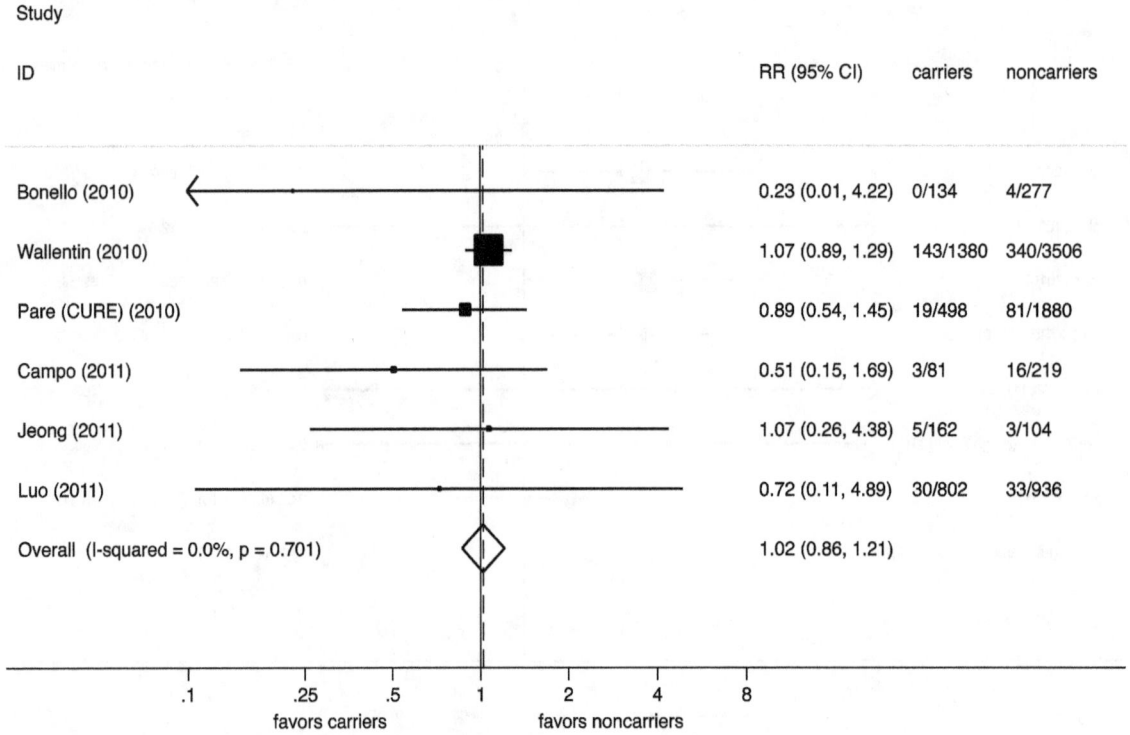

Study ID	RR (95% CI)	carriers	noncarriers
Bonello (2010)	0.23 (0.01, 4.22)	0/134	4/277
Wallentin (2010)	1.07 (0.89, 1.29)	143/1380	340/3506
Pare (CURE) (2010)	0.89 (0.54, 1.45)	19/498	81/1880
Campo (2011)	0.51 (0.15, 1.69)	3/81	16/219
Jeong (2011)	1.07 (0.26, 4.38)	5/162	3/104
Luo (2011)	0.72 (0.11, 4.89)	30/802	33/936
Overall (I-squared = 0.0%, p = 0.701)	1.02 (0.86, 1.21)		

favors carriers   favors noncarriers

Abbreviations: CI = confidence interval; LOF = loss-of-function; RR = relative risk.
The solid squares (and horizontal lines) indicate the RR of bleeding events (and the corresponding 95% CI) for individual studies. The affected numbers of carriers or noncarriers are shown to the right of the plot. The size of the squares is proportional to the weight of each study in the meta-analysis. The dashed vertical line represents the summary RR, with the open diamond showing the corresponding CI. The solid line indicates an RR of 1.

Information on the predictive value of gain-of-function alleles for bleeding events was reported in six studies with nonoverlapping populations of patients with ischemic heart disease.[79,88,109,118-120] Studies were large (minimum sample size = 300); however, they represented a minority of the 57 studies reporting clinical outcomes. The summary RR for all bleeding events comparing carriers of any loss-of-function allele versus noncarriers was 1.51 (95% CI 1.08, 2.11); p=0.016. Overall, there was moderate (and statistically significant) between-study heterogeneity ($P_Q = 0.088$; $I^2 = 48$ percent). Figure 17 presents the meta-analysis results, along with study-specific event rates.

Figure 17. Meta-analysis of bleeding events comparing carriers and noncarriers of gain-of-function CYP2C19 alleles

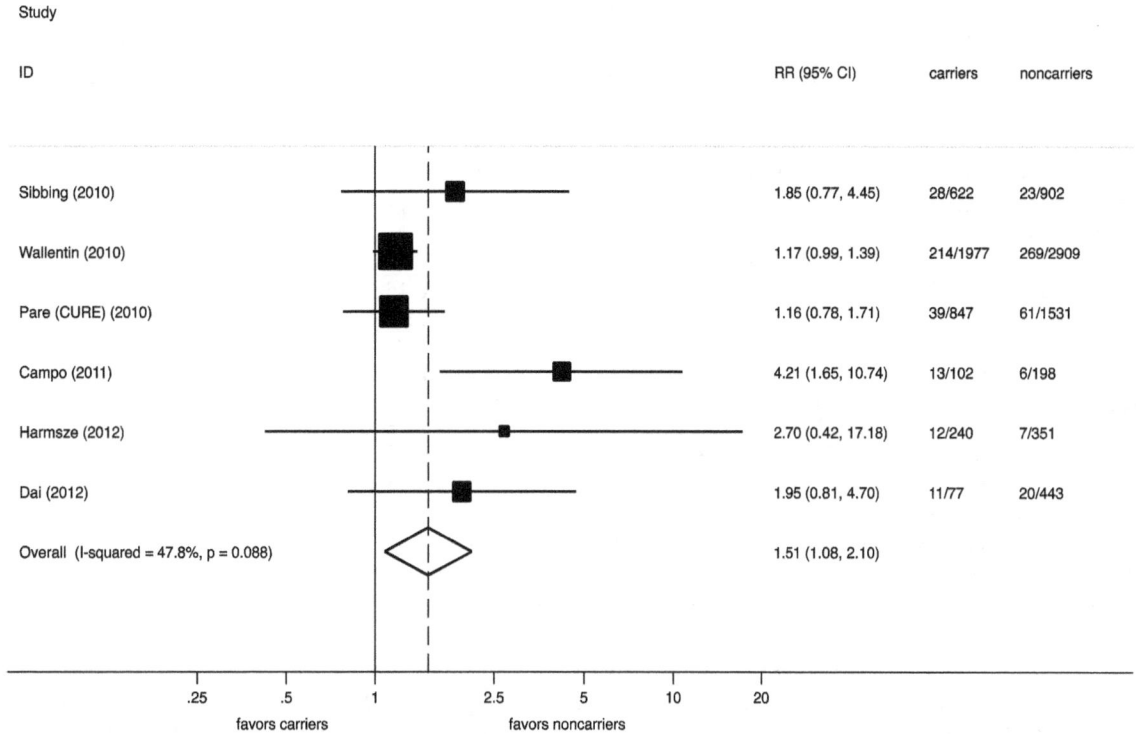

Bleeding events, GOF carriers vs. noncarriers

Study ID	RR (95% CI)	carriers	noncarriers
Sibbing (2010)	1.85 (0.77, 4.45)	28/622	23/902
Wallentin (2010)	1.17 (0.99, 1.39)	214/1977	269/2909
Pare (CURE) (2010)	1.16 (0.78, 1.71)	39/847	61/1531
Campo (2011)	4.21 (1.65, 10.74)	13/102	6/198
Harmsze (2012)	2.70 (0.42, 17.18)	12/240	7/351
Dai (2012)	1.95 (0.81, 4.70)	11/77	20/443
Overall (I-squared = 47.8%, p = 0.088)	1.51 (1.08, 2.10)		

Abbreviations: CI = confidence interval; GOF = gain-of-function; RR = relative risk.
The solid squares (and horizontal lines) indicate the RR of bleeding events (and the corresponding 95% CI) for individual studies. The affected numbers of carriers or noncarriers are shown to the right of the plot. The size of the squares is proportional to the weight of each study in the meta-analysis. The dashed vertical line represents the summary RR, with the open diamond showing the corresponding CI. The solid line indicates an RR of 1.

Other Clinical Outcomes

Seven studies reported information on five additional clinical outcomes (1 on urgent revascularization of any vessel and on a composite of "ischemic endpoints related to stent thrombosis;"[121] 1 on urgent revascularization (no additional details provided)[100]; 3 on target vessel revascularization throughout the study period;[90] 1 on any revascularization; and one on a composite of benefits and harms, termed "net clinical benefit"[118]). All studies assessed the effect of loss-of-function alleles; one also assessed gain of function alleles. Generally event rates were higher among carriers of loss-of-function alleles (results were statistically significant only in 3 cases[121]). These outcomes were not considered adequately homogeneous for further quantitative synthesis; study specific results have been summarized in Appendix D.

Sensitivity Analyses to Alternative Genetic Models

The majority of studies presented results only under a dominant genetic model. To evaluate the robustness of our findings to alternative genetic models, when possible, we repeated the analyses assuming a recessive or additive genetic model. Such analyses were possible for the outcomes of stent thrombosis and MACE and only for the effect of LOF alleles. Table 4 summarizes our findings. Generally, these results are supportive of the analyses using a dominant model, because they also indicate significant association between LOF alleles and adverse clinical outcomes. Effect sizes using both models are larger than those under the additive model, however this observation alone does not imply that any one model is more likely to be true. Further, I^2 values were higher under the recessive and additive models, suggesting that the average effect is less representative of the individual studies. Of particular note is also the very limited number of studies providing evidence for comparisons under a recessive or additive model (maximum of 9 and 11 as compared to a total of 25 and 17 nonoverlapping studies providing data on MACE and stent thrombosis for the dominant model, respectively).

Table 4. Sensitivity analysis to alternative genetic models

Genetic	Outcome	Number of studies	RR (95% CI)	p-value	P_Q; I^2
Recessive	MACE	9	1.85 (1.19 to 2.86)	0.006	0.152; 33.3%
	Stent thrombosis	11	2.40 (1.61 to 3.57)	<0.001	0.215; 24.0%
Additive	MACE	6	1.54 (1.11 to 2.14)	0.010	0.001; 77.1%
	Stent thrombosis	9	1.77 (1.44 to 2.18)	<0.001	0.135; 35.4%

Abbreviations: CI = confidence interval; MACE = major adverse cardiovascular event; RR = relative risk.
Additive model estimates for each individuals study were obtained from studies reporting at least one event in each genotype category using generalized linear models with an appropriate link function (logit for case-control studies and log for longitudinal studies) and binomial variance. Meta-analysis estimates were then obtained using a random effects model.

For LOF alleles, under a recessive genetic model, we also evaluated prognostic performance using bivariate meta-analysis of sensitivity and specificity (Figure 18). For MACE the summary sensitivity was 0.10 (95% CI 0.04, 0.24) and the summary specificity was 0.94 (95% CI 0.90, 0.97). For stent thrombosis the summary sensitivity was 0.10 (95% CI 0.06, 0.17) and the summary specificity was 0.96 (95% CI 0.93, 0.97). The estimates for sensitivity are lower and the estimates for specificity are higher compared to those obtained under the dominant model, for both outcomes.

Figure 18. Prognostic performance under a recessive model for CYP2C19*2 LOF variants

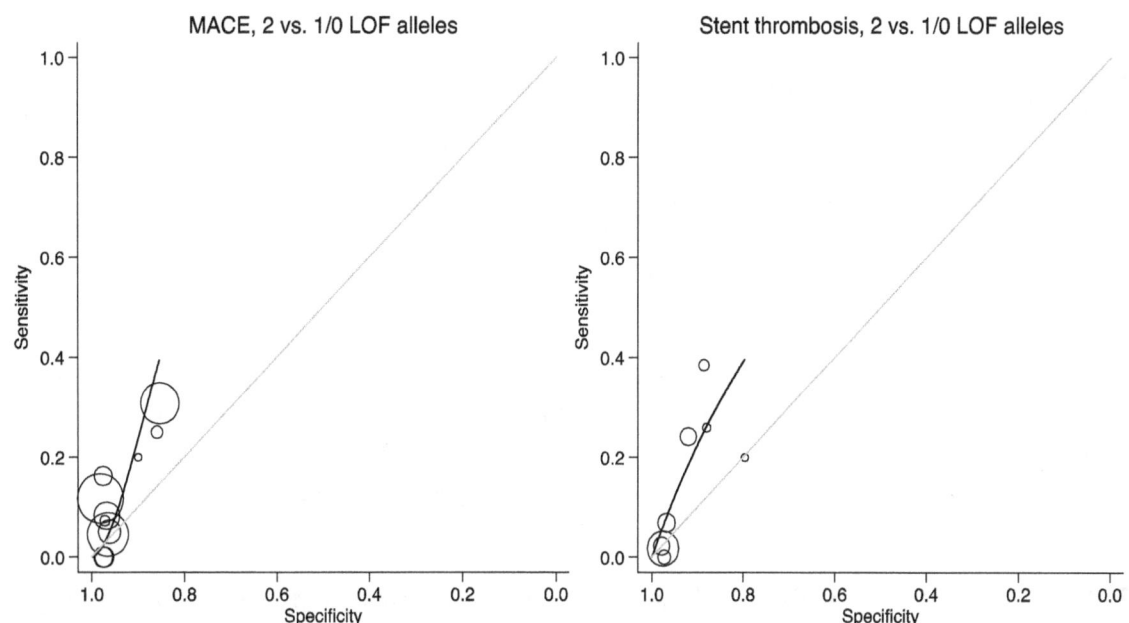

Abbreviations: LOF = loss-of-function alleles; MACE = major adverse cardiovascular events.
Bivariate meta-analysis of sensitivity and specificity for predicting MACE (left panel) and stent thrombosis (right panel). Black solid lines show the fitted summary receiver operating characteristic curves for each meta-analysis; gray solid lines indicate the chance diagonal. Individual studies are shown as bubbles with size proportional to sample size.

Intermediate Outcome: Platelet Reactivity

Seventy-four studies used the results of CYP2C19 genetic testing to predict intermediate outcomes of platelet reactivity, either as a continuous variable or according to a threshold of reactivity (e.g., high vs. low). The assays used to measure platelet reactivity are described in detail later in the Results section (see Key Question 2a and Appendix D). Several studies used more than one assay as a method for outcome ascertainment, with platelet reactivity measured with light-transmission aggregometry (LTA) in 43 studies (58 percent), VerifyNow P2Y12 in 33 (45 percent), the VASP assay in 17 (23 percent), and other assays in 10 studies (14 percent). All studies used ADP as the agonist of interest. Detailed information about the assays used and study-level results of platelet reactivity as a continuous outcome are presented in Appendix D.

Platelet Reactivity as a Continuous Outcome

Sixty-one studies reported on the effect of genotype on platelet reactivity as a continuous outcome. Reactivity was commonly assessed using LTA, the VASP assay, or VerifyNow P2Y12.

Studies generally showed that the mean or median reactivity was higher among clopidogrel-treated patients with one or two loss-of-function alleles compared to those with no loss-of-function alleles. The followup periods differed across the studies (from a few hours to more than 1 year after clopidogrel loading) and measurements were obtained using different assays and different calculation methods (e.g., absolute within-patient change from baseline, percent change within patient, or absolute value at last followup). Furthermore, the genotype groupings employed were also variable. Finally, the studies used different statistical tests and made different parametric assumptions for their comparisons. Because of the extensive differences among studies and the often incomplete reporting of numerical information we did not perform meta-analyses for studies using continuous measurements of reactivity as the outcome of interest.

Platelet Reactivity as a Categorical Outcome

Thirty-nine studies reported on the effect of genotype on platelet reactivity as a categorical outcome. Reactivity was commonly assessed using LTA, the VASP assay, or VerifyNow P2Y12.

Studies generally showed that platelet reactivity above the threshold used (or in higher quantiles compared to lower quantiles of reactivity) was more common in clopidogrel-treated patients with one or two loss-of-function alleles than those with no loss-of-function alleles. As was true for studies assessing reactivity as a continuous outcome, results in studies of categories of reactivity were reported with different followup periods and measurements were obtained using different assays and different calculation methods (i.e., by discretizing absolute within-patient change from baseline, percent change within patient, or absolute reactivity values at last followup). Furthermore, genotype grouping was also variable. Because of these extensive differences among studies, we did not perform meta-analyses for studies using categorical measurements of reactivity as the outcome of interest.

Patient Populations Other Than Those With Ischemic Heart Disease

Only six studies reported results on the predictive value of CYP2C19 genotyping for clinical or intermediate outcomes in non–ischemic heart disease populations (three of mixed populations of coronary, cerebrovascular, and peripheral arterial disease; one of patients with cerebrovascular disease; one of a mixed population of patients with manifest atherothrombotic disease along with asymptomatic patients at high risk for atherothrombotic disease; one of patients with atrial fibrillation at risk for stroke). Detailed information on these studies is presented in Appendix D. These studies included very different clinical populations and reported information on diverse outcomes [2 clinical outcomes; 2 intermediate outcomes (platelet reactivity); 2 both].

Comparisons Between Genetic Testing for CYP2C19 Variants and Phenotypic Testing for Platelet Reactivity

Only four studies provided extractable information regarding the relative prognostic ability of genetic testing for CYP2C19 loss-of-function variants and phenotypic testing of platelet reactivity for MACE (4 studies) or stent thrombosis (3 studies).[82,88,95,111] These studies have been considered with regards to the prognostic value of genetic testing in the preceding sections of this chapter. To avoid duplication, the comparative data have been summarized qualitatively under Key Question 2b.

Risk of Bias for Studies Reviewed for Key Question 1b

The detailed assessment of 11 risk-of-bias items for studies evaluating the predictive ability of genetic testing regarding clinical outcomes or platelet reactivity is presented in Appendix D. Briefly, most studies used a longitudinal design (not case–control) and no studies had substantial loss-to-followup. Inappropriate exclusions were uncommon however information on blinding was often not reported (particularly for the index test) or not used. Using the arbitrary cutoff values based on the number of adequately addressed risk of bias items 12 studies were rated as quality "A," 88 studies were rated as quality "B," and 6 were rated as quality "C."

For outcomes for which we performed meta-analysis, we assessed differences between more precise (larger) and less precise (smaller) studies using the Egger regression-based test for small-study effects. Overall, we found a statistically significant difference between smaller and larger studies on the effect size for stent thrombosis, MACE, and bleeding events for loss-of-function carriers (see "P-Value" column in Table 3). Smaller studies had more extreme (larger) effect sizes as compared to larger studies. Although publication bias (i.e., selective publication of positive or extreme findings) is a potential explanation for these associations, other factors, such as "true" heterogeneity between smaller and larger studies, outcome reporting bias (in the case of stent thrombosis), chance, or other sources of bias could explain these results. Nonetheless, these results suggest that selective publication may have affected the available data and limits somewhat the strength of the conclusions that can be drawn (e.g., it contributed to our decision to grade the strength of evidence on MACE as moderate, rather than high).

Key Question 1c. What is the impact of modifying factors on the association between genetic test results and clinical outcomes?

We reviewed studies to identify any evidence that patient- or system-level factors or test characteristics could modify the predictive ability of genetic testing for CYP2C19 variants. Evidence of effect modification by person-level characteristics (e.g., age, sex, disease severity) is best obtained from comparisons within a given study (i.e., among subgroups of the patient population that were selected using the same criteria and managed in a similar way). Additional evidence on effect modification can be derived from exploratory comparisons across studies, by assessing study-level characteristics (e.g., the setting of care or study design characteristics) or characteristics of the overall patient population (e.g., populations selected on the basis of ancestry).[d] In the following sections we discuss each of these sources of information regarding effect modification separately.

Effect Modification Within Studies

In total, 20 studies (see Table 5) reported information on modification of the predictive effect of the genetic test by various factors. Eight of the studies used platelet reactivity as the outcome of interest and 12 reported information on clinical outcomes (adverse cardiovascular outcomes or bleeding events). We caution that, because only a small subset of the eligible studies provided information adequate to statistically assess effect modification, selective reporting is highly likely.

The 10 studies assessed a diverse set of potential modifiers. Five studied effect modification by proton-pump inhibitors;[122-124] three by ancestry (European vs. Latin American;[109] European vs. non-European; and European American vs. African American vs. other), five assessed gene–gene interactions (CYP2C19*2 and an ABCB1 variants;[110] CYP2C19*2 and *3 variants;[103] CYP2C19 *2 carrier status with PON1 variants in one; and multiple CYP2C19 variants and ITGB3 variants). The following modifiers were also evaluated: indication for clopidogrel use (acute coronary syndrome vs. stable angina),[125] whether patients were clopidogrel pre-treated or naïve upon study entry, whether patients required a loading dose or not (because they were on

---

[d]We refer to the information obtained from cross-study comparisons as "exploratory" because comparisons for given characteristics across studies may be confounded (by other study features). Our ability to statistically "control" for such differences is typically limited by the relatively small number of available studies available for meta-analysis.

chronic clopidogrel therapy),[103] the duration of clopidogrel therapy,[97] smoking status (number of cigarettes per day),[126] body-mass index (≥ 25 kg/m^2 vs. <25 kg/m^2),[123] and stent type (bare metal vs. drug eluting);[111] myocardial infarction subtype (ST-elevation or non-ST-elevation); clinical presentation (comparing a cohort of patients with myocardial infarction, ischemic stroke, or peripheral arterial disease vs. asymptomatic patients at high-risk for atherothrombotic events); history of PCI (yes vs. not); interactions with a large set of clinical and procedural factors; administration of polyunsaturated fatty acids; whether patients were on calcium channel blockers or their combination with PPIs; (five studies assessed more than two potential effect modifiers[103,123]).

Only two of the effects assessed was statistically significant (a multiplicative interaction between the *2 and *3 CYP2C19 alleles on on-clopidogrel platelet reactivity[103] and an interaction between symptomatic patients (CAPRIE-like cohort) and asymptomatic patients in the CHARISMA genetics substudy). Overall, the reported findings do not provide sufficient evidence to support (or exclude) a differential effect of CYP2C19 variants across any of the factors assessed in the studies we reviewed. The statistically significant findings are unlikely to indicate true effect medication, given the number of comparisons performed and potential for selective reporting across studies.

Table 5. Studies reporting information on effect modification

Author Year Country PMID Study Name (when available)	Patient Population	Antiplatelet Regimen	Effect Modifier	Summary of Findings*
Fernando[122] 2011 21696537 Australia NR	Patients with ACS treated with PCI with stent implantation; all patients were participants in a randomized cross-over trial of esomeprazole 40 mg vs. placebo	Aspirin (100 mg/d) and clopidogrel (75 mg/d)	Esomeprazole (40 mg/d) [the study drug]	After 6 w of exposure to each study drug, extensive metabolizers (those with no LOF alleles, i.e., no CYP2C19*2 allele) showed a significant mean reduction from baseline (−8% for PRI by VASP assay, −8.5 AUC units by aggregometry, −37 PRU by VerifyNow; p<0.01 for all comparisons) in platelet reactivity with esomeprazole vs. placebo. In poor or intermediate metabolizers (with at least one CYP2C19*2 allele) the mean reduction was nonsignificant (−8.73% for PRI, p=0.157; −3 AUC units for aggregometry, p=0.566; 39 PRU by VerifyNow, p=0.139) with esomeprazole vs. placebo.
Harmsze[125] 2010 19934793 Netherlands NR	Patients with CAD undergoing PCI with stent implantation	Clopidogrel "maintenance therapy" and aspirin (80 mg/d)	Indication for PCI with stent placement: ACS or stable angina	ORs for stent thrombosis: *For patients undergoing PCI for ACS* Carrier of *2 vs. not, OR=2.0 (95% CI, 1.1 to 4.5) Carrier of *3 vs. not, OR=2.9 (95% CI, 1.0 to 9.3) *For patients undergoing PCI for stable angina* Carrier of *2 vs. not, OR=1.7 (95% CI, 0.9 to 4.1) Carrier of *3 vs. not, OR=1.2 (95% CI, 0.4 to 6.5) Interaction p-value for the effect of *2 over PCI indication=0.97 Interaction p-value for the effect of *3 over PCI indication=0.18

49

Table 5. Studies reporting information on effect modification (continued)

Author Year Country PMID Study Name (when available)	Patient Population	Antiplatelet Regimen	Effect Modifier	Summary of Findings*
Harmsze[103] 2010 20833683 Netherlands NR	Patients undergoing elective stent implantation	All patients received aspirin (80–100 mg/d); 297 patients were on chronic clopidogrel (maintenance dose of 75 mg/d) and 131 patients received a clopidogrel loading dose of 300 mg upon study entry	Clopidogrel treatment status (maintenance treatment vs. loading dose); assessment of gene–gene interaction	Mean difference between carriers and noncarriers of CYP2C19*2 allele stratified by clopidogrel treatment group, using different assays (unadjusted results): *Clopidogrel maintenance treatment* LTA ADP 5 µmol/L: 6.7 (95% CI, 3.6 to 9.8) LTA ADP 20 µmol/L: 6.3 (95% CI, 3.4 to 9.3) VerifyNow PRU: 35.1 (95% CI, 17.2 to 53.0) *Clopidogrel loading dose* LTA ADP 5 µmol/L: 7.8 (95% CI, 3.9 to 12.6) LTA ADP 20 µmol/L: 7.4 (95% CI, 3.3 to 11.6) VerifyNow PRU: 37.5 (95% CI, 16.5 to 58.5) z-score p-values for effect modification (calculated): nonsignificant for all comparisons OR for *2 carriers vs. noncarriers for predicting poor response (>70% aggregation on LTA ADP 20 µmol/L) to antiplatelet treatment (unadjusted results): *Maintenance treatment, LTA ADP 20 µmol/L* OR=3.7 (95% CI, 2.0, 6.9) *Loading, LTA ADP 20 µmol/L* OR=3.7 (95% CI, 2.0, 6.9) z-score p-value for interaction: >0.99 Multiplicative interaction between *2 and *3 variants for poor response: *LTA ADP 20 µmol/L* 0.1 (95% CI, 0.004 to 0.79); p=0.033 *VerifyNow PRU* 0.1 (95% CI, 0.002 to 0.7); p=0.035

50

Table 5. Studies reporting information on effect modification (continued)

Author Year Country PMID Study Name (when available)	Patient Population	Antiplatelet Regimen	Effect Modifier	Summary of Findings*
Liu[126] 2010 21163112 China NR	Patients undergoing elective stent implantation for stable angina	Clopidogrel (300 mg loading dose and 75 mg/d maintenance dose) and aspirin (300 mg/d)	Smoking status (≥10 cigarettes/d)	p=0.671 for interaction between smoking status and *2 carrier status for predicting poor response by LTA (≤10% reduction in baseline aggregation at 24 h) in a logistic regression model
Maeda[123] 2011 21178986 Japan NR	Patients with CAD undergoing PCI	Aspirin (100 mg/d) and clopidogrel (75 mg/d) for >4 w	PPI treatment vs. not; BMI≥25 kg/m²	CYP2C19 genotype effect (mean residual % on-clopidogrel reactivity) stratified by PPI status: *On PPI* Two LOF alleles: n=2, mean=36.0, SD=8.5 One LOF allele: n=13, mean=27.5, SD=9.9 No LOF allele: n=14, mean=22.7, SD=7.6 *Not on PPI* Two LOF alleles: n=14, mean=33.5, SD=8.0 One LOF allele: n=33, mean=25.7, SD=9.0 No LOF allele: n=25, mean=17.7, SD=8.4 Interaction p-values (calculated with inverse variance-weighted least-squares regression): for one LOF allele × PPI=0.466 for two LOF alleles × PPI=0.724

CYP2C19 genotype effect (mean residual % on-clopidogrel reactivity) stratified by BMI status: *BMI≥25 kg/m²* Two LOF alleles: n=4, mean=36.0, SD=8.7 One LOF allele: n=16, mean=25.9, SD=9.8 No LOF allele: n=9, mean=24.4, SD=7.4 *BMI<25 kg/m²* Two LOF alleles: n=14, mean=33.1, SD=4.3 One LOF allele: n=14, mean=26.4, SD=8.5 No LOF allele: n=14, mean=17.1, SD=8.9 Interaction p-values (calculated with inverse variance-weighted least-squares regression): for one LOF allele × PPI=0.071 for two LOF alleles × PPI=0.347 |

51

Table 5. Studies reporting information on effect modification (continued)

Author Year Country PMID Study Name (when available)	Patient Population	Antiplatelet Regimen	Effect Modifier	Summary of Findings*
Pare[109] 2010 20979470 Multiple countries CURE	Patients with NSTE ACS in the clopidogrel-treated arm of the CURE randomized trial	Aspirin and clopidogrel (75 mg/d)	Race/ethnicity (European ancestry vs. Latin American Ancestry)	Interaction p-value for the predictive value of genotype group (intermediate/poor metabolizer vs. extensive/ultra metabolizer) between ancestry groups (calculated with chi-square test for heterogeneity): *For the first primary composite outcome* (cardiovascular death, nonfatal MI, or stroke)=0.682 *For another first primary composite outcome* (cardiovascular death, nonfatal MI, stroke, recurrent ischemia, or hospitalization for unstable angina)=0.722 *For major bleeding*=0.678

Table 5. Studies reporting information on effect modification (continued)

Author Year Country PMID Study Name (when available)	Patient Population	Antiplatelet Regimen	Effect Modifier	Summary of Findings*
Simon[124] 2011 21262992 France FAST-MI	Patients admitted to intensive care unit for definite AMI within 48 h after symptom onset with available DNA; patients had to be PPI-naïve at study entry for the main analysis	Clopidogrel-based treatment	PPI therapy (yes vs. no)	Estimate for PPI group vs. no-PPI group (adjusted for GRACE score, sex, and cardiovascular risk factors) *OR for in-hospital death, MI, or stroke* No variant allele, OR=0.68 (95% CI, 0.37 to 1.25) One variant allele, OR=0.34 (95% CI, 0.11 to 1.08) Two variant alleles, OR=1.05 (95% CI, 0.03 to 34.6) Interaction p-value across groups=0.547 [calculated with chi-square test for heterogeneity] *HR for death, MI, or stroke in hospital survivors receiving clopidogrel at 1 year* No variant allele, 1.13 (95% CI, 0.74 to 1.74 One variant allele, 1.02 (95% CI, 0.44 to 2.40) Two variant alleles, 0.25 (95% CI, 0.02 to 3.58) Interaction p-value across groups=0.527 calculated with chi-square test for heterogeneity] Overall interaction effect: For the short-term outcome, p=0.57 For the 1-year outcome, p=0.64
Simon[110] 2009 19106083 France FAST-MI	Patients admitted to intensive care unit for definite AMI within 48 h after symptom onset with available DNA	Clopidogrel-based treatment (mean clopidogrel loading dose 300 mg; mean maintenance dose 75 mg/d)	ABCB1 genotype (rs1045642) [carrier of at least one T allele vs. none]	p=0.99 for interaction between CYP2C19 and ABCB1 for the composite outcome of death, nonfatal MI, or stroke at 1 yr

53

Table 5. Studies reporting information on effect modification (continued)

Author Year Country PMID Study Name (when available)	Patient Population	Antiplatelet Regimen	Effect Modifier	Summary of Findings*
Trenk[111] 2008 18482659 Germany EXCELSIOR	Patients undergoing elective PCI with stent placement	Clopidogrel (600 mg loading dose) and aspirin (100 mg) for ≥5 d before the procedure	Stent type (BMS vs. DES)	OR for CYP2C19*2 carriers vs. noncarriers for death or MI at 1 yr *Patients with ≥ 1 DES* OR=1.60 (95% CI, 0.35 to 7.32) *Patients with BMS only* OR=0.30 (95% CI, 0.07 to 1.34) Interaction p-value=0.118 [calculated with chi-square test for heterogeneity]
Yamamoto[97] 2011 21168310 Japan NR	Patients undergoing cardiac catheterization at time of diagnosis of stable CAD	Aspirin (100 mg/d) and clopidogrel (75 mg/d)	Days on clopidogrel-based therapy (<7 vs. ≥7)	CYP2C19 genotype effect (on-clopidogrel reactivity in AU*min by LTA ADP 20 mol/L) stratified by days on treatment: *<7 d* Two LOF alleles: n=12, mean=3186, SD=1595 One LOF allele: n=32, mean=4655, SD=1380 No LOF allele: n=25, mean=5663, SD=1385 *≥7 d* Two LOF alleles: n=13, mean=3007, SD=1541 One LOF allele: n=19, mean=3490, SD=1392 No LOF allele: n=22, mean=4674, SD=824 Interaction p-value [calculated with inverse variance-weighted least-squares regression] For one LOF allele × PPI=0.106 For two LOF alleles × PPI=0.212

54

Table 5. Studies reporting information on effect modification (continued)

Author Year Country PMID Study Name (when available)	Patient Population	Antiplatelet Regimen	Effect Modifier	Summary of Findings*
Bhatt[85] 2012 22450429 Multinational CHARISMA	Patients with manifest atherothrombotic disease (coronary, cerebrovascular, or peripheral artery) or patients at high risk for atherothrombotic disease	Aspirin (75 to 162 mg/d) and clopidogrel (75 mg/d)	Ethnicity (Asian vs. non-Asian) PCI subcohort vs. non-PCI subcohort "CAPRIE-like" cohort vs. others (CAPRIE-like was defined as the subgroup of patients with MI, ischemic stroke, or symptomatic PAD)	*Prognostic effect under dominant model for LOF alleles for the MACE (defined as first occurrence of non-fatal or fatal MI, non-fatal or fatal stroke, or cardiovascular death):* - European ancestry: OR=1.28 (95% CI, 0.89 to 1.83) - Asian or African ancestry: OR=1.80 (95% CI, 0.55 to 5.92) Interaction p-value=0.58 - CAPRIE-like cohort (only among patients of European ancestry): OR=1.38 (95% CI, 0.88 to 2.17) - Others (only among patients of European ancestry): OR=1.14 (95% CI, 0.63 to 2.07) Interaction p-value=0.61 - PCI-subcohort (only among patients of European ancestry): OR=0.72 (95% CI, 0.28 to 1.80) - Non-PCI subcohort: OR=1.43 (95% CI, 0.96 to 2.13) Interaction p-value=0.18

Table 5. Studies reporting information on effect modification (continued)

Author Year Country PMID Study Name (when available)	Patient Population	Antiplatelet Regimen	Effect Modifier	Summary of Findings*
				Prognostic effect under dominant model for LOF alleles for the MACE (defined as first occurrence of non-fatal or fatal MI, non-fatal or fatal stroke, cardiovascular death, hospitalization for unstable angina, TIA, or revascularization procedure): - European ancestry: OR=1.06 (95% CI, 0.83 to 1.34) - Asian or African ancestry: OR=1.18 (95% CI, 0.49 to 2.85) Interaction p-value=0.82 - CAPRIE-like cohort (only among patients of European ancestry): OR=1.17 (95% CI, 0.86 to 1.59) - Others (only among patients of European ancestry): OR= 0.92 (95% CI, 0.64 to 1.35) Interaction p-value=0.35 - PCI-subcohort (only among patients of European ancestry): OR=0.80 (95% CI, 0.51 to 1.26) - Non-PCI subcohort: OR=1.20 (95% CI, 0.90 to 1.59) Interaction p-value=0.14

Table 5. Studies reporting information on effect modification (continued)

Author Year Country PMID Study Name (when available)	Patient Population	Antiplatelet Regimen	Effect Modifier	Summary of Findings*
				Prognostic effect under dominant model for LOF alleles for major GUSTO bleeding: - European ancestry: OR=1.13 (95% CI, 0.71 to 1.79) - Asian or African ancestry: OR=0.85 (95% CI, 0.15 to 4.81) Interaction p-value=0.76 - CAPRIE-like cohort (only among patients of European ancestry): OR=1.70 (95% CI, 0.97 to 2.98) - Others (only among patients of European ancestry): OR=0.55 (95% CI, 0.24 to 1.28) Interaction p-value=0.03 - PCI-subcohort (only among patients of European ancestry): OR=1.81 (95% CI, 0.68 to 4.83) - Non-PCI subcohort: OR=0.99 (95% CI, 0.59 to 1.67) Interaction p-value=0.29

57

Table 5. Studies reporting information on effect modification (continued)

Author Year Country PMID Study Name (when available)	Patient Population	Antiplatelet Regimen	Effect Modifier	Summary of Findings*
				Prognostic effect under dominant model for LOF alleles for all GUSTO bleeding: - European ancestry: OR=0.76 (95% CI, 0.63 to 0.92) - Asian or African ancestry: OR=0.82 (95% CI, 0.36 to 1.86) Interaction p-value=0.87 - CAPRIE-like cohort (only among patients of European ancestry): OR=0.76 (95% CI, 0.59 to 0.98) - Others (only among patients of European ancestry): OR=0.76 (95% CI, 0.57 to 1.00) Interaction p-value=0.97 - PCI-subcohort (only among patients of European ancestry): OR=0.84 (95% CI, 0.59 to 1.20) - Non-PCI subcohort: OR= 0.74 (95% CI, 0.59 to 0.92) Interaction p-value= 0.54

Table 5. Studies reporting information on effect modification (continued)

Author Year Country PMID Study Name (when available)	Patient Population	Antiplatelet Regimen	Effect Modifier	Summary of Findings*
				Prognostic effect under dominant model for GOF alleles for the MACE (defined as first occurrence of non-fatal or fatal MI, non-fatal or fatal stroke, or cardiovascular death): - European ancestry: OR=0.94 (95% CI, 0.66 to 1.34) - Asian or African ancestry: OR=0.58 (95% CI, 0.15 to 2.25) Interaction p-value=0.50 - CAPRIE-like cohort (only among patients of European ancestry): OR= 0.82 (95% CI, 0.53 to 1.29) - Others (only among patients of European ancestry): OR=1.17 (95% CI, 0.66 to 2.07) Interaction p-value=0.35 - PCI-subcohort (only among patients of European ancestry): OR= 0.58 (95% CI, 0.24 to 1.38) - Non-PCI subcohort: OR=1.04 (95% CI, 0.71 to 1.54) Interaction p-value=0.23

Table 5. Studies reporting information on effect modification (continued)

Author Year Country PMID Study Name (when available)	Patient Population	Antiplatelet Regimen	Effect Modifier	Summary of Findings*
				Prognostic effect under dominant model for GOF alleles for the MACE (defined as first occurrence of non-fatal or fatal MI, non-fatal or fatal stroke, cardiovascular death, hospitalization for unstable angina, TIA, or revascularization procedure): - European ancestry: OR=0.98 (95% CI, 0.78 to 1.23) - Asian or African ancestry: OR= 1.55 (95% CI, 0.64 to 3.74) Interaction p-value=0.32 - CAPRIE-like cohort (only among patients of European ancestry): OR= 0.87 (95% CI, 0.64 to 1.16) - Others (only among patients of European ancestry): OR= 1.17 (95% CI, 0.82 to 1.66) Interaction p-value=0.95 - PCI-subcohort (only among patients of European ancestry): OR=1.02 (95% CI, 0.68 to 1.52) - Non-PCI subcohort: OR= 0.97 (95% CI, 0.74 to 1.27) Interaction p-value=0.86

Table 5. Studies reporting information on effect modification (continued)

Author Year Country PMID Study Name (when available)	Patient Population	Antiplatelet Regimen	Effect Modifier	Summary of Findings*
				Prognostic effect under dominant model for GOF alleles for major GUSTO bleeding: - European ancestry: OR= 0.91 (95% CI, 0.59 to 1.42) - Asian or African ancestry: OR=0.35 (95% CI, 0.04 to 3.09) Interaction p-value=0.40 - CAPRIE-like cohort (only among patients of European ancestry): OR=0.80 (95% CI, 0.45 to 1.42) - Others (only among patients of European ancestry): OR=1.11 (95% CI, 0.56 to 2.20) Interaction p-value=0.47 - PCI-subcohort (only among patients of European ancestry): OR=0.91 (95% CI, 0.33, 2.51) - Non-PCI subcohort: OR=0.90 (95% CI, 0.55, 1.48) Interaction p-value=0.98

Table 5. Studies reporting information on effect modification (continued)

Author Year Country PMID Study Name (when available)	Patient Population	Antiplatelet Regimen	Effect Modifier	Summary of Findings*
				Prognostic effect under dominant model for GOF alleles for all GUSTO bleeding: - European ancestry: OR= 1.10 (95% CI, 0.93 to 1.31) - Asian or African ancestry: OR=0.61 (95% CI, 0.26 to 1.45) Interaction p-value=0.19 - CAPRIE-like cohort (only among patients of European ancestry): OR= 1.02 (95% CI, 0.81 to 1.28) - Others (only among patients of European ancestry): OR=1.23 (95% CI, 0.95 to 1.60) Interaction p-value=0.29 - PCI-subcohort (only among patients of European ancestry): OR=1.13 (95% CI, 0.81 to 1.56) - Non-PCI subcohort: OR=1.10 (95% CI, 0.90 to 1.34) Interaction p-value=0.89 [all results were calculated; data to evaluate effect modification under other genetic models were NR]

Table 5. Studies reporting information on effect modification (continued)

Author Year Country PMID Study Name (when available)	Patient Population	Antiplatelet Regimen	Effect Modifier	Summary of Findings*
Cayla 2011 22028352 France ONASSIT	Case-control study of patients with definite stent thrombosis and controls identified in a local PCI database (1:2 matched for age and sex)	Cases and controls were on dual antiplatelet therapy	Interactions were tested between "independent clinical and angiographic factors" (acute PCI, complex lesions, LVEG <40%, DM, use of PPI, clopidogrel loading dose) and genetic variants (CYP2C19) Gene-gene interaction (CYP2C19 variants with ABCB1 and ITGB3)	All analyses were for the outcome of stent thrombosis. None of the interactions were statistically significant (all p>0.05). The exact p-value was reported only for the interaction of CYP2C19 and high-clopidogrel dose: p=0.46.
Collet 2011 21511218 France CLOVIS-2	Patients with MI before the age of 45, screened from the AFIJI multicenter registry.	Patients were on maintenance aspirin (75 mg/d) and/or clopidogrel (75 mg/d) for ≥3 mo. They were randomized to an open-label loading dose of 300 or 900 mg of clopidogrel in a 2-period crossover fashion. Clopidogrel maintenance treatment (75 mg) was continued for ≥21 d before patients were crossed over to the alternate loading dose of clopidogrel.	Clopidogrel pre-treatment status (naive vs. pre-treated)	The p-value for interaction between pre-treatment status and CYP2C19*2 carriage was not statistically significant for the relative reduction in residual platelet aggregation after both loading doses (p=0.76 for the 300 mg loading dose and p=0.62 for the 900 mg loading dose).

Table 5. Studies reporting information on effect modification (continued)

Author Year Country PMID Study Name (when available)	Patient Population	Antiplatelet Regimen	Effect Modifier	Summary of Findings*
Delaney 2011 22190063 USA BioVU biobank	Patients started on antiplatelet therapy after MI or PCI with stent placement	Patients receiving clopidogrel on discharge	Ethnicity (European American vs. African American)	Prognostic effect under dominant model for the *2 allele for MACE (defined as all-cause mortality, MI, revascularization, or stroke) European Americans, OR=1.39 (95% CI, 0.96 to 2.01) African Americans, OR=2.46 (95% CI, 0.86 to 7.07) Others, OR=3.00 (95% CI, 0.14 to 64.26) P-for interaction = 0.55 [calculated] Prognostic effect under dominant model for the *17 allele for MACE (defined as all-cause mortality, MI, revascularization, or stroke) European Americans, OR=0.85 (95% CI, 0.60 to 1.21) African Americans, OR=1.31 (95% CI, 0.46 to 3.79) Others, OR=0.54 (95% CI, 0.02 to 14.35) P-for interaction = 0.72 [calculated]
Gajos 2012 22623230 Poland NR	Patients with stable CAD who underwent successful PCI with stent placement	Clopidogrel (600 mg loading dose; 75 mg/d maintenance) + aspirin 75 mg/d for 1 mo	1000 mg of omega-3 PUFA (460 mg of eicosapentaenoic acid + 380 mg docosahexaenoic acid) vs. 1000 mg of soybean oil in a single capsule (placebo); exposure to the effect modifier was randomized	Interaction p-value at 30 d (maximum followup) using LTA ADP 5 µmol/L to assess outcomes=0.17 [calculated] Interaction p-value at 30 d (maximum followup) using LTA ADP 20 µmol/L to assess platelet reactivity=0.36 [calculated]

64

Table 5. Studies reporting information on effect modification (continued)

Author Year Country PMID Study Name (when available)	Patient Population	Antiplatelet Regimen	Effect Modifier	Summary of Findings*
Harmsze 2011 21854540 Netherlands POPular	Patients with established coronary artery disease scheduled for elective PCI with stent implantation	Prior to PCI, all patients were pretreated with clopidogrel (75 mg/d therapy for >5 days or a loading dose of 300mg >24h before PCI or 600 mg >4h before PCI) + aspirin (80-100 mg/d for >10 d. Maintenance treatment was with clopidogrel (75 mg/d) + aspirin (80-100 mg/d)	Calcium channel blockers (yes vs. not) PPIs (yes vs. not) CCB + PPIs (yes vs. not)	For predicting MACE, defined as all-cause death, non-fatal MI, stent thrombosis, or ischemic stroke at 1 yr) [all results were calculated]: - Interaction p-value comparing the effect of *2 carriership among patients receiving CCBs vs. not=0.16 - Interaction p-value comparing the effect of *2 carriership among patients receiving PPIs vs. not=0.30 - Interaction p-value comparing the effect of *2 carriership among patients receiving CCBs + PPIs vs. not=0.69
Hsu 2011 21144850 Taiwan NR	Patients with atherosclerotic disease (ischemic heart disease or stroke) and gastroduodenal ulcer who underwent endoscopy for dyspeptic symptoms while receiving clopidogrel	Patients had received clopidogrel for ≥2 wk (75 mg/d or 37.5 mg/d) and required long term antiplatelet therapy; during the study all patients received clopidogrel 75 mg/d; patients with H. pylori infection also received antibiotic treatment following a standardized scheme	PPI administration (20 mg/d esomeprazole vs. no PPI) for 6 mo; exposure to the modifier was randomized	Prognostic effect (dominant model for *2 allele) for MACE (defined as unstable angina, acute MI, ischemic stroke, or vascular death): - among patients in the esomeprazole group: OR=4.23 (95% CI, 0.20 to 91.92) - among patients in the control group: OR=7.00 (95% CI, 0.35 to 141.00) Interaction p-value=0.82 [calculated results]
Hulot 2011 21972404 France CLOVIS-2	Patients with MI before the age of 45, screened from the AFIJI multicenter registry. A total of 292 male patients were genotyped for CYP2C19*2. *2/*2 and *2/*1 patients were asked to participate in the trial. Age- and gender-matched CYP2C19 *1/*1 (noncarriers) from the AFIJI program were then recruited with a 1:1 ratio for each *2/*1 and a 2:1 ratio for each *2/*2 patient who was willing to participate.	Clopidogrel loading dose of 300 or 900 mg (crossover RCT). Clopidogrel maintenance treatment (75 mg) was continued for ≥21 days before patients were crossed over to the alternate loading dose group	Gene-gene interaction (CYP2C19 *2 carrier effect by PON1 variants; 2 variants were genotyped, Q192R and L55M)	The study reported that "no significant interactions between the tested CYP2C19 and PON1 genetic variants were observed" for pharmacodynamic endpoints. No additional results were reported.

Table 5. Studies reporting information on effect modification (continued)

Author Year Country PMID Study Name (when available)	Patient Population	Antiplatelet Regimen	Effect Modifier	Summary of Findings*
Jaitner 2012 22298798 Germany NR	Patients undergoing PCI with stent placement and receiving dual antiplatelet therapy; 2 cohorts, a prospective PCI cohort and a registry of stent thrombosis cases were analyzed	Patients received clopidogrel (600 mg) and aspirin (500 mg) loading doses; post-PCI patients received clopidogrel (2×75 mg/d for the remainder of hospitalization, up to three days, followed by clopidogrel 75 mg/d for 6 to 12 mo) + aspirin (2×100 mg/d indefinitely)	Gene-gene interaction (CYP2C19 *2 carrier effect by ABCB1 3435TT genotype)	The p-value for interaction for the outcome of stent thrombosis was 0.51 in multivariate analyses that adjusted for multiple clinical and procedural factors. No additional results were reported.
Jeong 2011 22045970 S. Korea NR	Patients with AMI admitted to a single academic center who did not experience in-hospital death and did not need emergent bypass operation	Patients received loading with aspirin (300 mg) + clopidogrel (600 mg); maintenance therapy was with aspirin (200 mg/d for 1 mo, followed by 100–200 mg/d indefinitely) + clopidogrel (75 mg/d for ≥1 yr); patients on intensified antiplatelet therapy (cilostazol or high-dose clopidogrel) were excluded	MI subtype (STEMI vs. NSTE-MI)	Prognostic effect under dominant mode for the LOF alleles (*2 or *3) for MACE (defined as cardiovascular death, MI, or stroke): NSTE-MI, OR= 2.63 (95% CI, 0.29 to 24.25) STEMI, OR= 4.85 (95% CI, 0.58 to 40.53) Interaction p-value=0.697 [calculated results]

Prognostic effect under dominant mode for LOF alleles (*2 or *3) for TIMI major or minor bleeding: NSTE-MI, OR=1.95 (95% CI, 0.20 to 19.26) STEMI, OR=0.64 (95% CI, 0.09 to 4.67) Interaction p-value=0.472 [calculated results] |

Abbreviations: ACS = acute coronary syndromes; ADP = adenosine diphosphate; AU = aggregation units; AUC = area under the curve; BMI = body-mass index; BMS = bare-metal stent; CAD = coronary artery disease; CI = confidence interval; CURE = Clopidogrel in Unstable Angina to Prevent Recurrent Events trial; d = day(s); DES = drug-eluting stent; EXCELSIOR = Impact of Extent of Clopidogrel-Induced Platelet Inhibition During Elective Stent Implantation on Clinical Event Rate; FAST-MI = French Registry on Acute ST-elevation and non ST-elevation Myocardial Infarction; GOF = gain-of-function; GRACE = Global Registry of Acute Coronary Events; h = hours; LOF = loss-of-function; LTA = light-transmission aggregometry; MI = myocardial infarction; NA = not applicable; NR = not reported; NSTE = non-ST-elevation; OR = odds ratio; PCI = percutaneous coronary intervention; PPI = proton-pump inhibitor; PRI = platelet reactivity index; PRU = platelet reactivity units; SD = standard deviation; PUFA = polyunsaturated fatty acids; VASP = vasodilator-stimulated phosphoprotein; w = weeks.

"Calculated" indicates that the result was not reported by the article's authors; rather, we derived the result from reported raw data.
*The description "calculated values" indicates that the results are based on statistical procedures we conducted in cases where studies provided sufficient statistics for the assessment of effect modification but did not assess its statistical significance.

Effect Modification Across Studies

On the basis of the availability of data from studies considered eligible for Key Question 1b, we assessed the following characteristics as potential modifiers of the predictive effect of genetic testing for CYP2C19 by performing comparisons across studies using subgroup analysis: disease subtype (acute coronary syndromes vs. mixed coronary artery disease populations), setting of care (PCI vs. other), race or ethnicity (white vs. East Asian), duration of followup (≤30 days vs. >30 days); and year when enrollment was started (continuous variable). Meta-regressions were performed for only the two outcomes that were reported in 10 or more studies—major adverse cardiovascular events and stent thrombosis—and for only carriers versus noncarriers of CYP2C19 loss-of-function alleles.

Table 6 summarizes the findings of our meta-regression analyses for the outcome of stent thrombosis and Table 7 summarizes findings for the composite endpoint of MACE.

Table 6. Meta-regression results for study-level effect modifiers of the predictive value of genetic testing for CYP2C19 variants in patients with ischemic heart disease: stent thrombosis

Effect Modifier	Groups Compared	No. of Studies	RR (95% CI) Within Subgroup	rRR (95% CI); P-Value
All studies	NA	17	1.52 (1.17 to 1.97)	NA
ACS vs. ischemic heart disease	Other ischemic heart disease or mixed	10	1.54 (1.07, 2.20)	0.98 (0.58 to 1.65); 0.936
	ACS	7	1.51 (1.03 to 2.19)	
Race or ethnicity	Whites	14	1.44 (1.10 to 1.88)	3.49 (1.00 to 12.19); 0.050
	East Asians	3	5.02 (1.48 to 17.03)	
Followup	Longitudinal	13	1.62 (1.15 to 2.27)	0.86 (0.51 to 1.46); 0.579
	Case–control or case-cohort	4	1.39 (0.93 to 2.09)	
Duration of followup	>30 d	12	1.41 (1.07 to 1.86)	2.73 (0.39 to 19.19); 0.313
	≤30 d	1	3.86 (0.56 to 26.63)	
Enrollment start year	(continuous variable)	14	NA	0.96 (0.87 to 1.06); 0.472

Abbreviations: ACS = acute coronary syndromes; CI = confidence interval; d = day(s); NA = not applicable; RR = relative risk; rRR = relative RR (between groups).

Results across all studies are provided for comparison. For stent thrombosis, all patients had to undergo percutaneous coronary intervention, so results by setting of care are not presented. One study did not report the year enrollment was started.

Table 7. Meta-regression results for study-level effect modifiers of the predictive value of genetic testing for CYP2C19 variants in patients with ischemic heart disease: MACE

Effect Modifier	Groups Compared	No. of Studies	RR (95% CI) Within Subgroup	rRR (95% CI); P-Value
All studies	NA	25	1.20 (1.04 to 1.39)	NA
ACS vs. ischemic heart disease	Other ischemic heart disease or mixed	13	1.44 (1.08 to 1.92)	0.80 (0.58 to 1.10); 0.175
	ACS	12	1.11 (0.95 to 1.30)	
PCI vs. other clinical settings	Other	15	1.25 (1.03 to 1.52)	0.91 (0.65 to 1.29); 0.599
	PCI	10	1.13 (0.88 to 1.46)	
Race or ethnicity	Whites	19	1.10 (0.97 to 1.24)	1.96 (1.21 to 3.18); 0.006
	East Asians	5	2.54 (1.45 to 4.44)	
Duration of follow-up	>30 d	22	1.21 (1.03 to 1.41)	0.93 (0.42 to 2.06); 0.859
	≤30 d	1	1.14 (0.60 to 2.17)	
Enrollment start year	(continuous variable)	17	NA	1.06 (0.99, 1.13); 0.109

Abbreviations: ACS = acute coronary syndromes; CI = confidence interval; d = days; NA = not applicable; PCI = percutaneous coronary intervention; RR = relative risk; rRR = relative RR (between groups).
Results across all studies are provided for comparison. All eligible studies were longitudinal (cohort studies), so results by study design are not presented.

For all factors other than ethnicity, considering both within-study and across studies analyses, there is insufficient information to support or exclude the presence of substantial modification of the predictive effect of CYP2C19 variants by any of the investigated factors. Meta-regression analyses (both for stent thrombosis and MACE) suggested that the effect of LOF alleles may be more extreme among individuals of East Asian Ethnicity; however, this finding needs to be interpreted with caution given the relatively small number of publications reporting on individual of East Asian ethnicity and the potential for confounding by other factors that differ between studies conducted in populations of different ethnicities.

Key Question 2a. What is the analytic validity (technical test performance) of the various assays used in phenotypic testing of platelet reactivity?

Eligible Studies for Key Question 2a

We identified 105 studies reporting information on the analytic validity of assays for measuring platelet reactivity; details about the design and results of individual studies are provided in Appendix E. We also reviewed 20 FDA 510(k) summaries on phenotypic testing assays (see Appendix C). Studies had intermediate sample sizes (median sample size=120; 25th percentile=93; 75th percentile=255) and were published between 2002 and 2012 (median publication year=2009). Seventeen studies (16 percent) were conducted in the United States, 58 (55 percent) in Europe, and 30 (29 percent) elsewhere. All studies enrolled patients with ischemic (atherothrombotic) vascular disease. The six most commonly assessed assays (with some studies assessing more than one) were LTA (in 71 studies; 68 percent), the VerifyNow P2Y12 assay (in 46 studies, 44 percent), the VASP assay (in 37 studies, 35 percent), the Multiplate analyzer (in 18 studies; 17 percent), the PFA device (in 10 studies; 10 percent), and thromboelastography (in 6 studies; 6 percent). The vast majority of studies used ADP as the agonist to stimulate platelets (in order to assess reactivity).

None of the 20 FDA 510(k) summaries on phenotypic tests of platelet reactivity reported relevant analyses (either no data were reported or the population or agonist used in test was not of interest, the analytic validity results were not reported for clopidogrel [rather, for a comedication], or the sample size was <10).

We organized studies reporting information relevant to analytic validity into four groups: analytic performance, interassay agreement, test reliability and assay variation, and correlations between assays applied to the same sample. No other aspect of analytic validity was evaluated in studies considered eligible for this review. Table 8 summarizes the information provided by each study type and the number of relevant publications included in our report. In subsequent sections we summarize key findings pertaining to each of these outcomes.

Overall there appeared to be low to moderate agreement between assays. Agreement was generally greater between measurements obtained with the same assay using different agonist concentrations than between different assays. Studies were generally of low methodological quality and poorly reported. Only 1 of the 11 items capturing risk of bias and completeness of reporting ("providing adequate details on the testing method" to allow for replication of test results) was satisfactorily addressed across studies. Detailed results regarding the quality items are presented at the end of this section.

Figure 19 presents an evidence map (a weighted scatter plot of tests and outcomes considered in the eligible studies) of studies assessing pairs of tests for analytic accuracy, agreement, or correlation (studies of these outcomes need to assess at least two tests). Only a minority of these studies reported information on analytic performance or test agreement, whereas a large number provided correlation results. Most of the studies reported test agreement or correlations between measurements obtained with different assays (e.g., LTA versus the VASP assay, VerifyNow, or the Multiplate analyzer); comparisons between measurements performed using the same assay with different agonist concentrations were also commonly reported.

Table 8. Studies reporting information relevant to analytic validity

Analytic Validity Category	Relevant Information	Assays Evaluated (no. of studies; % of total studies)
Analytic performance (analytic accuracy, sensitivity, specificity)	These studies used a reference standard test against which the analytic performance of one or more index tests is assessed. In theory, the reference standard test can also be considered to have non-negligible measurement error (i.e., to be a "tarnished" reference standard); however, in all the studies we reviewed, the analytic reference standards were considered to be "gold standards" (i.e., to have no measurement error).	Total=12 studies LTA (9; 75%) VASP assay (4; 33%) VerifyNow P2Y12 (6; 50%) Multiplate analyzer (4; 33%) PFA (3; 25%) TEG (1; 8%) Plateletworks (0; 0%) Others (3; 25%)
Interassay agreement	These studies assessed the amount of agreement (concordance) between measurements of the same sample obtained with different assays. Agreement can be assessed between continuous measurements or using nominal or ordinal classifications (e.g., by discretizing continuous measurements by applying a threshold).	Total=40 studies LTA (31; 78%) VASP assay (16; 40%) VerifyNow P2Y12 (23; 58%) Multiplate analyzer (11; 28%) PFA (7; 18%) TEG (2; 5%) Plateletworks (2; 5%) Others (7; 18%)
Assay reliability (variability)	These studies assessed the reliability of assays during repeat testing and provided estimates of the variation of results when testing was repeated across different batches of analytes or portions of the same sample. The studies we reviewed typically expressed results as coefficients of variation.*	Total=43 studies LTA (24; 56%) VASP assay (16; 37%) VerifyNow P2Y12 (12; 28%) Multiplate analyzer (5; 12%) PFA (6; 14%) TEG (1; 2%) Plateletworks (0; 0%) Others (6; 14%)
Correlation between measurements obtained by different assays	Many of these studies reported correlations (typically Spearman or Pearson) between measurements obtained from the same sample. (These correlations were reported to support claims regarding interassay agreement; we discuss in the text why some methods for calculating correlations are not appropriate for this purpose.)	Total=72 studies LTA (58; 81%) VASP assay (31; 43%) VerifyNow P2Y12 (36; 50%) Multiplate analyzer (16; 22%) PFA (6; 8%) TEG (5; 7%) Plateletworks (4; 6%) Others (18; 25%)

Abbreviations: LTA = light-transmission aggregometry; PFA = Platelet Function Analyzer; TEG = thromboelastography; VASP = vasodilator-stimulated phosphoprotein assay using flow cytometry. "Other" denotes less commonly assessed assay types.

See Appendix E for a complete list of assays used in the included studies. Studies could have used more than one assay.

*The coefficient of variation is generally defined as the ratio of a measure of dispersion over a measure of central tendency.[127]

The most commonly used definition is the ratio of the estimated standard deviation (SD) over the sample mean ($\bar{x}$): $CoV = \frac{SD}{\bar{x}}$.

Figure 19. Evidence map of studies reporting information on the analytic validity of phenotypic assays

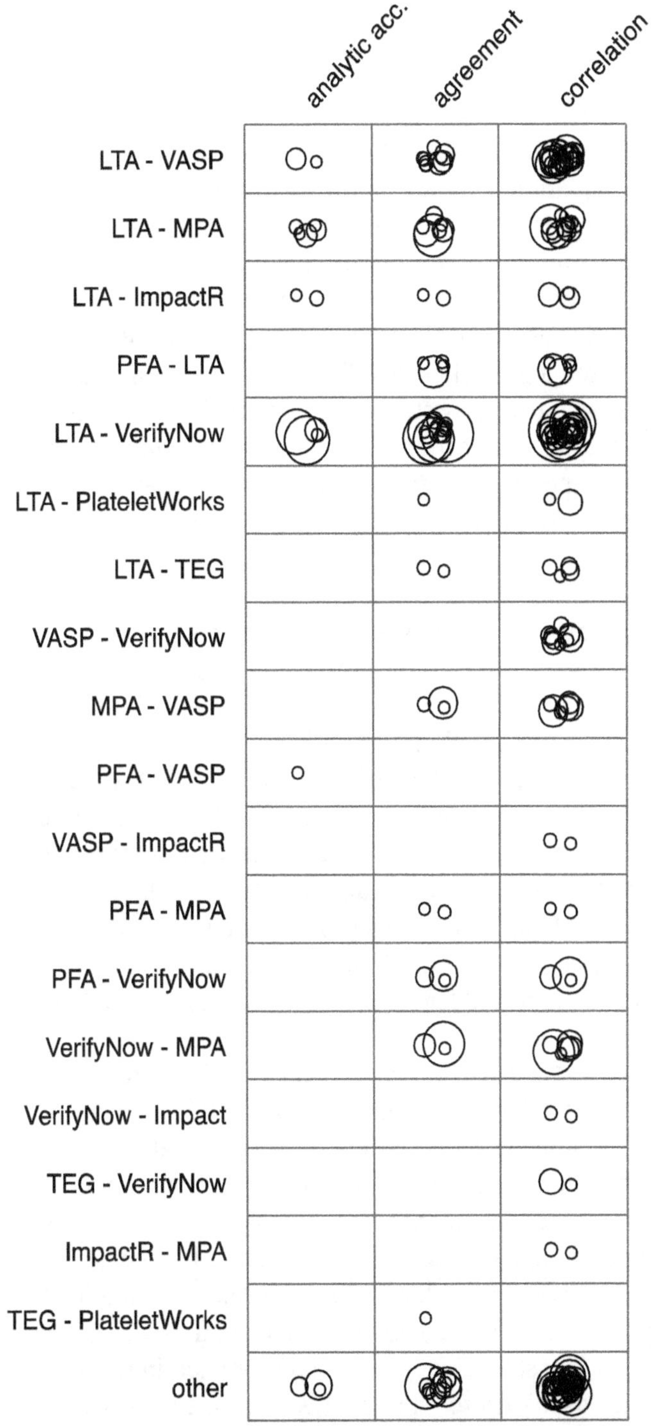

Abbreviations: Acc = accuracy; LTA = light-transmission aggregometry; MPA = Multiplate analyzer; PFA = Platelet Function Analyzer; TEG = thromboelastography; VASP = vasodilator-stimulated phosphoprotein. "Other" denotes pairs of assays where at least one of the assays was used in fewer than five studies or comparisons between measurements obtained with the same assay (e.g., using different agonist concentrations). Each circle represents a study; the size of the circle increases with increasing sample size, and location of circles within boxes is random. The assays used are described in detail in Appendix E.

Findings on the Analytic Validity of Platelet Reactivity Assays

Analytic Performance

Only a small number of studies (n=12) provided information on analytic performance. In these studies, LTA (eight studies), the VASP assay (two studies), or the Multiplate analyzer (one study) was considered as "gold standard" tests. In one study the reference standard test was platelet-receptor expression after ADP stimulation, assessed by flow cytometry. Reported analytic sensitivities ranged between 0.35 and 1.00; reported specificities ranged between 0.42 and 0.95. In studies reporting results across multiple cutoff values, a tradeoff between sensitivity and specificity was apparent (as expected). Overall, results were indicative of poor agreement between classifications (e.g., "high reactivity" vs. "low reactivity") obtained by the pairs of tests assessed when one of the tests was considered a gold standard. We did not perform meta-analyses of test performance metrics because only a few studies were available for each index test–reference standard pair and because studies used different thresholds to define positive and negative results. Detailed information on the populations included, assays used, analyses performed, and study results are presented in Appendix E.

Interassay Agreement

Forty studies provided information on interassay agreement. The most commonly assessed pairs of tests were LTA and VerifyNow (14 studies), LTA and the VASP assay (9 studies), and LTA and the Multiplate analyzer (7 studies). Information on the included populations, assays used, thresholds applied, and study results are presented in Appendix E.

Fourteen studies evaluated interassay agreement on the basis of continuous measurements by various assays (using valid methods, such as Bland–Altman analyses[128] or Lin's concordance correlation coefficient[129]—i.e., major axis regression). Thirty-three of the studies reported agreement on the basis of dichotomizing platelet reactivity values using various thresholds; 29 of these reported or allowed for the calculation of kappa statistics (98 estimates in total). Across all comparisons reported, the median kappa value was 0.40 (25th percentile=0.23; 75th percentile=0.53). Only four (4 percent) of the reported kappa values were higher than 0.8 (a commonly used threshold for "excellent" agreement[130]), 15 (15 percent) of the values were between 0.6 and 0.8 (considered indicative of "substantial" agreement), 28 (29 percent) were between 0.4 and 0.6 (considered to indicate "moderate" agreement), and 51 (53 percent) were lower than 0.4 (indicating "poor to fair" agreement). Overall these results indicate that disagreements are relatively common between measurements obtained by different assays or by using different agonist concentrations within the same assays.

Figure 20 presents histograms of reported kappa values (chance corrected agreement statistics), suggesting that overall, agreement was somewhat lower between LTA and the VASP assay than between LTA and the VerifyNow P2Y12 assay. Quantitative synthesis of kappa statistics was not performed because only a few studies were available for each index test–reference standard pair and because studies used different thresholds to define positive and negative results.

Figure 20. Histograms of kappa values between methods for measurement of platelet reactivity

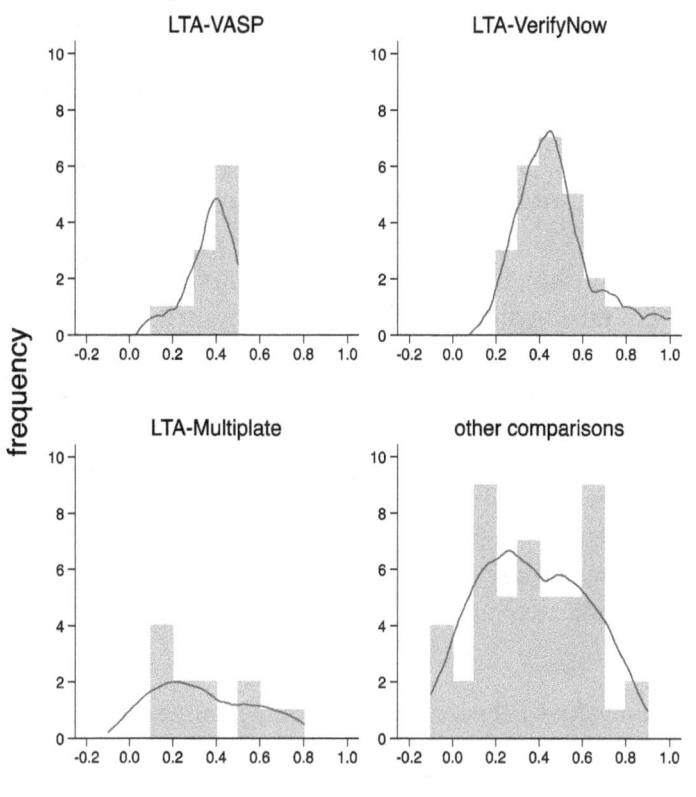

kappa estimates

Abbreviations: LTA = light-transmission aggregometry; VASP = vasodilator-stimulated phosphoprotein.
"Frequency" refers to the number of studies. Black solid lines are kernel densities fitted over the distribution of kappa values.
Each panel shows at least 10 reported kappa values.

Assay Reliability

Forty-three studies reported information on assay variability. The information reported about the experimental designs used to obtain the reported results was limited (e.g., >90 percent of the studies did not report the number of replicate samples). Variability or coefficient-of-variation results were less than 10 percent in all but two studies. One study used the intraclass correlation coefficient for repeat measurements to assess the reliability of measurements using LTA, the VASP assay, the Multiplate analyzer, and the INNOVANCE assay.

All extracted assay reliability results are presented in Appendix E. These results need to be interpreted with caution, give the poor reporting of study methods and the fact that multiple studies were published by a limited number of investigative teams (there was no way to ascertain whether the studied populations are the same or similar).

Correlation Between Measurements Used as a Method To Assess Agreement

Pearson or Spearman correlation coefficients are poor metrics for assessing agreement between measurements.[e] Correlation values are informative only in extreme cases: for example,

---

[e]Briefly, these coefficients are suboptimal for assessing agreement because: (1) correlations measure association and not agreement; (2) correlations are independent of scale of measurement, whereas agreement is not; (3) significant correlation results are likely when the range of measurements is wide, regardless of agreement; (4) the test for the

a Pearson correlation coefficient very close to 1 (or −1) indicates that the values of one assay can be linearly transformed to those of the other. More appropriate methods for assessing agreement between continuous measurements are available, such as the Bland–Altman approach[128] and Lin's concordance correlation coefficient.[129] Studies using the Bland–Altman method have been discussed above (see Interassay Agreement).

Of the 72 studies reporting correlation values, only one used Lin's concordance correlation coefficient,[131] reporting a high correlation ($\rho=0.97$) between observed and estimated platelet inhibition for the VerifyNow assay (comparing the change between pre- and post-treatment measurements with the change between post-treatment measurements and those from the TRAP channel of the device). The vast majority of the remaining studies reported Spearman or Pearson correlation coefficients, used linear regression (which in the simple bivariate case of two measurements is equivalent to the Pearson correlation), or did not report the calculation method employed. Detailed results from each comparison reported in the reviewed studies are presented in Appendix E. Given that the majority of correlation estimates reported had an absolute value lower than 0.9 (90% percent of the 290 values reported) the results indicate that the association between measurements obtained using different methods is relatively poor. However, given the inappropriateness of the methods used (for the purpose of assessing agreement), even high correlation values would not be considered indicative of good agreement. Figure 21 presents histograms of reported correlation values.

Figure 21. Histogram of reported correlation values between methods for measurement of platelet reactivity

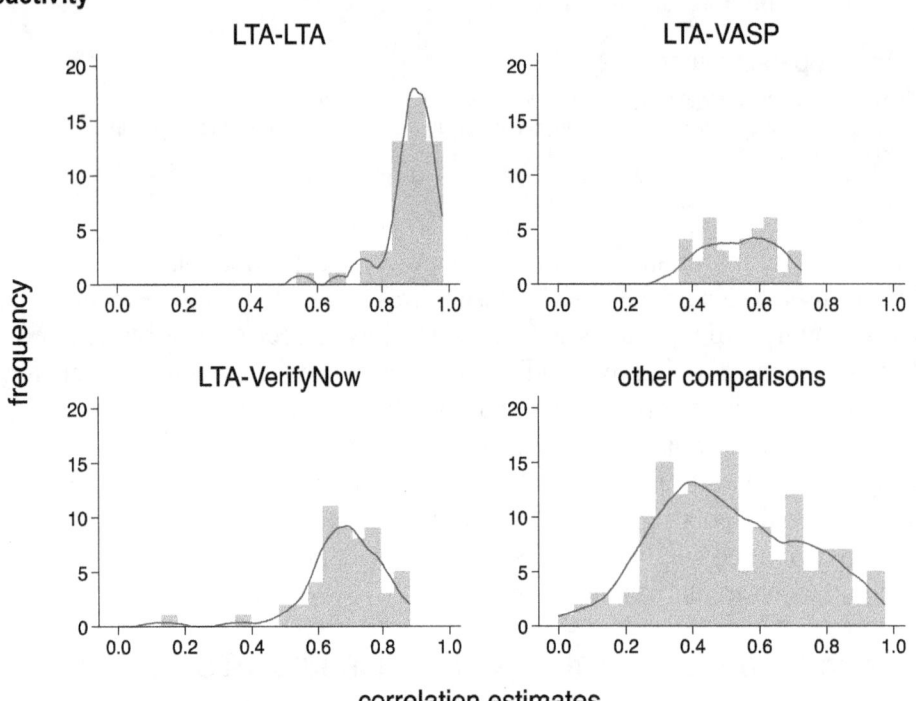

Abbreviations: LTA = light-transmission aggregometry; VASP = vasodilator-stimulated phosphoprotein.
"LTA-LTA" denotes comparisons between LTA assays using different agonists or different agonist concentrations. "Frequency" refers to the number of studies. Black solid lines are kernel densities fitted over the distribution of correlation values. Each panel shows at least 20 reported correlation values.

null hypothesis of no correlation is irrelevant to the question of agreement; and (5) even high correlation values (>0.95) do not imply good agreement. For additional discussion, see Bland and Altman 1986.[128]

Risk of Bias and Completeness of Reporting for Studies Reviewed for Key Question 2a

Studies reporting on assay variability were extremely poorly reported (in all but three studies, no information was provided on the study design, selection criteria, or measurement methods used; in over 90 percent of the studies, the number of replicate samples used for analyses was not reported). Thus it was impossible to assess the risk of bias of these studies. In addition, as mentioned in the preceding section, correlation estimates are practically uninformative for assessing agreement between assays. For these reasons, we limited the assessment of study quality to the 43 studies that reported information on analytic test performance or interassay agreement.

Appendix D includes our assessment of 11 items related to risk of bias and completeness of reporting of studies presenting information on test agreement or analytic performance (including the single study reporting Lin's concordance correlation coefficient[131] and studies using the Bland-Altman method). All but 1 of the 35 studies (a study published as a letter to the editor[132]) provided adequate descriptions of the assays used. Information on the use of positive or negative controls was poorly reported. About half the studies did not report the criteria for positive, negative, or indeterminate results; no study reported the limits of detection or assay linearity range. Only a minority of studies assessed reproducibility of results on repeat testing, and no study assessed reproducibility across operators, instruments, reagent lots, or over time. Only one study was conducted as part of a multilaboratory collaboration[133]; however, it did not provide details on the standardization procedures followed.

Key Question 2b. What is the clinical validity (predictive accuracy) of phenotypic testing for predicting intermediate and clinical outcomes in patients who are receiving clopidogrel therapy?

Eligible Studies for Key Question 2b

The studies included in our review all involved administration of clopidogrel, although the populations varied in their indications for use of the drug. Of the 128 studies addressing Key Question 2b, the vast majority (122 studies) were of patients with ischemic heart disease; four studies enrolled patients with cerebrovascular disease, one study enrolled patients with peripheral artery disease; and one study enrolled a mix of patients with ischemic heart disease cerebrovascular disease and peripheral arterial disease. Among studies of patients with ischemic heart disease, 43 enrolled patients with acute coronary syndromes; the remaining either included patients with chronic stable coronary artery disease (71 studies) or mixed populations with chronic and acute presentations (8 studies). Of the 122 studies enrolling patients with ischemic heart disease, 113 (93 percent) included predominantly (>80 percent of the included population) patients undergoing PCI; 2 (2 percent), patients undergoing angiography; 5 (4 percent), patients undergoing a combination of PCI, CABG and medical treatments; and 2 (2 percent), patients being treated with medical therapy without undergoing a procedure. The majority of studies were of patients receiving dual antiplatelet therapy with clopidogrel in combination with aspirin; when loading doses were used, the aspirin loading dose ranged between 250 and 500 mg and the clopidogrel loading dose ranged between 300 mg and 900 mg. Maintenance doses were between 81 mg and 325 mg for aspirin and 75 mg and 150 mg for clopidogrel. Detailed information on the selection criteria, settings, and treatment strategies (including adjunctive treatments) is presented under subsequent sections addressing each test for platelet reactivity separately.

Overall, studies had intermediate to large sample sizes (median=205, 25th percentile=97, 75th percentile=606, minimum=15, maximum=2849). They had been conducted in recent years (median year of enrollment start was 2006). In 120 studies providing relevant information the median of the mean or median age was 65 years (range 47 to 83 years). Patients had a relatively high burden of risk factors for coronary artery disease (which are associated with adverse cardiovascular outcomes): the median proportion of patients with dyslipidemia was 60 percent (in 98 studies; range 11 - 100 percent); with hypertension, 67 percent (in 108 studies; range 18 - 92 percent); with diabetes mellitus, 29 percent (in 113 studies; range 0 -100 percent); who used tobacco, 31 percent (in 108 studies; range 6 - 75 percent). All studies were longitudinal cohort studies (as per our inclusion criteria for this Key Question).

Studies reported information on a variety of tests for measuring platelet reactivity. The prognostic ability of a single platelet reactivity assay was evaluated in 107 of the 128 studies, whereas 21 studies evaluated two or more assays (15 studies evaluated two assays, 5 studies evaluated three assays, and 1 study evaluated four assays). The assays used included those based on the principle of LTA (55 studies; 43 percent), the VerifyNow P2Y12 assay (38 studies; 30 percent), the VASP assay (19 studies; 15 percent), the Multiplate analyzer assay (18 studies; 14 percent), the PFA-100 assay (11 studies; 9 percent), thromboelastography (6 studies; 5 percent), and other tests (9 studies; 7 percent). Detailed information on each test is presented separately under the discussion of individual tests for platelet reactivity.

Overall, studies were of moderate quality. Based on our assessment of 11 items derived from the QUADAS-2 instrument and using arbitrary thresholds based on the number of items considered as adequately addressed, 35 of the studies were rated "A," 81 were rated "B," and 12 were rated "C." We caution that this aggregate risk-of-bias rating can be misleading, especially in the presence of poor reporting. A more detailed discussion of risk of bias, focusing on the individual items assessed, is presented later in this chapter.

In the following sections we discuss studies by outcomes reported, for each individual test, grouped by the patient populations enrolled. When study designs, assays, and outcome definitions were considered sufficiently similar across three or more studies, we performed meta-analyses to synthesize findings (using data from nonoverlapping populations). (Please see the Methods section for additional details on how we assessed potential population overlap.) Based on the results of our review on the analytic validity of assays for measuring platelet reactivity (presented under Key Question 2a of this report), we did not combine information across different assays or different agonist concentrations.

Results from subgroup and effect-modification analyses for studies relevant to Key Question 2b are presented under Key Question 2c. Table 9 summarizes information on the patient populations and outcomes assessed in the studies considered eligible for Key Question 2b.

Table 9. Populations and outcomes in studies for Key Question 2b, according to test used

Test Used (Total Number of Studies; Studies by Patient Population)	All-Cause Death	CV Death	ACS	ST	Stroke	Bleeding	MACE	Other Clinical Outcomes	Platelet Reactivity
LTA (total = 55; IHD = 53; PAD = 1; IHD, CVD, PAD = 1)	IHD = 13 [low]	IHD = 9 [low]	IHD = 18 [low]	IHD = 19 [low]	IHD = 12 [low]	IHD = 7 [insufficient]	IHD = 37 [low] IHD, CVD, PAD = 1 [insufficient]	IHD = 8 [insufficient]	IHD = 11 [insufficient] PAD = 1 [insufficient]
VerifyNow P2Y12 (total = 38; IHD = 35; CVD = 3)	IHD = 10 [low]	IHD = 7 [moderate]	IHD = 19 [low]	IHD = 15 [low]	IHD = 8 [insufficient]	IHD = 12 [low]	IHD = 24 [moderate]	IHD = 7 [insufficient] CVD = 3 [insufficient]	IHD = 4 [insufficient]
VASP (total = 19; IHD = 18; IHD, CVD, PAD = 1)	IHD = 4 [insufficient]	IHD = 6 [insufficient]	IHD = 6 [low]	IHD = 10 [low]	IHD = 1 [insufficient]	IHD = 1 [insufficient]	IHD = 8 [low] IHD, CVD, PAD = 1 [insufficient]	IHD = 4 [insufficient]	IHD = 7 [insufficient]
Multiplate analyzer (total = 18; IHD = 17; CVD = 1)	IHD = 6 [insufficient]	IHD = 5 [insufficient]	IHD = 9 [insufficient]	IHD = 10 [insufficient]	IHD = 3 [insufficient]	IHD = 9 [insufficient]	IHD = 13 [insufficient] CVD = 1 [insufficient]	IHD = 6 [insufficient]	IHD = 2 [insufficient]
TEG (total = 6; IHD = 6)	IHD = 2 [insufficient]	No studies	IHD = 2 [insufficient]	IHD = 1 [insufficient]	IHD = 1 [insufficient]	IHD = 3 [insufficient]	IHD = 4 [insufficient]	No studies	No studies
PFA-100 (total = 11; IHD = 10; IHD, CVD, PAD = 1)	IHD = 2 [insufficient]	IHD = 2 [insufficient]	IHD = 5 [insufficient]	IHD = 3 [insufficient]	IHD = 1 [insufficient]	IHD = 1 [insufficient]	IHD = 9 [low] IHD, CVD, PAD = 1 [insufficient]	IHD = 2 [insufficient]	IHD = 1 [insufficient]
Other (total = 9; IHD = 9)	IHD = 3 [insufficient]	No studies	IHD = 3 [insufficient]	IHD = 1 [insufficient]	IHD = 1 [insufficient]	IHD = 2 [insufficient]	IHD = 6 [insufficient]	IHD = 3 [insufficient]	IHD = 3 [insufficient]

Abbreviations: ACS = acute coronary syndromes; CV = cardiovascular; CVD = cerebrovascular disease; IHD = ischemic heart disease; LTA = light-transmission aggregometry; MACE = major adverse cardiovascular events; PAD = peripheral arterial disease; PFA = Platelet Function Analyzer; ST = stent thrombosis; TEG = thromboelastography; VASP = vasodilator-stimulated phosphoprotein.
Numbers indicate the number of available studies for each test–outcome combination in the population specified. (Studies could have involved more than one combination.) The ratings in brackets reflect our assessment of the strength of evidence for each test–outcome association.

77

LTA

Fifty-five studies reported information on the predictive ability of platelet reactivity measured by LTA. Of these, 53 included patients with ischemic heart disease, one included patients with peripheral arterial disease, and one included a mix of patients with ischemic heart disease and peripheral artery disease. None of the studies included patients with cerebrovascular disease. Detailed information on selection criteria, settings, and treatment strategies (including adjunctive treatments) used in these studies is presented in Appendix E.

Overall, studies using LTA to measure platelet reactivity employed variable metrics, such as percent change of reactivity within a patient (termed "inhibition of platelet aggregation") or absolute values of on-clopidogrel reactivity at a single timepoint (termed "residual platelet reactivity"). Furthermore, the cutoff values for defining increased reactivity varied across studies, even among studies using the same metric. We decided not to perform meta-analyses for studies assessing platelet reactivity using LTA because for all outcomes considered, the heterogeneity in metrics and cutoff values would result in the inclusion of only a select subset of studies for each comparison. Instead, we narratively summarized study results and performed qualitative synthesis for each reported outcome.

Ischemic Heart Disease

Fifty-three studies included patients with ischemic heart disease and reported information on the predictive value of platelet reactivity measured by LTA.[134,13595,111,117,136-182] Of these, 47 studies assessed the value of the test for predicting clinical outcomes; and 11, for predicting platelet reactivity during followup (4 studies reported both clinical and intermediate outcomes). Thirty-eight of the 53 studies enrolled patients with chronic stable coronary artery disease, 12 enrolled patients with acute coronary syndromes, and three studies enrolled mixed populations with chronic and acute presentations.

Clinical Outcomes

All-Cause Mortality

Thirteen studies reported information on the ability of platelet reactivity measured by LTA to predict all-cause mortality.[111,137,140,141,143,150,156,160,163,165,180-182] Most studies used ADP as the agonist to assess reactivity. One study used ADP in combination with arachidonic acid (AA) to assess the response to both clopidogrel and aspirin.[141] Thresholds for defining "positive" results were based on prior literature (or other sources external to the study) in 8 studies; derived from the observed study data in two studies; and not explicitly reported in three studies. Studies had variable sample sizes, ranging from 100 to 1058 enrolled patients. Of the 13 studies reporting relevant information on all-cause mortality, 10 did not report statistically significant results (6 studies reported higher rates of death in patients with higher reactivity and four did not report any deaths); additionally, three studies reported statistically significantly higher risk of deaths due to any cause in patients with high reactivity compared to those with low reactivity. In summary, reviewed studies suggested an association between increased platelet reactivity by LTA and all-cause mortality in patients with ischemic heart disease; however, results were inconclusive as heterogeneity between the studies prevents pooling of results.

Cardiovascular Mortality

Nine studies reported information on the ability of platelet reactivity measured by LTA to predict cardiovascular mortality.[142,150,153,155,167,173,174,182,183] All studies used ADP as the agonist for measuring platelet reactivity. One study used ADP in combination with AA to assess the response to both clopidogrel and aspirin.[155] Thresholds for defining "positive" results were based on prior literature (or other sources external to the study) in seven studies, derived from the observed study data in one study,[142] and not explicitly reported in one study.[153] Studies had variable sample sizes, ranging from 106 to 1058 patients. Of the nine studies reporting relevant information, five reported a statistically significantly higher risk of death among patients with high platelet reactivity and four found no significant association when comparing patients with high reactivity versus those with low reactivity. In summary, reviewed studies suggest an association between increased platelet reactivity by LTA and cardiovascular death in patients with ischemic heart disease; however, results were inconclusive, as heterogeneity between the studies prevented our pooling the results.

Acute Coronary Syndromes

Eighteen studies reported information on the ability of platelet reactivity measured by LTA to predict acute coronary syndromes.[111,137,140-143,150,153,156,160,165,167,172-175,182,184] All studies used ADP as the agonist to assess platelet reactivity. One study used ADP in combination with AA to assess the response to both clopidogrel and aspirin.[141] Thresholds for defining "positive" results were based on prior literature (or other sources external to the study) in 11 studies, derived from the observed study data in three studies, and were not explicitly reported in four studies. Studies had variable sample sizes, enrolling 26 to 1058 patients. Of the 18 studies reporting relevant information, ten reported statistically significant associations between increased reactivity and myocardial infarction and eight did not reach statistical significance. In summary, results were inconclusive regarding the association between increased platelet reactivity as measured by LTA and acute coronary syndrome risk in patients with ischemic heart disease.

Stent Thrombosis

Nineteen studies reported information on the ability of platelet reactivity measured by LTA to predict stent thrombosis.[95,111,138,140-142,148,153-156,160,167,169,170,173,174,180,183] Three publications report data from the same population.[95,154,155] The longest available followup was considered for these studies. All studies used ADP as the agonist; two studies used ADP in combination with AA to assess the response to both clopidogrel and aspirin.[141,155] Thresholds for defining high platelet reactivity were based on prior literature (or other sources external to the study) in nine studies, were derived from the observed study data in four studies, and were not explicitly reported in six studies. The numbers of patients included in the studies ranged from 105 to 1058. Of the 16 studies reporting relevant information, 12 reported statistically significant associations between increased reactivity and stent thrombosis; 4 did not report statistically significant results; one did not report any stent thrombosis events. Taken together, studies suggested an association between increased platelet reactivity (as measured by LTA) and increased risk of stent thrombosis in patients with ischemic heart disease.

MACE

Thirty-seven studies reported information on the ability of platelet reactivity measured by LTA to predict composites of major adverse cardiovascular events for clopidogrel-treated patients with ischemic heart disease. Three studies reported data from the same population.[95,154,155] The longest followup was considered for these studies. All studies used ADP as the agonist to measure platelet reactivity; two studies used ADP in combination with AA to assess the response to both clopidogrel and aspirin.[141,155] Thresholds for defining "positive" results were based on prior literature (or other sources external to the study) in 17 studies, were derived from the observed study data in 13 studies, and were not explicitly reported in 7 studies. Studies had variable sample sizes, ranging from 90 to 1335 enrolled patients. Of the 33 studies reporting relevant information, 30 reported statistically significant associations between increased platelet reactivity and risk of MACE; only 3 did not find a statistically significant association. In summary, the majority of reviewed studies suggested an association between increased platelet reactivity by LTA and MACE in patients with ischemic heart disease.

Stroke

Twelve studies reported information on the ability of platelet reactivity measured by LTA to predict stroke.[137,140,141,150,153,156,160,165,167,174,182,183] All studies used ADP as the agonist to measure reactivity. One study also used ADP in combination with AA to assess the response to both clopidogrel and aspirin.[141] Thresholds for defining "positive" results were based on prior literature (or other sources external to the study) in nine studies, were derived from the observed study data in two studies, and were not explicitly reported in one study.[153] Sample sizes ranged from 100 to 1058 patients. Of the 12 studies reporting relevant information on stroke, 10 did not report statistically significant results. One study reported that clopidogrel nonresponders had higher stroke risk than patients who were low responders or normal responders.[167] One study reported a significantly higher stroke risk in patients who were either clopidogrel nonresponders or clopidogrel and aspirin nonresponders than responders to both drugs or to aspirin alone.[141] In summary, reviewed studies did not suggest an association between increased platelet reactivity as measured by LTA and stroke in patients with ischemic heart disease; however, results were inconclusive, as heterogeneity in reactivity measurements prevented our conducting quantitative synthesis and study specific estimates had wide CIs, indicating considerable uncertainty.

Bleeding Events

Seven studies reported information on the ability of platelet reactivity measured by LTA to predict bleeding events.[137,145,148,163,167,181,183] All studies used ADP as the agonist for measuring reactivity. Thresholds for defining "positive" results were based on prior literature (or other sources external to the study) in four studies and were not explicitly reported in two studies. Sample sizes ranged from 100 to 1058 patients. Of the seven studies reporting relevant information on bleeding events, five did not report statistically significant associations; one study did not report any events;[181] one study reported significantly higher bleeding rate in "hyper-responders" (i.e., patients with ADP-induced aggregation <40%).[148] In summary, the studies did not suggest an association between increased platelet reactivity as measured by LTA and bleeding events in patients with ischemic heart disease; however, results were considered inconclusive because of between-study heterogeneity in reactivity measurements that precluded quantitative synthesis.

Other Clinical Outcomes

Eight studies reported information on the ability of platelet reactivity measured by LTA to predict other clinical outcomes.[111,137,143,156,160,167,173,181] Seven studies reported target-vessel revascularization as an outcome,[111,137,143,156,160,173,181] two reported non–target-vessel revascularization as an outcome,[137,160] one reported on recurrent ischemia,[167] and two reported on rehospitalization for ischemia.[137,160] All studies used ADP as the assay to measure platelet reactivity. Thresholds for defining "positive" results were based on prior literature (or other sources external to the study) in six studies, were derived from the observed study data in one study,[160] and were not explicitly reported in one study.[143] Sample sizes were variable, ranging from 96 to 802 patients. Of the seven studies reporting information on target-vessel revascularization, four did not report statistically significant associations; one study did not report any events;[181] and, two reported significantly higher event rates of target-vessel revascularization among patients with increased platelet reactivity. Two studies on non–target-vessel revascularization and two studies on recurrent ischemia also reported significantly higher event rates among patients with increased platelet reactivity. In summary, reviewed studies did not provide sufficient evidence for an association between increased platelet reactivity as measured by LTA and target-vessel revascularization, non–target-vessel revascularization, or recurrent ischemia.

Intermediate Outcome: Platelet Reactivity During Followup

Reactivity as a Continuous Outcome

Eight studies[134,136,144,167,168,171,176,177] reported on the predictive value of baseline on-clopidogrel platelet reactivity measured by LTA on platelet reactivity as a continuous outcome assessed during subsequent followup timepoints. In these studies reactivity was assessed using LTA in six studies (75 percent); the VASP assay in one (12.5 percent); and flow cytometry in one (12.5 percent).

Five of the studies enrolled patients with acute coronary syndromes,[136,144,168,171,177] whereas three studies[134,167,176] enrolled patients with chronic ischemic heart disease. Seven studies were conducted in the setting of interventional cardiac procedures (four with PCI and two with PCI with stenting); one study treated patients with medical therapy.

Studies generally showed that the mean or median reactivity was higher among clopidogrel-treated patients who were classified either as nonresponders or as slow responders at baseline, as compared to responders. Results were reported for different followup periods (ranging from a few hours post clopidogrel loading to a followup of 1 year) and measurements were obtained using different assays and different calculation methods (percent change within a patient or absolute value at last followup). All of the six studies reported that platelet reactivity during followup was statistically significantly higher among patients with high baseline reactivity compared to those with low or normal baseline reactivity. Because of the extensive between-study differences we did not perform meta-analyses for studies using reactivity as the outcome of interest.

Reactivity as a Categorical Outcome

Three studies[157,162,164] reported information on the association between baseline reactivity measured by LTA and platelet reactivity during followup reported as a categorical outcome. In two studies reactivity (during followup) was assessed using LTA only[157,164]; in one study it was assessed using 3 different assays (LTA, VASP and VerifyNow P2Y12).[162] Cutoff values for assessing reactivity were variable (among studies using the same assay). Two studies explicitly provided the rationale for selecting a specific cutoff.[162,164] In both, the cutoff value was based on prior literature (i.e., information external to the dataset where the cutoff value was applied). All studies enrolled patients with chronic ischemic heart disease. Two studies were conducted in the setting of interventional cardiac procedures,[162,164] whereas one included patients managed medically.[157] One of the studies reported data in graphical form which was not amenable to quantitative analysis.[164] When 20 μmol/L ADP was used as an agonist at baseline measurement, response status was not significantly associated with platelet reactivity after 30 days of followup (using LTA or VerifyNow). Increased baseline reactivity by LTA was significantly associated with platelet reactivity during followup measured by the VASP assay. When 5 μmol/L ADP was used as an agonist at baseline measurement, platelet reactivity by LTA was significantly associated with reactivity after 30 days of followup.

In summary, while studies suggested an association between increased platelet reactivity at baseline (measured by LTA) and subsequent platelet reactivity measurements (with different assays), the results are inconclusive due to sparseness of the data.

Patients With Peripheral Arterial Disease

Intermediate Outcome: Platelet Reactivity During Followup

Reactivity as a Categorical Outcome

One study[185] reported on the effect using LTA on platelet reactivity as a categorical outcome for clopidogrel-treated patients with peripheral artery disease. In this study, both baseline and follow up measurements were performed with LTA. The cutoff value used to assess nonresponsiveness was based on prior literature (i.e., information external to the dataset where the cutoff value was applied). The study showed that baseline LTA reactivity was statistically significantly associated with the of responding patients after a median followup of 17.5 months.

Mixed Patient Population With Ischemic Heart Disease and Peripheral Arterial Disease

One study included a mix of patients with ischemic heart disease and peripheral arterial disease and reported information on the predictive value of platelet reactivity measured by LTA.[186] The study recruited 534 patients with chronic stable coronary artery disease on clopidogrel and assessed the value of the test for predicting the first occurrence of MACE. The study also assessed the value of the VASP and PFA-100 test for predicting the first occurrence of the same outcome. The results from these tests are reported under the respective sections.

Clinical Outcomes

MACE

The study reported information on the ability of platelet reactivity measured by LTA to predict MACE (defined as acute myocardial infarction, unstable angina, hospitalization for revascularization, acute limb ischemia, ischemic stroke, transient ischemic attack, or cardiovascular death.[186] The study reported results for LTA using two ADP concentrations (5 μmol/L and 20 μmol/L) with different cut-offs (>42 percent and >55 percent, respectively) to identify high reactivity. The thresholds for defining "positive" results were based on prior literature. Of the 771 enrolled patients, 534 were taking clopidogrel at the time of platelet testing. Increased reactivity did not adversely affect MACE-free survival (for ADP 5 μmol/L, HR=1.40; 95% CI=0.88, 2.23; p-value=0.16; for ADP 20 μmol/L ADP, HR=1.29; 95% CI=0.86, 1.94; p-value=0.22). In summary, the study did not suggest an association between increased platelet reactivity as measured by LTA and MACE in a mixed population of patients with ischemic heart disease and peripheral artery disease. This result is inconclusive because of the limited available data.

VerifyNow P2Y12

Thirty-eight studies reported information on the predictive ability of the VerifyNow P2Y12 assay. Of these, 35 studies included patients with ischemic heart disease and three studies included patients with cerebrovascular disease. None of the studies included patients with peripheral arterial disease or other populations receiving clopidogrel-based antiplatelet therapy. Detailed information on the selection criteria, settings, and treatment strategies (including adjunctive treatments) is presented in Appendix E.

Patients With Ischemic Heart Disease

Thirty-five studies included patients with ischemic heart disease and reported information on the predictive value of the VerifyNow P2Y12 assay (this assay uses ADP as the agonist to assess reactivity).[88,140,141,180,183,187-216] Of these, 33 assessed the value of the test for predicting clinical outcomes and four for predicting platelet reactivity during followup (two studies reported both clinical and platelet reactivity outcomes). Of the 35 studies, 21 enrolled patients with chronic stable coronary artery disease, 12 enrolled patients with acute coronary syndromes, and two enrolled mixed populations with chronic and acute presentations.

Clinical Outcomes

All-Cause Mortality

Ten studies reported information on the ability of the VerifyNow P2Y12 assay to predict all-cause mortality for patients receiving clopidogrel-based treatment.[88,140,141,180,187,203,209,211-213] One study used a combination of ADP and AA (in different assays) to define a population of combined clopidogrel and aspirin responders.[141] Thresholds for defining "positive" results were based on prior literature (or other sources external to the study) in six of the studies and derived from the observed study data in two of the studies (two of the studies used both approaches). Studies were generally large; sample sizes ranged from 181 to 2849 patients. Seven of the 10 studies did not report a statistically significant association between platelet reactivity (measured by the VerifyNow assay) and all-cause mortality; two studies did not report any events; and, one study reported a significant association between platelet reactivity (measured by the VerifyNow assay) and all-cause mortality.

Figure 22 presents a meta-analysis of the five studies that used ADP as the agonist and defined high platelet reactivity based on platelet reactivity units. The summary RR was 1.21 (95% CI, 0.83 to 1.77); p=0.313, indicating no significant association between high platelet reactivity and all-cause mortality. There was little evidence of between study heterogeneity (P_Q = 0.902; I^2 = 0 percent). The five studies not included in the meta-analysis did not report a significant association between higher platelet reactivity and increased all-cause mortality.

Figure 22. Meta-analysis of all-cause mortality comparing patients with high versus low reactivity measured using the VerifyNow P2Y12 assay

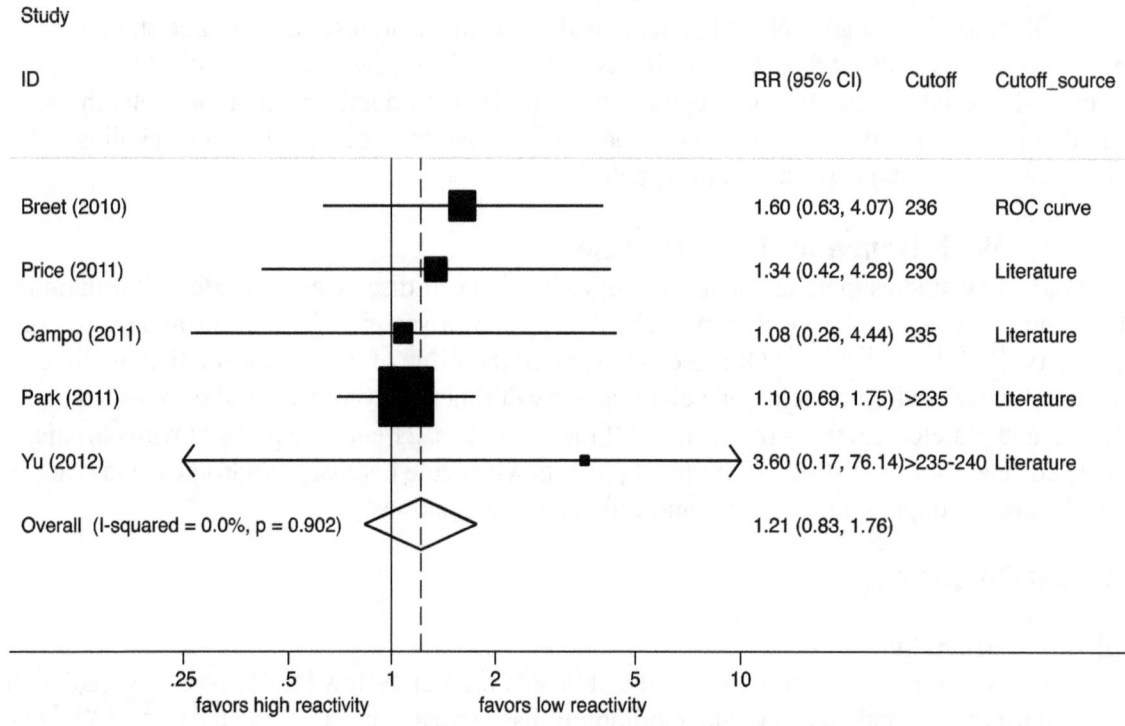

Abbreviations: CI = confidence interval; ROC curve = receiver-operating-characteristic curve analysis; RR = relative risk. Cutoff values, expressed in platelet reactivity units, are shown for high (above the cutoff) and low (below the cutoff) reactivity; the source of the cutoff value is also shown. The solid squares (and horizontal lines) indicate the RR of all-cause mortality (and the corresponding 95% CI) for individual studies. The size of the squares is proportional to the weight of each study in the meta-analysis. The dashed vertical line represents the summary RR, with the open diamond showing the corresponding CI. The solid line indicates an RR of 1.

Cardiovascular Mortality

Seven studies reported information on the ability of the VerifyNow P2Y12 assay to predict cardiovascular mortality for patients receiving clopidogrel-based treatment.[183,193,195,199,202,203,210] The assay uses ADP as the agonist to assess reactivity. Thresholds for defining "positive" results were based on prior literature (or other sources external to the study) in five of the 7 studies and derived from the observed study data in two of the studies. Studies had moderate to large sample sizes, ranging from 110 to 1691 included patients.

Figure 23 presents a meta-analysis of the four studies that used cutoff values based on platelet reactivity units (meta-analysis was not performed for three other studies using percent platelet inhibition to define reactivity and two of the studies using platelet reactivity units were considered to overlap). The summary RR was 2.50 (95% CI, 1.28 to 4.87); p=0.007, indicating a significant association between high platelet reactivity and cardiovascular mortality. There was little evidence of between study heterogeneity (P_Q = 0.527; I^2 = 0 percent). The three studies not included in the meta-analysis did not report a significant association between higher platelet reactivity and increased cardiovascular mortality.

Figure 23. Meta-analysis of all-cause mortality comparing patients with high versus low reactivity measured using the VerifyNow P2Y12 assay

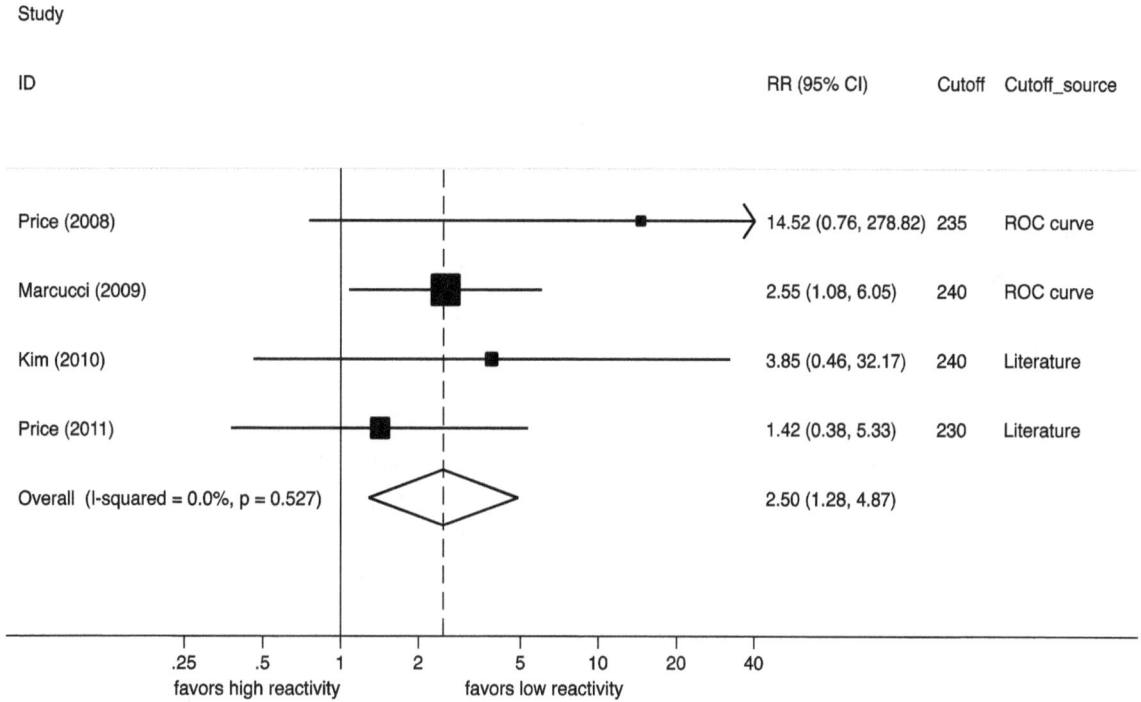

CV mortality, high vs. low reactivity

Abbreviations: CI = confidence interval; ROC curve = receiver-operating-characteristic curve analysis; RR = relative risk. Cutoff values, expressed in platelet reactivity units, are shown for high (above the cutoff) and low (below the cutoff) reactivity; the source of the cutoff value is also shown. The solid squares (and horizontal lines) indicate the RR of cardiovascular mortality (and the corresponding 95% CI) for individual studies. The size of the squares is proportional to the weight of each study in the meta-analysis. The dashed vertical line represents the summary RR, with the open diamond showing the corresponding CI. The solid line indicates an RR of 1.

Acute Coronary Syndromes

Nineteen studies reported information on the ability of the VerifyNow P2Y12 assay to predict myocardial infarction[189,194,196-198,206,209-213] or acute coronary syndromes over a longer followup[140,141,183,187,193,199,202,203] for patients receiving clopidogrel-based treatment. One study used a combination of ADP and AA (in different assays) to define a population of combined clopidogrel and aspirin responders.[141] Thresholds for defining "positive" results were based on prior literature (or other sources external to the study) in 10 studies; derived from the observed study data in 7 studies; and it was not explicitly reported in two studies. Studies were generally large; sample sizes ranged from 110 to 2849. Because of heterogeneity in the study populations, and the metrics and thresholds used to define increased platelet reactivity, we did not perform meta-analyses of predictive ability for this group of studies. Of the six studies reporting information on periprocedural myocardial infarctions, four studies reported a statistically significant association between higher reactivity levels and periprocedural events and two did not report statistically significant results. Of the eight studies reporting information on acute coronary syndromes during followup, four reported a statistically significant association between increased reactivity and risk of acute coronary syndromes, two did not report statistically significant results, and one reported that patients with low response to both aspirin and

85

clopidogrel had significantly higher risks compared to patients with adequate response. Taken together, studies suggested an association between increased platelet reactivity by VerifyNow and both periprocedural and non-periprocedural acute coronary syndromes in patients with ischemic heart disease.

Stent Thrombosis

Fifteen studies reported information on the ability of the VerifyNow P2Y12 assay to predict stent thrombosis for patients receiving clopidogrel-based treatment.[88,140,141,180,183,187,193,195,202,203,209-213] Thresholds for defining "positive" results were based on prior literature (or other sources external to the study) in 11 of the 15 studies and derived from the observed study data in four of the studies. Studies were generally large; sample sizes ranged from 110 to 2849. Of the 15 studies reporting relevant information, 11 did not report statistically significant results and produced relatively wide CIs, indicating substantial uncertainty around estimates of the RR; four studies reported statistically significant associations between high reactivity with risk of stent thrombosis. Because of heterogeneity in the metrics used to define platelet reactivity meta-analysis was possible only for six studies that use the same metrics and cut-offs for reactivity (Figure 24). The summary RR was 1.67 (95% CI, 0.80 to 3.47); p=0.172. There was some evidence of between study heterogeneity ($P_Q = 0.159$; $I^2 = 37$ percent). Considering all studies, there was weak evidence to support an association between increased platelet reactivity by VerifyNow and stent thrombosis in patients with ischemic heart disease; more definitive results could not be reached because of heterogeneity in metrics used that precluded further synthesis of all studies.

Figure 24. Meta-analysis of stent thrombosis comparing patients with high versus low reactivity measured using the VerifyNow P2Y12 assay

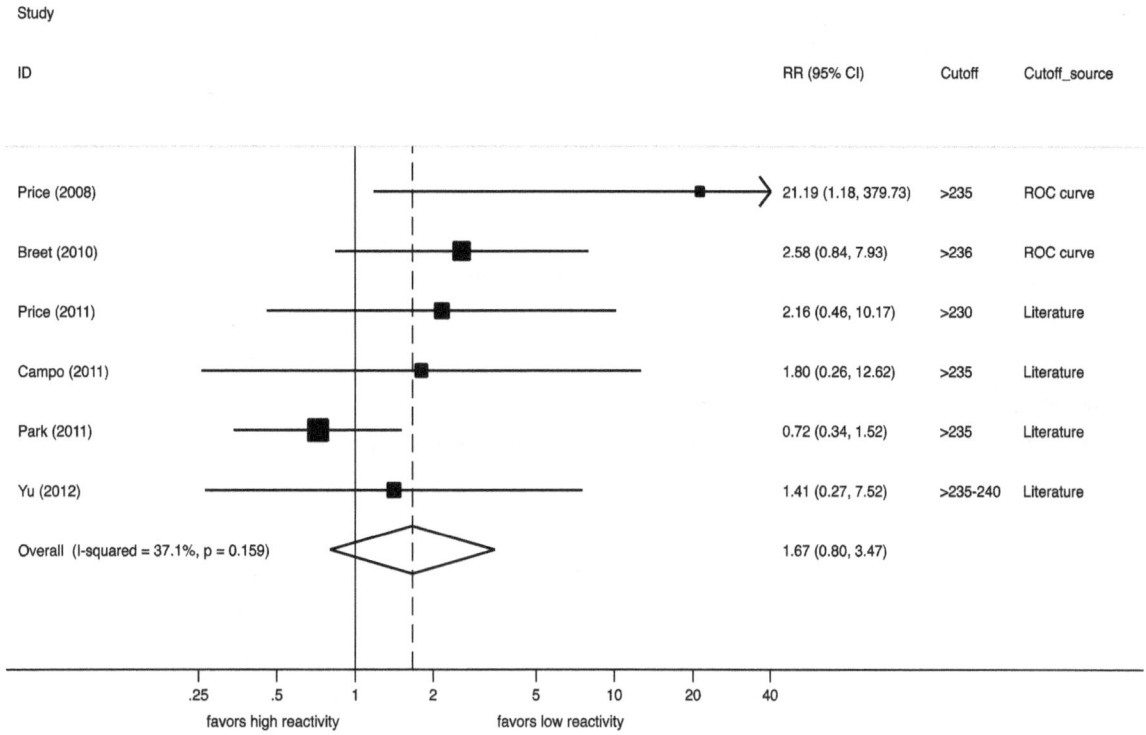

Stent thrombosis, high vs. low reactivity

Abbreviations: CI = confidence interval; ROC curve = receiver-operating-characteristic curve analysis; RR = relative risk. Cutoff values, expressed in platelet reactivity units, are shown for high (above the cutoff) and low (below the cutoff) reactivity; the source of the cutoff value is also shown. The solid squares (and horizontal lines) indicate the RR of cardiovascular mortality (and the corresponding 95% CI) for individual studies. The size of the squares is proportional to the weight of each study in the meta-analysis. The dashed vertical line represents the summary RR, with the open diamond showing the corresponding CI. The solid line indicates an RR of 1.

MACE

Twenty-four studies reported information regarding the ability of the VerifyNow P2Y12 assay to predict MACE for patients receiving clopidogrel-based treatment. One study used a combination of ADP and AA (different assays) to define a population of combined clopidogrel and aspirin responders[141]. Of the 23 remaining studies, 13 enrolled nonoverlapping patients populations and used cutoff values for platelet reactivity based on platelet reactivity units (the 10 studies not included in meta-analysis used other metrics to define platelet reactivity, had overlapping patient populations, or did not provide adequate data for inclusion). The summary RR was 2.48 (95% CI, 1.86 to 3.32); p<0.001 with evidence of moderate heterogeneity (P_Q = 0.045; I^2 = 44 percent). Results from the meta-analysis are presented in Figure 25. Among the 10 studies not included in the meta-analysis, five used percentage of platelet inhibition to define platelet reactivity, two used substantially different cutoffs, two did not provide adequate data for inclusion, and one overlapped with another publication that had larger sample size. Among the five studies that used percentage of platelet inhibition to define platelet reactivity, four studies reported significantly higher rates of MACE at 6 months to a year in those with a low response to clopidogrel; one study reported lower rates of MACE at 30 days in those with a low response to clopidogrel.

Figure 25. Meta-analysis of major adverse cardiovascular events comparing patients with high versus low reactivity measured using the VerifyNow P2Y12 assay

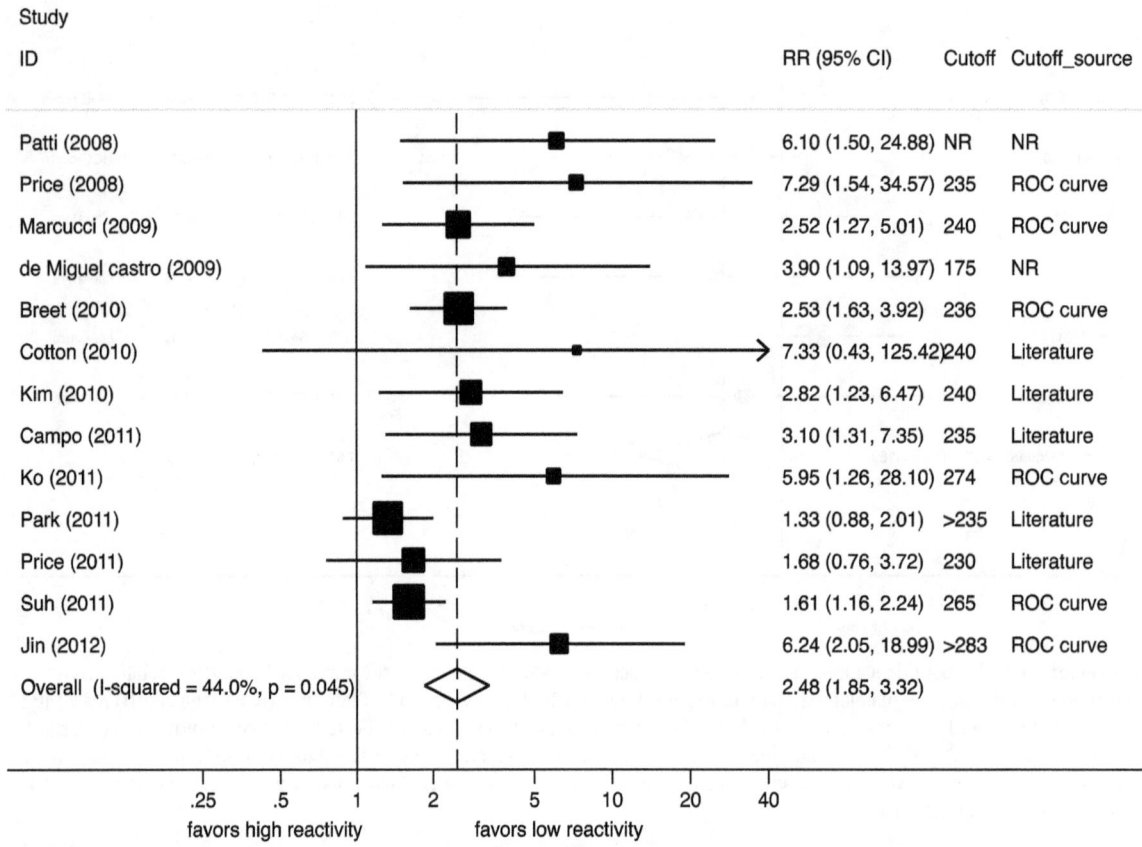

MACE, high vs. low reactivity

Study ID	RR (95% CI)	Cutoff	Cutoff_source
Patti (2008)	6.10 (1.50, 24.88)	NR	NR
Price (2008)	7.29 (1.54, 34.57)	235	ROC curve
Marcucci (2009)	2.52 (1.27, 5.01)	240	ROC curve
de Miguel castro (2009)	3.90 (1.09, 13.97)	175	NR
Breet (2010)	2.53 (1.63, 3.92)	236	ROC curve
Cotton (2010)	7.33 (0.43, 125.42)	240	Literature
Kim (2010)	2.82 (1.23, 6.47)	240	Literature
Campo (2011)	3.10 (1.31, 7.35)	235	Literature
Ko (2011)	5.95 (1.26, 28.10)	274	ROC curve
Park (2011)	1.33 (0.88, 2.01)	>235	Literature
Price (2011)	1.68 (0.76, 3.72)	230	Literature
Suh (2011)	1.61 (1.16, 2.24)	265	ROC curve
Jin (2012)	6.24 (2.05, 18.99)	>283	ROC curve
Overall (I-squared = 44.0%, p = 0.045)	2.48 (1.85, 3.32)		

.25   .5   1   2   5   10   20   40

favors high reactivity   favors low reactivity

Abbreviations: CI = confidence interval; MACE = major adverse cardiovascular events; NR = not reported; ROC curve = receiver-operating-characteristic curve analysis; RR = relative risk.
Cutoff values, expressed in platelet reactivity units, are shown for high (above the cutoff) and low (below the cutoff) reactivity; the source of the cutoff value is also shown. The solid squares (and horizontal lines) indicate the RR of major adverse cardiovascular events (and the corresponding 95% CI) for individual studies. The size of the squares is proportional to the weight of each study in the meta-analysis. The dashed vertical line represents the summary RR, with the open diamond showing the corresponding CI. The solid line indicates an RR of 1.

Stroke

Eight studies reported information on the ability of the VerifyNow P2Y12 assay to predict strokes for patients receiving clopidogrel-based treatment.[140,141,183,187,193,211-213] One study used a combination of ADP and AA (different assays) to define a population of combined clopidogrel and aspirin responders.[141] Thresholds for defining "positive" results were based on prior literature (or other sources external to the study) in six of the eight studies; and derived from the observed study data in two studies.[140,212] Studies were generally large; sample sizes ranged from 110 to 1069. Because of heterogeneity in the metrics used to define platelet reactivity we did not perform meta-analyses of predictive ability for this group of studies. Seven studies using ADP as the agonist did not report statistically significant associations. The eighth study did not find a statistically significant difference in the risk of stroke between patients with low response to both aspirin and clopidogrel compared to patients with adequate response.

Bleeding Events

Thirteen studies reported information regarding the ability of the VerifyNow P2Y12 assay to predict bleeding events for patients receiving clopidogrel-based treatment. Of these, five studies reported results based on percent inhibition or used different cutoff values for reactivity; thus they were not considered adequately similar for meta-analysis. Of the remaining seven studies one reported that no events were observed (regardless of reactivity status), leaving six nonoverlapping studies for meta-analysis (four reported information on bleeding events regardless of severity and four reported information on major bleeding events).

Figure 26 presents meta-analysis results for all bleeding events combined. The summary RR was 1.09 (95% CI, 0.88 to 1.37); p=0.421, with little evidence for heterogeneity (P_Q = 0.738; I^2 =0 percent). Figure 27 presents meta-analysis results for major bleeding events. The summary RR was 0.85 (95% CI, 0.32 to 2.25); p=0.738, with evidence of moderate heterogeneity (P_Q = 0.074; I^2 = 57 percent).

Figure 26. Meta-analysis of bleeding events comparing patients with high versus low reactivity measured using the VerifyNow P2Y12 assay

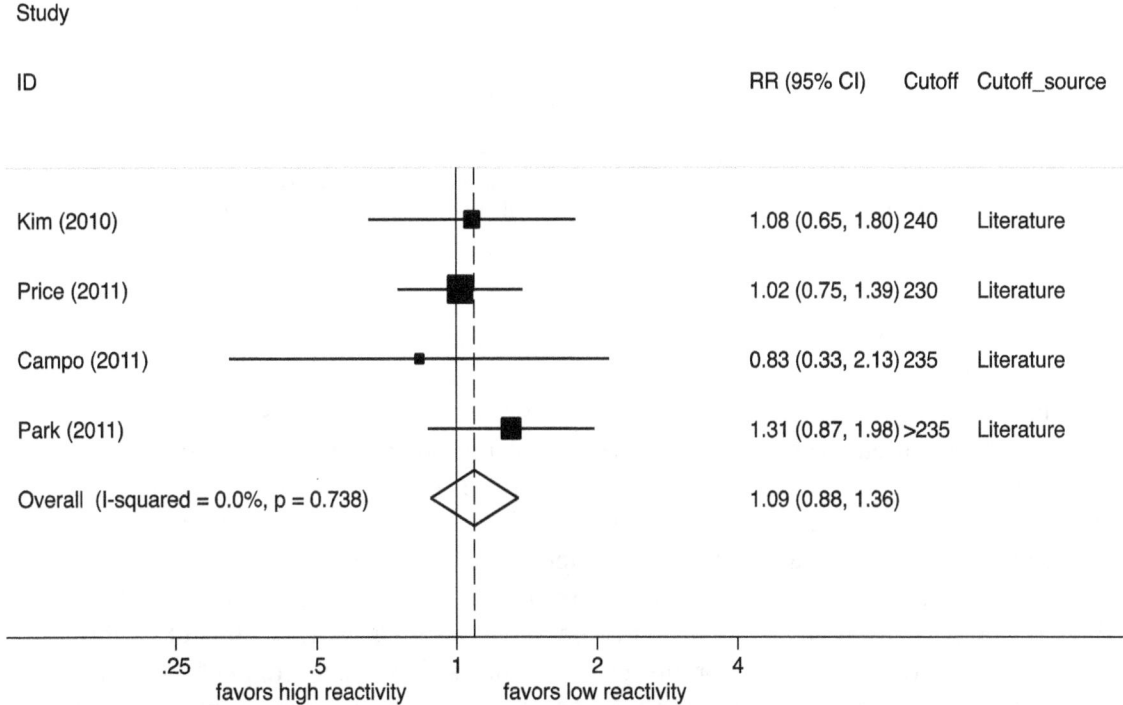

All bleeding events, high vs. low reactivity

Abbreviations: CI = confidence interval; ROC curve = receiver-operating-characteristic curve analysis; RR = relative risk. Cutoff values, expressed in platelet reactivity units, are shown for high (above the cutoff) and low (below the cutoff) reactivity; the source of the cutoff value is also shown. The solid squares (and horizontal lines) indicate the RR of bleeding events (and the corresponding 95% CI) for individual studies. The size of the squares is proportional to the weight of each study in the meta-analysis. The dashed vertical line represents the summary RR, with the open diamond showing the corresponding CI. The solid line indicates an RR of 1.

Figure 27. Meta-analysis of major bleeding events comparing patients with high versus low reactivity measured using the VerifyNow P2Y12 assay

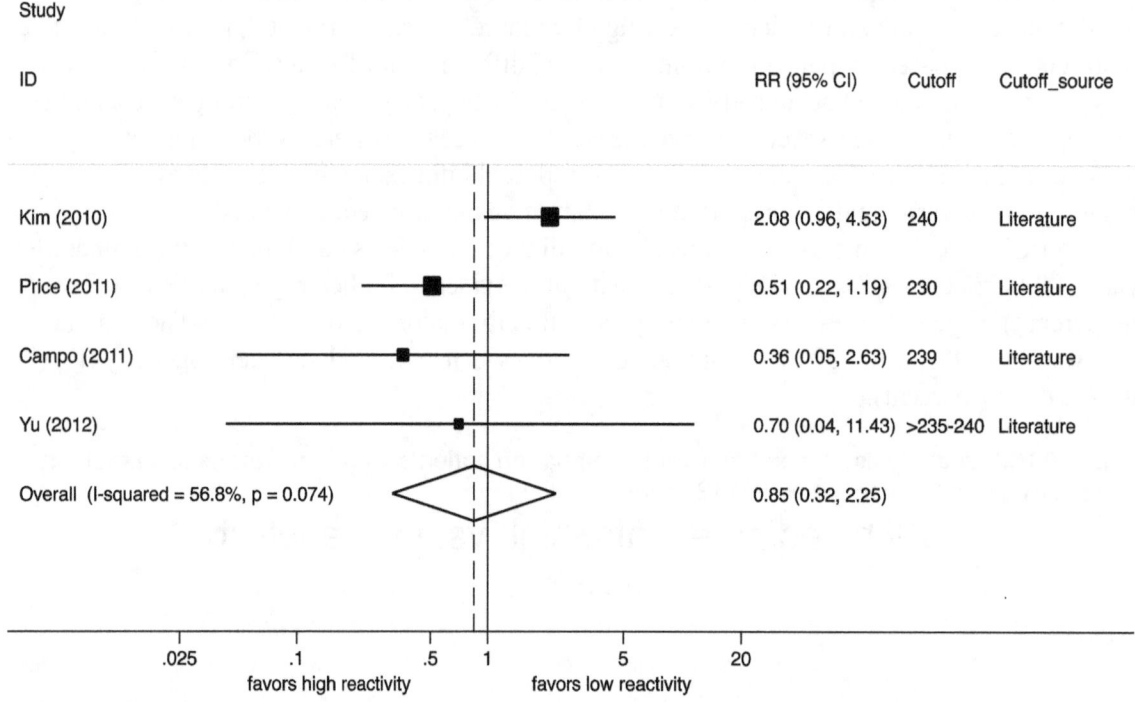

Major bleeding, high vs. low reactivity

Abbreviations: CI = confidence interval; ROC curve = receiver-operating-characteristic curve analysis; RR = relative risk. Cutoff values, expressed in platelet reactivity units, are shown for high (above the cutoff) and low (below the cutoff) reactivity; the source of the cutoff value is also shown. The solid squares (and horizontal lines) indicate the RR of major bleeding events (and the corresponding 95% CI) for individual studies. The size of the squares is proportional to the weight of each study in the meta-analysis. The dashed vertical line represents the summary RR, with the open diamond showing the corresponding CI. The solid line indicates an RR of 1.

Other Clinical Outcomes

Seven studies reported information on the ability of the VerifyNow P2Y12 assay to predict other clinical outcomes.[193,199,201,209-212] Five studies reported information on target level revascularization,[193,199,209-212] and two studies on a composite of PCI entry-site complications such as hematoma, pseudoaneurysm, arteriovenous fistula, and bleeding[201] or hematoma >10 cms.[209] Thresholds for defining "positive" results were derived from the observed study data in four of the studies and based on prior literature (or other sources external to the study) in four studies (one study used both approaches). The metrics used to define positive results were calculated differently across studies. Studies were generally large; sample sizes ranged from 110 to 2849. Because of heterogeneity in the outcomes and thresholds used, we did not perform meta-analyses of predictive ability for this group of studies. Two studies did not report any statistically significant associations; one study reported a statistically significant association between increased platelet reactivity and risk of PCI entry-site complications.

Intermediate Outcome: Platelet Reactivity During Followup

Reactivity as a Continuous Outcome

One study[188] reported information on the predictive value of baseline platelet reactivity status (ascertained with the VerifyNow P2Y12) on platelet reactivity during followup measured as a continuous outcome. In this study, baseline reactivity was assessed using the VerifyNow assay. The study enrolled patients with acute coronary syndromes[188] and was conducted in the setting of interventional cardiac procedures—a mix of PCI and PCI with stenting.[188] The study reported that patients with poor response at baseline had significantly higher reactivity 1 month after PCI compared to those with adequate response.

Reactivity as a Categorical Outcome

Three studies[88,191,215] reported information on the value of baseline platelet reactivity status (ascertained using VerifyNow P2Y12) for predicting platelet reactivity during followup as a categorical outcome. In both studies, baseline reactivity was assessed using the VerifyNow assay. Cutoff values and metrics for defining reactivity were variable; two studies study used absolute reactivity as the metric with a cutoff value derived from literature.[88,215] The other study used the percent within-patient change to define reactivity.[191] Two studies enrolled patients with chronic ischemic heart disease; one study enrolled patients with acute MI;[215] and all were conducted in the setting of interventional cardiac procedures.

Results were reported for different followup periods (ranging from a 7 days to 6 months). Response status during followup in all studies was measured by the same assays that were used at baseline. One of the studies reported a 100 percent sensitivity of baseline response status in predicting status at 7 day status;[191] two other studies reported a statistically significant difference in platelet reactivity during followup comparing nonresponders and responders at baseline.[88,215]

In summary, while suggested an association between platelet reactivity at baseline and measurement obtained during followup, results were inconclusive due to the small number of available studies.

Patients With Cerebrovascular Disease

Three studies[217-219] included patients with cerebrovascular disease and reported information on the predictive value of the VerifyNow assay on clinical outcomes. No studies reported information on the predictive value of the VerifyNow assay on platelet reactivity during followup. All three studies were conducted in the setting of interventional procedures (stent implantation and coil embolization).

Clinical Outcomes

Studies reported information on the ability of the VerifyNow P2Y12 assay to predict only clinical outcomes for clopidogrel-treated patients with cerebrovascular disease. No studies reported information on the ability of the VerifyNow P2Y12 assay to predict platelet reactivity as a continuous or categorical outcome for clopidogrel-treated patients with cerebrovascular disease.

Three studies[217-219] reported information on the ability of the VerifyNow P2Y12 assay to predict various clinical outcomes. One study reported outcomes such as intraprocedural thrombosis, thromboembolic event, good function score on modified Rankin Scale, good function Glasgow Outcome Score;[219] another reported procedure-related thromboembolism and procedure-related aneurysm perforation[218]; the third study reported thromboembolic complications of the procedure.[217] Thresholds for defining "positive" results were not explicitly reported in any of the studies. The metrics used to define positive results were calculated differently across studies. Studies were small; sample sizes ranged from 52 to 186. Because of heterogeneity in the thresholds used, we did not perform meta-analyses of predictive ability for this group of studies. The results from two studies indicated that increased reactivity was statistically significantly associated with increased event rates of the outcomes being studied; another study reported 75 percent sensitivity for clopidogrel resistance to predict thromboembolic events.

VASP Assay With Flow Cytometry

Nineteen studies reported information on the predictive ability of the VASP assay.[82,138,149,180,186,220-233] Eighteen studies included patients with ischemic heart disease; and one included a mixed population of patients with ischemic heart disease and peripheral artery disease. Detailed information on the selection criteria, settings, and treatment strategies (including adjunctive treatments) is presented in Appendix E.

Patients With Ischemic Heart Disease

Eighteen studies included patients with ischemic heart disease and reported information on the predictive value of the VASP assay. Of these, 13 assessed the value of the test for predicting clinical outcomes and six for predicting platelet reactivity during followup (1 study reported both clinical and platelet reactivity outcomes). Of the 18 studies, eight enrolled patients with acute coronary syndromes, five enrolled patients with chronic stable coronary artery disease, and five enrolled mixed populations with chronic and acute presentations.

All-Cause Mortality

Four studies reported information on the ability of the VASP assay to predict all-cause mortality for patients receiving clopidogrel-based treatment.[180,223,224,227] The assay uses ADP as the agonist to assess reactivity. Thresholds for defining "positive" results were based on prior literature (or other sources external to the study) in three of the studies;[180,224,227] and derived from the observed study data in one study.[223] Studies were generally large; sample sizes ranged from 200 to 460. Three studies reported statistically significant association of higher mortality with high platelet reactivity or low response to clopidogrel (however, we assumed that all of the studies enrolled overlapping patient populations on the basis of their population base and enrollment periods); one study reported no events.[180] In summary, data suggested an association between increased platelet reactivity by VASP and all-cause mortality in patients with ischemic heart disease; however, results were inconclusive due to limited effective information size.

Cardiovascular Mortality

Six studies reported information on the ability of the VASP assay to predict all-cause mortality for patients receiving clopidogrel-based treatment. Two of the studies were conducted in overlapping patient populations (on the basis of study base and enrollment periods). Figure 28 presents a meta-analysis of the remaining four studies that used cutoff values based on platelet reactivity units (meta-analysis was not performed for the other two studies using percent platelet inhibition to define reactivity). The summary RR was 2.42 (95% CI, 0.86 to 6.82); p=0.095. There was little evidence of between study heterogeneity ($P_Q = 0.616$; $I^2 = 0$ percent). Even though the test for heterogeneity was not statistically significant, studies produced point estimates that ranged from protective effects to very large increases in risk. Results were imprecise and confidence intervals could not exclude a clinically significant predictive effect.

Figure 28. Meta-analysis of cardiovascular mortality comparing patients with high versus low reactivity measured using the VASP assay with flow cytometry

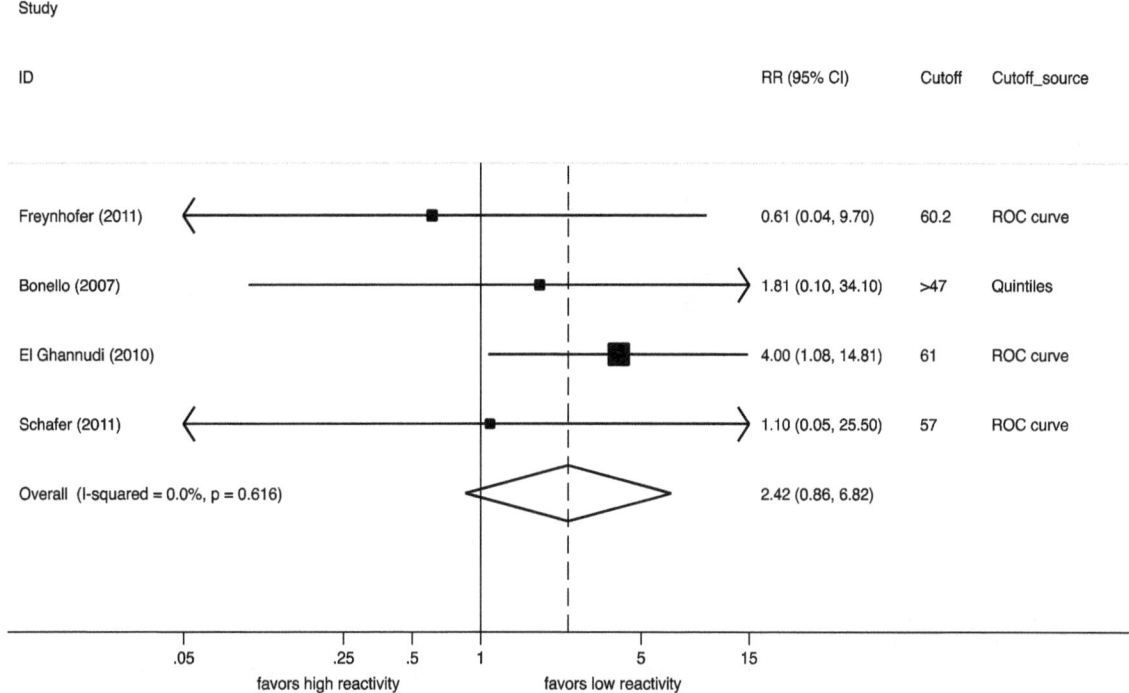

CV death, high vs. low reactivity

Abbreviations: CI = confidence interval; CV = cardiovascular; ROC curve = receiver-operating-characteristic curve analysis; RR = relative risk; VASP = vasodilator-stimulated phosphoprotein.
Cutoff values, expressed in platelet reactivity units, are shown for high (above the cutoff) and low (below the cutoff) reactivity; the source of the cutoff value is also shown. The solid squares (and horizontal lines) indicate the RR of CV mortality (and the corresponding 95% CI) for individual studies. The size of the squares is proportional to the weight of each study in the meta-analysis. The dashed vertical line represents the summary RR, with the open diamond showing the corresponding CI. The solid line indicates an RR of 1.

Acute Coronary Syndromes

Six studies reported information on the ability of the VASP assay to predict acute coronary syndromes for patients receiving clopidogrel-based treatment. One study reported that no events occurred regardless of platelet reactivity status. Of the remaining five studies, three reported on overlapping populations (on the basis of study base and enrollment periods). Figure 29 presents a meta-analysis of the three studies (one study contributed separate estimates by diabetes status). The summary RR was 1.47 (95%, CI 0.77 to 2.79); p=0.246, indicating that the association between high platelet reactivity and acute coronary syndromes was not statistically significant. There was little evidence of between-study heterogeneity ($P_Q = 0.372$; $I^2 = 0$ percent).

Figure 29. Meta-analysis of acute coronary syndromes comparing patients with high versus low reactivity measured using the VASP assay with flow cytometry

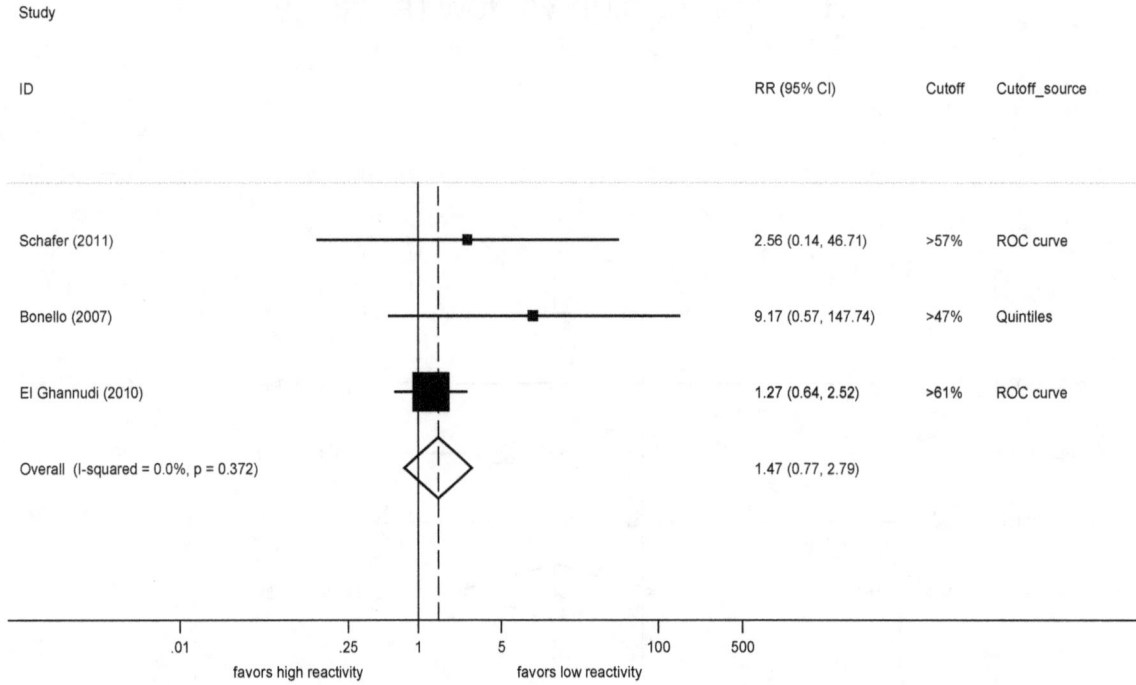

Acute coronary syndromes, high vs. low reactivity

Study ID	RR (95% CI)	Cutoff	Cutoff_source
Schafer (2011)	2.56 (0.14, 46.71)	>57%	ROC curve
Bonello (2007)	9.17 (0.57, 147.74)	>47%	Quintiles
El Ghannudi (2010)	1.27 (0.64, 2.52)	>61%	ROC curve
Overall (I-squared = 0.0%, p = 0.372)	1.47 (0.77, 2.79)		

.01 .25 1 5 100 500

favors high reactivity   favors low reactivity

Abbreviations: CI = confidence interval; ROC curve = receiver-operating-characteristic curve analysis; RR = relative risk, VASP = vasodilator-stimulated phosphoprotein.

Cutoff values, expressed in platelet reactivity units, are shown for high (above the cutoff) and low (below the cutoff) reactivity; the source of the cutoff value is also shown. The solid squares (and horizontal lines) indicate the RR of acute coronary syndromes (and the corresponding 95% CI) for individual studies. The size of the squares is proportional to the weight of each study in the meta-analysis. The dashed vertical line represents the summary RR, with the open diamond showing the corresponding CI. The solid line indicates an RR of 1.

Stent Thrombosis

Ten studies provided information on stent thrombosis (definite or probable, when study definitions were available). Two studies reported that no events were observed (regardless of platelet reactivity status). Of the remaining eight studies, one reported test performance data; and, three studies enrolled overlapping populations (on the basis of study base and enrollment periods; we used data from the publication reporting the largest number of events). Figure 30 presents a meta-analysis of the four nonoverlapping studies. The summary RR was 3.37 (95% CI, 1.59 to 7.11); p=0.015, indicating a significant association between high platelet reactivity and stent thrombosis. There was little evidence of between-study heterogeneity ($P_Q = 0.487$; $I^2 = 0$ percent).

Figure 30. Meta-analysis of stent thrombosis comparing patients with high versus low reactivity measured using the VASP assay with flow cytometry

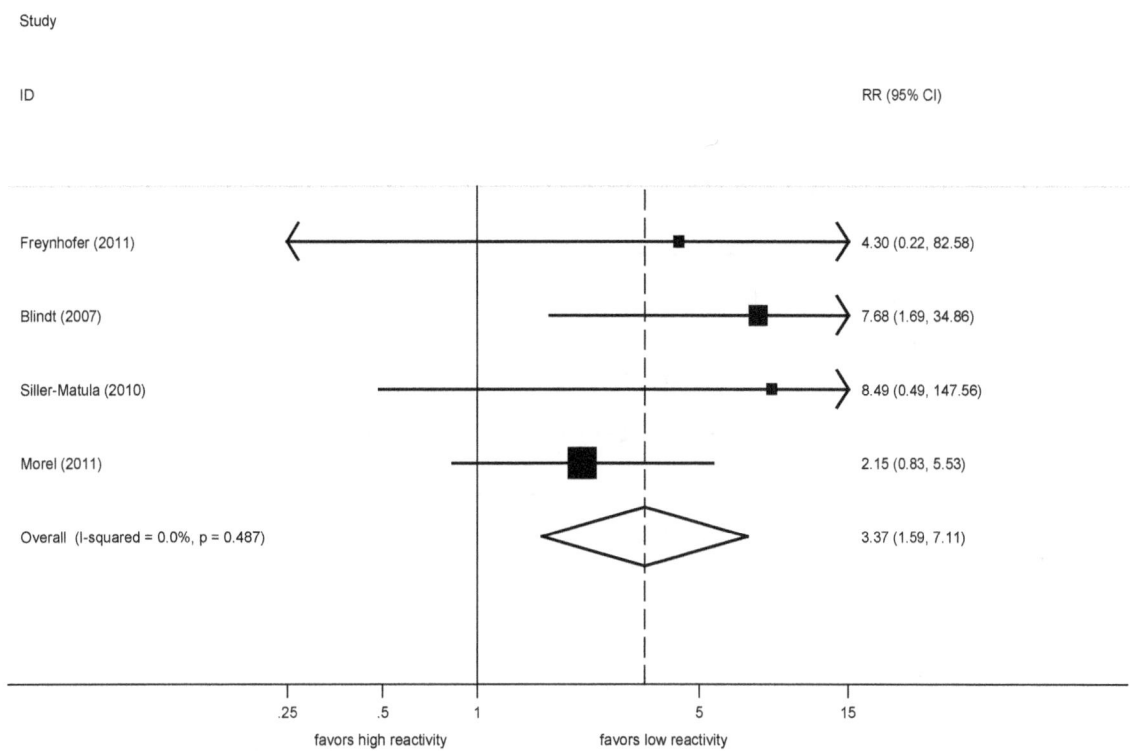

Stent thrombosis, high vs. low reactivity

Abbreviations: CI = confidence interval; ROC curve = receiver-operating-characteristic curve analysis; RR = relative risk, VASP = vasodilator-stimulated phosphoprotein.

The solid squares (and horizontal lines) indicate the RR of stent thrombosis (and the corresponding 95% CI) for individual studies. The size of the squares is proportional to the weight of each study in the meta-analysis. The dashed vertical line represents the summary RR, with the open diamond showing the corresponding CI. The solid line indicates an RR of 1.

MACE

Eight studies reported information on the ability of the VASP assay to predict MACE for patients receiving clopidogrel-based treatment. One study reported test performance data; and, two studies reported on overlapping patient populations based on source population and enrollment periods (in meta-analyses we included the publication reporting on the largest total number of cardiovascular events). Figure 31 presents a meta-analysis of the six nonoverlapping studies (one study contributed separate estimates by diabetes status). The summary RR was 2.57 (95% CI, 1.21 to 5.47); p=0.015, indicating a significant association between high platelet reactivity and major adverse cardiovascular events. There was evidence of moderate between-study heterogeneity (P_Q = 0.044; I^2 = 56 percent).

Figure 31. Meta-analysis of MACE comparing patients with high versus low reactivity measured using the VASP assay with flow cytometry

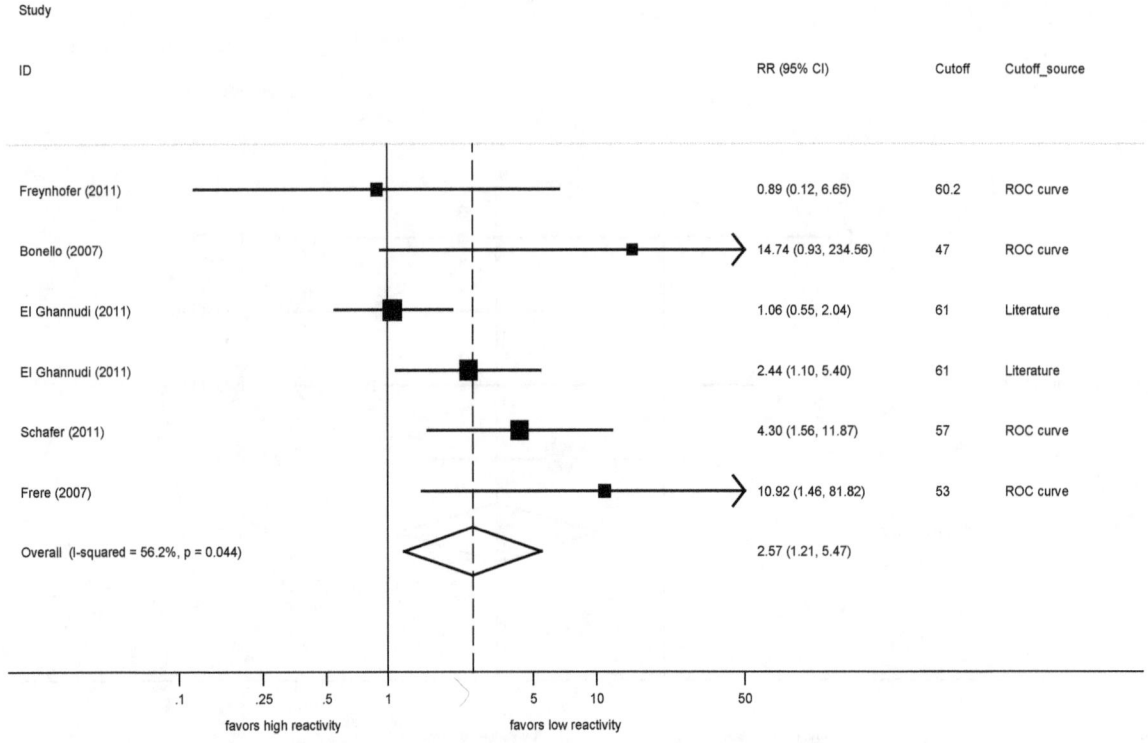

Abbreviations: CI = confidence interval; MACE = major adverse cardiovascular events; ROC curve = receiver-operating-characteristic curve analysis; RR = relative risk; VASP = vasodilator-stimulated phosphoprotein.
Cutoff values, expressed in platelet reactivity units, are shown for high (above the cutoff) and low (below the cutoff) reactivity; the source of the cutoff value is also shown. The solid squares (and horizontal lines) indicate the RR of major adverse cardiovascular events (and the corresponding 95% CI) for individual studies. The size of the squares is proportional to the weight of each study in the meta-analysis. The dashed vertical line represents the summary RR, with the open diamond showing the corresponding CI. The solid line indicates an RR of 1.

Stroke

One study reported information on the ability of the VASP assay to predict strokes for patients receiving clopidogrel-based treatment.[229] The study used ADP as an agonist to assess reactivity and the thresholds for defining "positive" results were derived from both the observed study data and from literature. The study enrolled 54 patients with acute ST elevation myocardial infarction admitted for a coronary intervention with a followup time of 12 months. This suggests an association between increased platelet reactivity by the VASP assay and stroke, but the result is inconclusive owing to insufficient information.

Other Clinical Outcomes

Four studies reported information on the ability of the VASP assay to predict other clinical outcomes for patients receiving clopidogrel-based treatment.[221,222,224,229] Target lesion revascularization was studied in three studies; other outcomes that were reported were the rates of followup interventions such as PCI and CABG surgery. All the studies used ADP as an agonist to assess reactivity. Thresholds for defining "positive" results were based on prior literature (or other sources external to the study) in two studies; they were not explicitly reported in one study; and they were derived from the observed study data and literature in the one study. Study sample sizes ranged from 54 to 436; followup time ranged from 6 to 12 months. Because of clinical heterogeneity across studies we did not perform meta-analyses of predictive ability. Of the three studies reporting information on target-vessel revascularization, two did not report statistically significant results and one study reported that no events occurred (regardless of reactivity status). The studies reporting on followup interventions documented statistically significantly increased rates of the intervention with increased reactivity.

Bleeding

One study reported information on the ability of the VASP assay to predict bleeding outcomes for patients receiving clopidogrel-based treatment.[233] The study used ADP as an agonist to assess reactivity with the thresholds for defining "positive" results being based on prior literature (or other sources external to the study). No bleeding events were observed, regardless of platelet reactivity status.

Intermediate Outcome: Platelet Reactivity During Followup

Reactivity as a Continuous Outcome

Two studies[226,232] reported information on the value of the VASP assay for predicting platelet reactivity during followup as a continuous outcome. In these two studies, reactivity at baseline was assessed using LTA with different concentrations of ADP as an agonist. Platelet reactivity was also assessed using P-selectin expression, platelet/monocyte conjugates, and platelet/neutrophil conjugates after ADP stimulation. The studies enrolled patients with acute coronary syndromes and was conducted in the setting of interventional cardiac procedures (PCI). The study showed that the patients with a poor response at baseline had significantly higher reactivity one month after PCI, compared to patients with adequate response at baseline, irrespective of the methods used to assess reactivity.

Reactivity as a Categorical Outcome

Five studies[220,222,226,228,230] reported information on the value of the VASP assay for predicting platelet reactivity during followup as a continuous outcome. In these studies reactivity during followup was assessed using the VASP assay in four studies and by LTA in one study. Three of the five studies enrolled patients with acute coronary syndromes,[220,222,228] whereas two studies[226,230] enrolled patients with chronic ischemic heart disease. All five studies were conducted in the setting of interventional cardiac procedures—three, in patients with PCI[226,228,230]; one, in patients with PCI with stenting[222]; and one, in patients with coronary angiography.[220]

Of the four studies with available data, three studies showed that the VASP assay was not a significant predictor of future platelet reactivity.[222,228,230] In one study, baseline reactivity measured with the VASP assay was significantly associated with response status at 1 month.[226] One study did not allow for conclusions because none of the patients at baseline could be categorized as nonresponders.[220]

Mixed Patient Population With Ischemic Heart Disease and Peripheral Artery Disease

One study included a mixed population of patients with ischemic heart disease and peripheral arterial disease and reported information on the predictive value of platelet reactivity measured by VASP.[186] The study recruited 534 chronic stable coronary artery disease patients treated with clopidogrel and assessed the value of the test for predicting the first occurrence of MACE. The study also assessed the value of the LTA and PFA-100 test for predicting the first occurrence of the same outcome. The results from these tests are reported under the respective sections.

Clinical Outcomes

MACE

One study reported information on the ability of platelet reactivity measured by VASP to predict MACE as defined by a composite of acute myocardial infarction, unstable angina, hospitalization for revascularization, acute limb ischemia, ischemic stroke, transient ischemic attack, or cardiovascular death.[186] ADP was used as the agonist to assess reactivity, with a cutoff >50 percent to indicate high reactivity.

The thresholds for defining "positive" results were based on prior literature. Of the 771 enrolled patients, 534 were taking clopidogrel at the time of platelet testing. The test results did not impact on MACE-free survival and the multivariate Cox regression did not report a significant higher risk of MACE with reactivity as measured by the VASP assay (HR = 1.06; 95% CI=0.73 to1.53; p-value = 0.77). In summary, the study does not suggest an association between increased platelet reactivity by VASP and MACE in a mixed population of patients with ischemic heart disease and peripheral artery disease; however, results were inconclusive due to paucity of data.

Multiplate Analyzer

Eighteen studies reported information on the predictive ability of the Multiplate analyzer assay. Of these, 17 included patients with ischemic heart disease and one included patients with cerebrovascular disease. No study enrolled patients with peripheral arterial disease. Detailed information on the selection criteria, settings, and treatment strategies (including adjunctive treatments) is presented in **Appendix E**.

Patients With Ischemic Heart Disease

Seventeen studies included patients with ischemic heart disease and reported information on the predictive value of the Multiplate analyzer assay.[82,194,215,225,230,231,234-244] Sixteen studies assessed the value of the test for predicting clinical outcomes and one for predicting platelet reactivity during followup. Ten of the 17 enrolled patients with chronic stable coronary artery disease; four studies enrolled patients with acute coronary syndrome; and the remaining included mixed populations with chronic coronary disease and acute coronary syndromes.

Clinical Outcomes

All-Cause Mortality

Six studies reported information on the ability of the Multiplate analyzer assay to predict all-cause mortality for patients receiving clopidogrel-based treatment.[234,236,237,240,242,243] Three studies appear to have been based on the same patient populations, reporting results at 30 days,[237] 6 months,[240] and 1 year of followup.[236] One study reported all cause death in two arms of the trial, where patients in each arm got different drugs (bivalirudin and abciximab) in addition to clopidogrel; these two arms are regarded as independent populations.[242] All the studies used ADP as an agonist to assess reactivity. One study also used ADP in combination with AA to assess the response to both clopidogrel and aspirin.[234] Thresholds for defining "positive" results were based on prior literature (or other sources external to the study) in the three studies of the same patient population[236,237,240]; they were derived from the observed study data and literature in the other three studies.[234,242,243] The three studies of the same patient population enrolled 1608 patients; the sample size in the other three studies ranged from 219 to 290 patients. Followup durations were in hospital to 12 months. Because of the limited number of studies in nonoverlapping populations we did not perform meta-analyses of predictive ability. Of the three studies conducted in the same patients, the study with the longest followup did not find a statistically significant difference in the risk of all-cause mortality among patients with high platelet reactivity;[236] one study with two independent trial arms[242] and one study in ACS patients[243] did not report a higher risk of all-cause mortality with higher reactivity. One study, reporting on groups stratified by a combination of high reactivity to both clopidogrel (using ADP as the agonist) and aspirin (using AA as the agonist), also did not report statistically significantly higher event rates in patient groups having high reactivity to clopidogrel only or to both clopidogrel and aspirin, as compared to the other groups.[234] In summary, the reviewed studies do not suggest an association between increased platelet reactivity by the Multiplate analyzer assay and all-cause mortality in patients with ischemic heart disease; however, results were inconclusive due to the limited number of studies in nonoverlapping patient populations providing information.

Cardiovascular Mortality

Five studies reported information on the ability of the Multiplate analyzer assay to predict cardiovascular mortality for patients receiving clopidogrel-based treatment.[82,225,235,236,240] Two studies reported information from the same patient population, with one reporting outcomes at 6 months of followup[240] and the other at 1 year.[236] All studies used ADP as the agonist to assess reactivity. One study also used ADP in combination with AA to evaluate both clopidogrel and aspirin.[235] Thresholds for defining "positive" results were based on prior literature (or other sources external to the study) in four studies;[82,225,236,240] they were not explicitly reported in the other study.[235] Study sample sizes ranged from 182 to 1608; followup time ranged from 6 to 14 months. Because of limited number of studies reporting on nonoverlapping population and the diversity of metrics used to define high platelet reactivity we did not perform meta-analyses of predictive ability. Of the two studies reporting information on the same patient population, the study with the longest followup did not find a statistically significant effect of platelet reactivity on the odds of cardiovascular mortality.[236] Two studies reported a significantly higher number of deaths in patients with high platelet reactivity.[82,225] The study that assessed both clopidogrel and aspirin response status reported a lower risk of death among clopidogrel nonresponders than among responders to at least one of the drugs, but the difference was not statistically significant.[235] In summary, reviewed studies do not provide sufficient evidence of an association between increased platelet reactivity by the Multiplate analyzer assay and cardiovascular mortality in patients with ischemic heart disease.

Acute Coronary Syndromes

Nine studies reported information on the ability of the Multiplate analyzer assay to predict myocardial infarction or other acute coronary syndromes for patients receiving clopidogrel-based treatment.[194,225,234-237,240,242,243] Three studies reported information from the same patient population over different followup durations.[236,237,240] One study reported MIs in two arms of the trial, where patients in each arm got different drugs (bivalirudin and abciximab) in addition to clopidogrel; these two arms are regarded as independent populations.[242] All studies used ADP as the agonist to assess reactivity. Two studies used ADP in combination with AA to assess response to both clopidogrel and aspirin.[234,235] Thresholds for defining "positive" results were based on prior literature (or other sources external to the study) in six studies,[225,236,240,242,243] were not explicitly reported in one study,[235] and in one study used both external sources and the observed study data.[234] Sample sizes ranged from 182 to 1608; followup time ranged from 6 to 14 months. Because of the limited number of nonoverlapping studies using similar metrics and cutoff values to define high platelet reactivity, we did not perform meta-analyses of predictive ability. Of the six studies reporting information on acute coronary syndrome risk stratified by reactivity status (using ADP as the agonist), four did not report statistically significant results and two reported that the risk myocardial infarction was higher in the group with low reactivity. Additionally, both studies that evaluated combined response to clopidogrel and aspirin reported that the association between dual nonresponsiveness and myocardial infarction risk was not statistically significant.[234,235] In summary, reviewed studies did not provide sufficient evidence of an association between increased platelet reactivity as measured by the Multiplate analyzer assay and myocardial infarction in patients with ischemic heart disease.

Stent Thrombosis

Ten studies reported information on the ability of the Multiplate analyzer assay to predict stent thrombosis for patients receiving clopidogrel-based treatment.[82,231,234,236-240,242,243] Two sets of studies appear to each have been based on one population–with three studies reporting results for the same population at different time points[236,237,240] and two other studies reporting on two different classifications of reactivity in another population.[238,239] One study reported stent thrombosis in two arms of the trial, where patients in each arm got different drugs (bivalirudin and abciximab) in addition to clopidogrel; these two arms are regarded as independent populations.[242]

The results of the studies with the longest followup were considered. All the studies used ADP as an agonist to assess reactivity. One study used ADP in combination with AA to assess the response to both clopidogrel and aspirin.[234] Thresholds for defining "positive" results were based on prior literature (or other sources external to the study) in seven studies[82,231,236,240,242,243] and were derived from the observed study data in two studies[238,239]; one study used both approaches.[234] Study sample sizes were variable, ranging from 30 to 2533 patients. Followup time was 1 day to 14 months. Because of the diversity of the metrics and cutoffs used to define high platelet reactivity, and substantial variability in followup durations, we did not perform meta-analyses of predictive ability.

In five of the seven studies, high on-clopidogrel platelet reactivity was significantly associated with a higher risk of stent thrombosis. In the study reported stent thrombosis in two arms of the trial, there was a significantly higher risk of stent thrombosis in both the arms, (bivalirudin and abciximab in addition to clopidogrel).[242] One study reported no events.[243] Overall, the studies provided weak evidence of an association between increased platelet reactivity (as measured by the Multiplate analyzer) and stent thrombosis in patients with ischemic heart disease; however, given the substantial clinical heterogeneity, the results are inconclusive.

MACE

Thirteen studies reported information on the ability of the Multiplate analyzer assay to predict MACE for patients receiving clopidogrel-based treatment.[82,194,225,234-242,244] Two sets of studies reported on overlapping patient populations: one set comprised three studies reporting results on the same population over different followup durations[236,237,240]; the second set comprised two studies employing two different classifications of reactivity on the same population.[238,239] In both cases, we based our conclusions on the studies with the longest followup duration. One study reported stent thrombosis in two arms of the trial, where patients in each arm got different drugs (bivalirudin and abciximab) in addition to clopidogrel; these two arms are regarded as independent populations.[242] The definitions of composite outcomes were variable across studies. All studies used ADP as the agonist to assess reactivity. Three studies used ADP in combination with AA to assess response to both clopidogrel and aspirin.[234,235,244] Thresholds for defining "positive" results were based on prior literature (or other sources external to the study) in six studies and not explicitly reported in two studies; they were derived from the observed study data and literature in six studies. Study sample sizes were variable, ranging from 106 to 2533 patients; followup durations ranged from 1 month to 14 months. Because of the diversity of the metrics and cutoff values used to define high platelet reactivity, and the substantial variability in followup durations, we did not perform meta-analyses of predictive ability for this group of studies.

Four studies reporting information on the predictive value of on-clopidogrel platelet reactivity (using ADP as the agonist) did not report statistically significant results; one study did reported no events. Among the three studies that evaluated a combination of clopidogrel and aspirin responders, both reported significantly higher rates of composite outcome events in patient groups with dual clopidogrel and aspirin nonresponse.[234,235,244] In summary, there was insufficient evidence to support an association between increased platelet reactivity measured by the Multiplate analyzer assay and composite clinical outcomes in patients with ischemic heart disease; however, given the heterogeneity in the studies, the results were inconclusive.

Stroke

Three studies reported information on the ability of the Multiplate analyzer assay to predict strokes for patients receiving clopidogrel-based treatment.[236,237,240] All three studies were based on the same patient population (1608 patients) and reported results over different followup durations. ADP was the agonist used to assess reactivity. Thresholds for defining "positive" results were based on prior literature (or other sources external to the study) in all studies. Followup duration ranged from 30 days to 12 months. The study reporting followup results at one year documented a statistically significant association between high platelet reactivity and ischemic stroke; the association was not statistically significant for hemorrhagic or overall stroke.[236]

Bleeding Events

Nine studies reported information on the ability of the Multiplate analyzer assay to predict bleeding events for patients receiving clopidogrel-based treatment.[82,236-243] Two sets of studies reported on overlapping patient populations: one set comprised three studies reporting results on the same population over different followup durations;[236,237,240] the second set comprised two studies employing two different classifications of reactivity on the same population.[238,239] In both cases we based our conclusions on the studies with the longest followup duration. One study reported stent thrombosis in two arms of the trial, where patients in each arm got different drugs (bivalirudin and abciximab) in addition to clopidogrel; these two arms are regarded as independent populations.[242] ADP was used as the agonist to assess reactivity. Thresholds for defining "positive" results were based on prior literature (or other sources external to the study) in six studies; they were derived from the observed study data and literature in three studies. Study sample sizes ranged from 106 to 2533 patients. Followup duration ranged from 30 days to 1 year. Because of the limited number of studies on nonoverlapping patient populations and diversity of the metrics and cutoff values used to define high platelet reactivity, we did not perform meta-analyses of predictive ability. Two studies reported no bleeding events in the study. Three studies did not find a statistically significant association between platelet reactivity measured by the Multiplate analyzer and risk of bleeding; the abciximab arm of the trial[242] and one other study reported that major bleeding risk was significantly higher in the group of patient with high on-clopidogrel reactivity.

Other Clinical Outcomes

Six studies reported information on the ability of the Multiplate analyzer assay to predict target lesion revascularization for patients receiving clopidogrel-based treatment[235-237,240,242,243] Three of the four studies reported results based on the same patient population at different followup durations.[236,237,240] We based our conclusions on the study with the longest followup duration. One study reported MIs in two arms of the trial, where patients in each arm got different drugs (bivalirudin and abciximab) in addition to clopidogrel; these two arms are regarded as independent populations.[242] All studies used ADP as an agonist to assess reactivity. One study also used ADP in combination with AA to assess the response to both clopidogrel and aspirin.[235] Thresholds for defining "positive" results were based on prior literature (or other sources external to the study) in five studies; they were not explicitly reported in one study. Study sample sizes ranged from 182 to 1608; followup time ranged from 1 to 14 months. Because of limited number of studies with nonoverlapping patient populations, we did not perform meta-analyses of predictive ability. One study reported no revascularization events in the study population.[243] Two studies did not find a statistically significant association between increased platelet reactivity and target lesion revascularization (using ADP as the agonist).[236,242] The study that assessed the impact of combined response to clopidogrel and aspirin on target lesion revascularization found a higher risk among patients exhibiting nonresponse (to both drugs).[235]

Intermediate Outcome: Platelet Reactivity During Followup

Reactivity as a Continuous Outcome

No studies reported information on the ability of the Multiplate analyzer assay to predict platelet reactivity as a continuous outcome for clopidogrel-treated patients with ischemic heart disease.

Reactivity as a Categorical Outcome

Two studies[215,230] reported on the effect of tests using the Multiplate analyzer assay on platelet reactivity as a categorical outcome. In this study, reactivity during followup was assessed using LTA with ADP as an agonist[230] and the other study used the Multiplate analyzer assay to assess platelet reactivity.[215] One study enrolled patients with chronic ischemic heart disease[230] and one study enrolled patients who had an MI.[215] Both studies were conducted in the setting of interventional cardiac procedures, specifically PCI. One study reported inadequate quantitative data to assess the predictive value of the Multiplate analyzer assay on platelet reactivity as a categorical outcome. One study reported a statistically significant difference in platelet reactivity during followup comparing nonresponders and responders at baseline.[215]

In summary, while suggestive of an association between platelet reactivity at baseline and measurement obtained during followup, results were inconclusive due to the small number of available studies.

Patients With Cerebrovascular Disease

One study reported information on the predictive value of the Multiplate analyzer assay for composite clinical outcomes among clopidogrel-treated patients with cerebrovascular disease.[245] No studies reported on the test's ability to predict platelet reactivity.

MACE

The study reported information on the ability of the Multiplate analyzer assay to predict composite MACE (transient intra-interventional thrombosis, transient ischemic attack, or cerebral infarction for clopidogrel-treated patients with cerebrovascular disease).[245] ADP was used as the agonist to assess reactivity. The rationale for selecting the threshold for defining a "positive" result was not explicitly reported in the study. This small study (n=50) reported that increased reactivity was statistically significantly associated with increased risk of the composite outcome.

Thromboelastography

Six studies reported information on the predictive ability of thromboelastography as an assay for measuring platelet reactivity. All five studies included patients with ischemic heart disease. No studies reporting information on this assay were conducted in other patient populations. Detailed information on the selection criteria, settings, and treatment strategies (including adjunctive treatments) is presented in **Appendix E**.

Patients With Ischemic Heart Disease

Six studies included patients with ischemic heart disease and reported information on the predictive value of thromboelastography.[137,159,161,188,246,247] Five studies assessed the value of the test for predicting clinical outcomes (all-cause mortality, acute coronary syndromes, composite cardiovascular outcomes, and bleeding events); one study assessed the value of the test for predicting platelet reactivity during followup.[247] Of the six studies, five enrolled patients with chronic stable coronary artery disease; the remaining study included patients with acute coronary syndromes.

Clinical Outcomes

All-Cause Mortality

Two studies reported on the predictive value of thromboelastography to predict all-cause mortality for patients receiving clopidogrel-based treatment.[137,247] In one study, reactivity was assessed using ADP as agonist[137] while the other study used ADP in combination with AA to assess the response to both clopidogrel and aspirin. Both studies enrolled patients with chronic stable coronary artery disease and was conducted in the setting of interventional cardiac procedures (PCI). One study reported that no deaths occurred (regardless of reactivity status) while the other study reported higher deaths in the group of people who exhibited higher reactivity to both clopidogrel and aspirin. There is insufficient information to assess the predictive ability of TEG for the outcome of all-cause mortality.

Acute Coronary Syndromes

Two studies reported on using thromboelastography to predict myocardial infarction for patients receiving clopidogrel-based therapy[137,247] In one study reactivity was assessed using ADP as agonist;[137] in the other study ADP was used in combination with in combination with AA to assess the response to both clopidogrel and aspirin. Both studies study enrolled patients with chronic stable coronary artery disease and was conducted in the setting of interventional cardiac procedures (PCI). Over a course of one year, both studies reported a higher risk of myocardial infarction among patients with high platelet reactivity; this difference was not statistically significant in one study[137] but was statistically significant in the other. [247]

Stent Thrombosis

One study reported information on using thromboelastography to predict stent thrombosis for patients receiving clopidogrel-based therapy[137,247] The study used ADP in combination with AA to assess the response to both clopidogrel and aspirin. The study enrolled 60 patients with chronic stable coronary artery disease. Over a course of one year, the study reported a significantly higher rate of stent thrombosis among patients with high platelet reactivity. This suggests an association between increased platelet reactivity by the TEG assay and stent thrombosis, but the result is inconclusive owing to insufficient information.

MACE

Four studies reported information on the ability of thromboelastography to predict MACE in patients receiving clopidogrel-based treatment.[137,159,161,188] Two of the studies reported information on the same patient population, with the one study reporting information after 6 months of followup[159] and the other after 36 months of followup.[161] We based our conclusions on the study with the longest followup. Definitions of composite clinical outcomes were different across studies. The studies conducted on the same population used thrombin and ADP as agonists;[159,161] the other two used ADP. Thresholds for defining "positive" results were based on prior literature (or other sources external to the study) in two studies and were derived from the observed study data in two studies. Study sample sizes ranged from 49 to 225 patients and followup time ranged from 6 months to 36 months. Because of the limited number of studies reporting on nonoverlapping patient population and the diversity of the cutoff values used to define high platelet reactivity, we did not perform meta-analyses of predictive ability. Two of the three studies reported that the risk of composite cardiovascular events was statistically significantly higher in groups identified as having high platelet reactivity when both ADP and thrombin were used as agonists.[137,161] The third study also reported significantly higher event rates in groups having high reactivity (using ADP as the agonist).[188] In summary, reviewed studies suggested an association between increased platelet reactivity by thromboelastography and composite adverse cardiovascular events in patients with ischemic heart disease; however, the evidence was limited by clinical heterogeneity across the few available studies.

Stroke

One study reported information on using thromboelastography to predict myocardial infarction for patients receiving clopidogrel-based therapy[137,247] The study used ADP in combination with AA to assess the response to both clopidogrel and aspirin. The study enrolled 60 patients with chronic stable coronary artery disease. Over a course of one year, the study reported no events regardless of the platelet reactivity status. This suggests no association between increased platelet reactivity by the TEG assay and stent thrombosis, but the result is inconclusive owing to insufficient information.

Bleeding Events

Three studies reported on using thromboelastography to predict bleeding events for patients receiving clopidogrel-based treatment.[137,246,247] In two studies, reactivity was assessed by thromboelastography using collagen and ADP as agonists[137,246] while the other study used ADP in combination with AA to assess the response to both clopidogrel and aspirin.[247] All studies enrolled patients with chronic stable coronary artery disease and were conducted in the setting of interventional cardiac procedures: PCI in one[137] and CABG surgery in the other.[246] One study assessed rates of intracranial hemorrhage in patients with high and low reactivity, and reported no events.[247] One study assessed major and minor bleeding events;[137] one study assessed post-operative transfusion requirement as an indicator for loss from bleeding.[246] The postoperative transfusion requirement was significantly higher with increased platelet reactivity[246]; the bleeding events did not differ statistically significantly between groups in the other study.[137] Overall, there was insufficient information to evaluate the predictive value of platelet reactivity as measured by thromboelastography and bleeding events in patients with ischemic heart disease.

PFA-100

Eleven studies reported information on the predictive ability of PFA-100 assay. Ten of the studies included patients with ischemic heart disease and one included a mix of patients with ischemic heart disease and peripheral artery disease. No relevant studies of this assay enrolled patients with cerebrovascular or peripheral arterial disease. Detailed information on the selection criteria, settings, and treatment strategies (including adjunctive treatments) is presented in Appendix E.

Patients With Ischemic Heart Disease

Ten studies included patients with ischemic heart disease and reported information on the predictive value of the PFA-100 assay.[82,140,154,230,248-253] One also assessed a variation of the PFA-100 assay called the INNOVANCE PFA P2Y assay.[140] Nine studies assessed the value of the test for predicting clinical outcomes and one for predicting platelet reactivity during followup. Of the ten studies, five enrolled patients with acute coronary syndromes[248-251,253]; the remaining five enrolled patients with chronic stable coronary artery disease.[82,140,154,230,252]

Clinical Outcomes

All-Cause Mortality

Two studies reported information on the ability of the PFA-100 and the INNOVANCE PFA P2Y assay to predict all-cause mortality for patients receiving clopidogrel-based treatment.[140,249] One study evaluated both assays;[140] the other study used only PFA-100.[249] All assays used collagen and ADP as agonists to assess reactivity. Thresholds for defining "positive" results were based on prior literature (or other sources external to the study) in one study; they were derived from the observed study data in the other. Study sample sizes were 612 and 1069 patients. Because of the limited number of available studies, we did not perform meta-analyses of predictive ability for this group of studies. Both studies reporting information on reactivity as measured by PFA-100 did not report statistically significant associations between reactivity status and all-cause mortality;[140,249] High on-treatment platelet reactivity as measured by INNOVANCE PFA P2Y assay was statistically significantly associated with risk of death.[140] The reviewed studies did not suggest an association between increased platelet reactivity by PFA-100 assay and all-cause mortality; however, data were very limited. Similarly, the association between increased platelet reactivity measured by the INNOVANCE PFA P2Y assay and all-cause mortality was supported by only a single study.

Cardiovascular Mortality

Two studies reported information on the ability of the PFA-100 assay to predict cardiac mortality for patients receiving clopidogrel-based treatment.[249,251] One study used two agonist combinations: collagen and epinephrine, and collagen and ADP to assess both aspirin and clopidogrel nonresponsiveness, respectively.[251] The other study used collagen and ADP as agonists.[249] Thresholds for defining "positive" results were based on prior literature (or other sources external to the study) in both studies. Study sample sizes were 125 and 612. Because of the limited number of available studies, we did not perform meta-analyses of predictive ability for this group of studies. One study reported that the risk of cardiac death was significantly higher among patients with high platelet reactivity while assessing clopidogrel responsiveness.[249] The other study, which assessed combined aspirin and clopidogrel responsiveness, reported that the risk of cardiac death was statistically significantly higher among patients with dual nonresponsiveness.[251] In summary, reviewed studies suggested an association between increased platelet reactivity by PFA-100 assay and cardiac mortality in patients with ischemic heart disease; however, results were inconclusive due to the limited number of publications and heterogeneity in the methods for reactivity assessment.

Acute Coronary Syndromes

Five studies reported information on the ability of the PFA-100 assay to predict acute coronary syndromes for patients receiving clopidogrel-based treatment.[140,248,249,251,252] One study used a combination of collagen and epinephrine, and collagen and ADP, to assess both aspirin and clopidogrel nonresponsiveness, respectively.[251] The other studies used collagen and ADP as agonists. Thresholds for defining "positive" results were based on prior literature (or other sources external to the study) in three studies; they were derived from the observed study data in one study; and not explicitly reported in one study. Study sample sizes ranged from 91 to 1069 patients. Because of the heterogeneity in the cutoff values used, we did not perform meta-analyses of predictive ability for this group of studies. Three studies did not report a statistically significant association between high reactivity as measured by PFA-100 and risk of myocardial infarction; the remaining two studies reported a statistically significantly higher risk of myocardial infarction among patients with high platelet reactivity. One study assessing high on-treatment platelet reactivity as measured by INNOVANCE PFA P2Y assay did find a statistically significant difference in the risk of myocardial infarction between groups.[140] In summary, studies did not suggest an association between increased platelet reactivity as measured by PFA-100 assay and acute coronary syndromes outcomes in patients with ischemic heart disease; however, results were inconclusive due to heterogeneity in the methods used to assess reactivity that precluded quantitative synthesis.

Stent Thrombosis

Three studies reported information on the ability of the PFA-100 and the INNOVANCE PFA P2Y assays to predict stent thrombosis for patients receiving clopidogrel-based treatment.[82,140,154] One study used measurements of platelet reactivity from both assays (used separately)[140]; one study used a combination of collagen and epinephrine, and collagen and ADP, to assess aspirin and clopidogrel nonresponsiveness, respectively;[154] the other study used ADP to assess clopidogrel responsiveness.[82] Thresholds for defining "positive" results were based on prior literature (or other sources external to the study) in two studies; they were derived from the observed study data in the other. Study sample sizes ranged from 402to 1069 patients. Because of the limited number of available studies, we did not perform meta-analyses of predictive ability. One study reported 100 percent sensitivity of PFA-100 assay to predict stent thrombosis;[154] one study reported a sensitivity of 0.7 to predict stent thrombosis;[82] the other study did not report a statistically significant association between platelet reactivity and stent thrombosis.[140]The association between high on-treatment platelet reactivity as measured by the INNOVANCE PFA P2Y assay with stent thrombosis was not statistically significant.[140] In summary, reviewed studies did not provide adequate evidence to support the association between increased platelet reactivity as measured by PFA-100 assay and stent thrombosis in patients with ischemic heart disease.

MACE

Nine studies reported information on the ability of the PFA-100 and the INNOVANCE PFA P2Y assays to predict MACE in patients receiving clopidogrel-based treatment.[82,140,154,248-253] Only one study used measurements of platelet reactivity from both assays (used separately);[140] the other studies used combinations of collagen and epinephrine and collagen and ADP to assess platelet reactivity. Thresholds for defining "positive" results were based on prior literature (or other sources external to the study) in four studies and were derived from the observed study data in three studies; one study used both approaches; and one did not explicitly report the rationale for selecting a cutoff value. Study sample sizes ranged between 71 and 1069 patients. Because of the limited number of available studies and heterogeneity in the methods used to define high platelet reactivity, we did not perform meta-analyses of predictive ability.

Seven of the nine studies using the PFA-100 assay reported statistically significant associations between increased platelet reactivity and increased risk of composite outcome events; the remaining two studies did not report statistically significant associations but produced effect sizes in the same direction (i.e., indicating an association between increased reactivity and higher risk of events). The association between high on-treatment platelet reactivity as measured by the INNOVANCE PFA P2Y assay with stent thrombosis was statistically significant indicating increased risk among patients with high on-clopidogrel reactivity.[140] In summary, the reviewed studies supported an association between increased platelet reactivity as measured by the PFA-100 assay and composite outcome events among patients with ischemic heart disease; however, the strength of these findings was limited by heterogeneity in definitions of increased reactivity that precluded quantitative synthesis.

Stroke

One study reported information on the ability of the PFA-100 assay to predict strokes for patients receiving clopidogrel-based treatment.[140] The study used collagen and ADP as an agonist. Thresholds for defining "positive" results were derived from the observed study data. The study enrolled 1069 patients who were undergoing PCI with stent implantation. This study did not report a statistically significant association between high reactivity as measured by PFA-100 and stroke at one year of followup. The result did not suggest an association between increased platelet reactivity by PFA-100 assay and stroke; however, results were inconclusive due to paucity of relevant information.

Bleeding Events

One study reported on the ability of the PFA-100 assay to predict bleeding events for patients receiving clopidogrel-based treatment.[248] In this study, reactivity was assessed using collagen and ADP as agonists. The study enrolled patients with acute coronary syndromes and was conducted in the setting of interventional cardiac procedures (PCI). The study reported that no bleeding events occurred (regardless of reactivity status).

Other Clinical Outcomes

Two studies reported information on the ability of the PFA-100 assay to predict miscellaneous clinical outcomes for patients receiving clopidogrel-based treatment.[248,251] The outcomes included: recurrent angina, arrhythmia, pulmonary edema, cardiogenic shock,[248] and rehospitalization for congestive heart failure.[251] One study used ADP and collagen as the agonist to assess reactivity;[248] the other used a combination of collagen and epinephrine, and collagen and ADP to assess both aspirin and clopidogrel nonresponsiveness.[251] The studies generally showed that higher reactivity was associated with higher risk of outcome events; however, the strength of evidence was limited by the small number of available studies and the heterogeneity in reactivity measurement methods .

Intermediate Outcome: Platelet Reactivity During Followup

Reactivity as a Continuous Outcome

No studies reported information on the ability of the PFA-100 assay to predict platelet reactivity as a continuous outcome among clopidogrel-treated patients with ischemic heart disease.

Reactivity as a Categorical Outcome

One study[230] reported on ability of the PFA-100 assay to predict platelet reactivity as a categorical outcome. In this study, reactivity at baseline was assessed using collagen and ADP as agonists. The study enrolled patients with chronic ischemic heart disease and was conducted in the setting of interventional cardiac procedures (PCI). Reactivity status, as measured by the PFA-100 assay at baseline, was not statistically significantly associated with response status during followup.

Mixed Patient Population With Ischemic Heart Disease and Peripheral Artery Disease

One study included a mixed population of patients with ischemic heart disease and peripheral artery disease and reported information on the predictive value of platelet reactivity measured by

PFA-100.[186] The study recruited 534 chronic stable coronary artery disease patients treated with clopidogrel and assessed the value of the test for predicting the first occurrence of MACE. The study also assessed the value of the LTA and VASP test for predicting the first occurrence of the same outcome. The results from these tests are reported under the respective sections.

Clinical Outcomes

MACE

One study reported information on the ability of platelet reactivity measured by PFA-100 to predict MACE (defined as acute myocardial infarction, unstable angina, hospitalization for revascularization, acute limb ischemia, ischemic stroke, transient ischemic attack, or cardiovascular death).[186] ADP was used as the agonist to assess reactivity, with a cutoff <190s of closing time to indicate high reactivity.

The thresholds for defining "positive" results were based on prior literature. Of the 771 enrolled patients, 534 were taking clopidogrel at the time of platelet testing. The test results did not impact on MACE-free survival and the multivariate Cox regression did not report a significant higher risk of MACE with reactivity measured by the PFA-100 assay (HR = 0.82; 95% CI = 0.57,1.19; p=0.30). In summary, the study does not suggest an association between increased platelet reactivity by PFA-100 and MACE in a mixed population of patients with ischemic heart disease and peripheral artery disease; however, results were inconclusive due to paucity of data.

Other Tests for Measuring Platelet Reactivity

Nine studies evaluated the predictive value of platelet reactivity by a diverse group of tests: one study used iron as an agonist[250]; two studies used the Plateletworks assay to measure reactivity[254,255]; one study used two separate assays (the Ichor Plateletworks and the Impact-R assay with ADP)[140]; one study only the Ichor Platelet works assay;[256] two studies used flow cytometry to assess ADP-stimulated P-selectin expression[157,179]; one study used a the results of two assays assessed jointly (LTA and the VerifyNow assay) to define platelet response[183]; and one study used a combination of three assays (conventional LTA, thromboelastography and Plateletworks assay).[257] All nine studies included patients with ischemic heart disease. None were conducted on other patient populations. Detailed information on the selection criteria, settings, and treatment strategies (including adjunctive treatments) is presented in **Appendix E.**

Patients With Ischemic Heart Disease

All nine studies using diverse tests for reactivity included patients with ischemic heart disease. Five of the seven studies assessed the value of the test for predicting clinical outcomes, and two for predicting platelet reactivity during followup. Four enrolled patients with acute coronary syndromes[250,254-256]; four included patients with chronic stable coronary artery disease[140,157,179,257]; and one enrolled mixed populations with chronic and acute presentations.[183]

Clinical Outcomes

All-Cause Mortality

Three studies reported information on all-cause mortality. One study used measurements of platelet reactivity from two assays—the Ichor Plateletworks and the Impact-R assay;[140]; one study used measure of reactivity by only the Plateletworks assay.[254] One study used the Ichor

Plateletworks assay to predict clinical outcomes in two arms of the trial, where patients in each arm got different drugs (tirofiban and abciximab) in addition to clopidogrel; these two arms are regarded as independent populations.[256] In all cases ADP was the agonist used to assess reactivity. Thresholds for defining "positive" results were based on prior literature (or other sources external to the study) in one study; they were derived from the observed study data in the other. Study sample sizes were 31 and 1069 patients. Because of limited number of available studies we did not perform meta-analyses of predictive ability. Of the three studies reporting relevant information on reactivity as measured by Plateletworks, one did not report a statistically significant association between platelet reactivity status and risk of death.[140] The second study reported that no deaths occurred, regardless of reactivity.[254] The third study did not report any events in the tirofiban and abciximab arms of the study.[256] The result did not suggest an association between increased platelet reactivity by the PlateletWorks assay and death. Platelet reactivity as measured by the Impact R assay was also not statistically significantly associated with risk of death.[140]

Acute Coronary Syndromes

Three studies reported information on acute coronary syndromes among patients receiving clopidogrel-based treatment. One study used the measure of platelet reactivity from two assays—the Ichor Plateletworks and the Impact-R assay[140]; one study used measure of reactivity by only the Plateletworks assay.[254] One study used the Ichor Plateletworks assay to predict clinical outcomes in two arms of the trial, where patients in each arm got different drugs (tirofiban and abciximab) in addition to clopidogrel; these two arms are regarded as independent populations.[256] In all cases ADP was the agonist used to assess reactivity. Thresholds for defining "positive" results were based on prior literature (or other sources external to the study) in one study; they were derived from the observed study data in one study. Study sample sizes were 31 and 1069 patients. Because of the limited number of available studies we did not perform meta-analyses. Of the three studies reporting information on reactivity as measured by the Plateletworks assay, two reported that not myocardial infarctions occurred, regardless of reactivity.[254,256] The other study reported that the risk of myocardial infarction was significantly higher among patients with high on-treatment platelet reactivity.[140] The result did not suggest an association between increased platelet reactivity by the PlateletWorks assay and myocardial infarction. Platelet reactivity as measured by Impact R ADP was not statistically significantly associated with myocardial infarction at 1 year.[140]

Stent Thrombosis

One study including 1069 patients reported information on stent thrombosis. The study used measurements of platelet reactivity from two assays—the Ichor Plateletworks and the Impact-R assay.[140] Both the assays used ADP as the agonist to assess reactivity. The threshold for defining "positive" results was derived from the observed study data. The study reported that the high platelet reactivity as measured by either Plateletworks or Impact R was not statistically significantly associated with stent thrombosis.

MACE

Six studies reported information on composite MACE (of varying definitions). One study used iron as an agonist in LTA and also used the Plateletworks assay;[250] one measured platelet reactivity using two assays—the Ichor Plateletworks and the Impact-R;[140] one study only the Ichor Platelet works assay;[256] one study used flow cytometry to assess ADP-stimulated P-selectin expression;[179] one study used a the joint results of two assays, conventional LTA and VerifyNow, to define platelet response; and one study used a combination of three assays—conventional LTA, thromboelastography, and Plateletworks—to categorize response to clopidogrel. Apart from the study using iron as an agonist, the other three studies used ADP as the agonist to assess reactivity. Thresholds for defining "positive" results were based on prior literature (or other sources external to the study) in one study, were derived from the observed study data in two study, and were not explicitly reported in three studies. Study sample sizes ranged from 30 to 1069 patients and followup durations ranged from 1 month to a year. Because of limited number of studies evaluating each test, we did not perform meta-analyses of predictive ability for this group of studies. Of the three studies reporting information on the predictive value of reactivity as measured by Plateletworks, one did not report any events regardless of the reactivity status;[256] one did not report a statistically significant difference between reactivity groups;[250] and one reported significantly higher risk the composite cardiovascular event among patients with high on-treatment platelet reactivity.[140] Platelet reactivity as measured by the Impact R assay was not statistically significant associated with outcome events.[140] Increased reactivity based on combined assay results (LTA and VerifyNow or LTA, thromboelastography, and PlateletWorks) was not significantly associate with increased event rates.

Stroke

One study reported information on the ability of Plateletworks and the Impact-R assay to predict strokes for patients receiving clopidogrel-based treatment. All the assays used ADP as the agonist to assess reactivity. Thresholds for defining "positive" results were derived from the observed study data in one study. The study enrolled 1069 patients undergoing PCI with stent implantation. This study did not find a statistically significant association between high reactivity as measured by either the Impact R or Plateletworks assay with stroke at 1 year of followup.

Bleeding Events

Two studies reported information on bleeding events for patients receiving clopidogrel-based treatment. One study used measurements of reactivity by the Plateletworks assay[254] and the other used two assays jointly—conventional LTA and VerifyNow assay—to assess platelet reactivity.[183] In all cases ADP was used as the agonist to assess reactivity. One study reported information on hematoma development as an outcome[254] while the other reported bleeding events.[183] Neither platelet reactivity as measured by the Plateletworks assay nor combined assessment with LTA and VerifyNow were statistically significantly associated with hematomas or bleeding events, respectively.

Other Clinical Outcomes

Three studies reported information on the ability of the different platelet function tests to predict bleeding events for patients receiving clopidogrel-based treatment. Two study used measurements of reactivity by the Plateletworks assay[254,256] and one used a combination of three assays—conventional LTA, thromboelastography, and Plateletworks assay—to categorize response to clopidogrel.[257] In all cases ADP was used as the agonist to assess reactivity. One study reported angina recurrence as an outcome;[254] one study reported rehospitalization rates for ischemia; one study reported rates of followup intervention, both PCI and CABG surgery.[257] Platelet reactivity measured with the Plateletworks assay and combined assessment with LTA, thromboelastography, and Plateletworks assays were not statistically significantly associated with the outcomes assessed.

Intermediate Outcome: Platelet Reactivity During Followup

Reactivity as a Continuous Outcome

No studies reported information on the ability of other tests of platelet reactivity to predict platelet reactivity as a continuous outcome for clopidogrel-treated patients with ischemic heart disease.

Reactivity as a Categorical Outcome

Three studies evaluated the predictive value of baseline platelet reactivity on platelet reactivity as a continuous outcome.[157,254,255] Two studies used the Plateletworks assay[254,255] and one study used flow cytometry to assess P-selectin expression.[157] Two of the three studies enrolled patients with acute coronary syndromes[254,255] while one study[157] enrolled patients with chronic ischemic heart disease. All three studies were conducted in the setting of interventional cardiac procedures—one PCI[254], one PCI with stent implantation,[157] and one CABG surgery.[255]

Results were reported with different followup periods (ranging from a one day to 30 days). Because of differences in the tests used, we did not perform meta-analyses for this group of studies. Baseline reactivity measured with Plateletworks and ADP-stimulated P-selectin expression was not statistically significantly associated with reactivity status during followup.

Studies Reporting Comparative Information on Test Performance

Comparisons Between Alternative Platelet Reactivity Tests

Several studies reported the application of two or more tests applied to the same population. However, no study was specifically designed and analyzed in a way to allow formal comparisons between tests. All studies evaluating multiple tests have been considered with regards to the individual tests they evaluated in the preceding sections of this chapter. Their risk of bias is discussed in the next section; overall, they did not differ substantially (in terms of risk of bias) from studies assessing only a single test. Twelve studies reported extractable information on clinical outcomes for at least two of the assessed tests. Complete information for the populations included, assays used, and study results are presented in Appendix E. Here, we focus on outcomes that were addressed by at least three comparative studies: major adverse cardiovascular events (composite outcome, ten studies) and stent thrombosis (four studies).[82,137,140,154,159,161,178,183,186,225] All studies were conducted in ischemic heart disease populations.

For each of these outcomes, we plotted the predictive effect sizes reported for each of the tests evaluated (grouped by study), along with information on the assay and threshold used (results have been organized by study to facilitate direct within-study, cross-assay comparisons). Unfortunately the data cannot be quantitatively synthesized, because when multiple assays are applied to the same patient population results for are likely to be correlated (because the population is shared and assays applied to the same sample produce correlated—if not identical—results) and because the within-study correlation of results cannot be accounted for using aggregate data extracted from the available published studies. Similar problems would be encountered for other measures of test performance, again due to the within-study correlation of reported effect sizes. In the Discussion section of the report we provide suggestions on how future research studies could provide additional information regarding comparative test performance.

MACE

Ten studies reported comparative information regarding the ability of assays for measuring platelet reactivity to predict major adverse cardiovascular events.[82,137,140,154,159,161,178,183,186,225] The most commonly used test was LTA, which was compared to various comparator tests (thromboelastography and VerifyNow P2Y12 were the most commonly used comparators). Results have been summarized in Figure 32. Overall, point estimates were similar between alternative test methods (within each study) and CIs were overlapping, suggesting that the predictive ability of the compared tests is fairly similar (i.e., the tests have similar abilities to discriminate between patients who will and those who will not experience events).

Figure 32. Comparative studies assessing the predictive ability of platelet-reactivity assays for major adverse cardiovascular events

Major adverse cardiovascular events

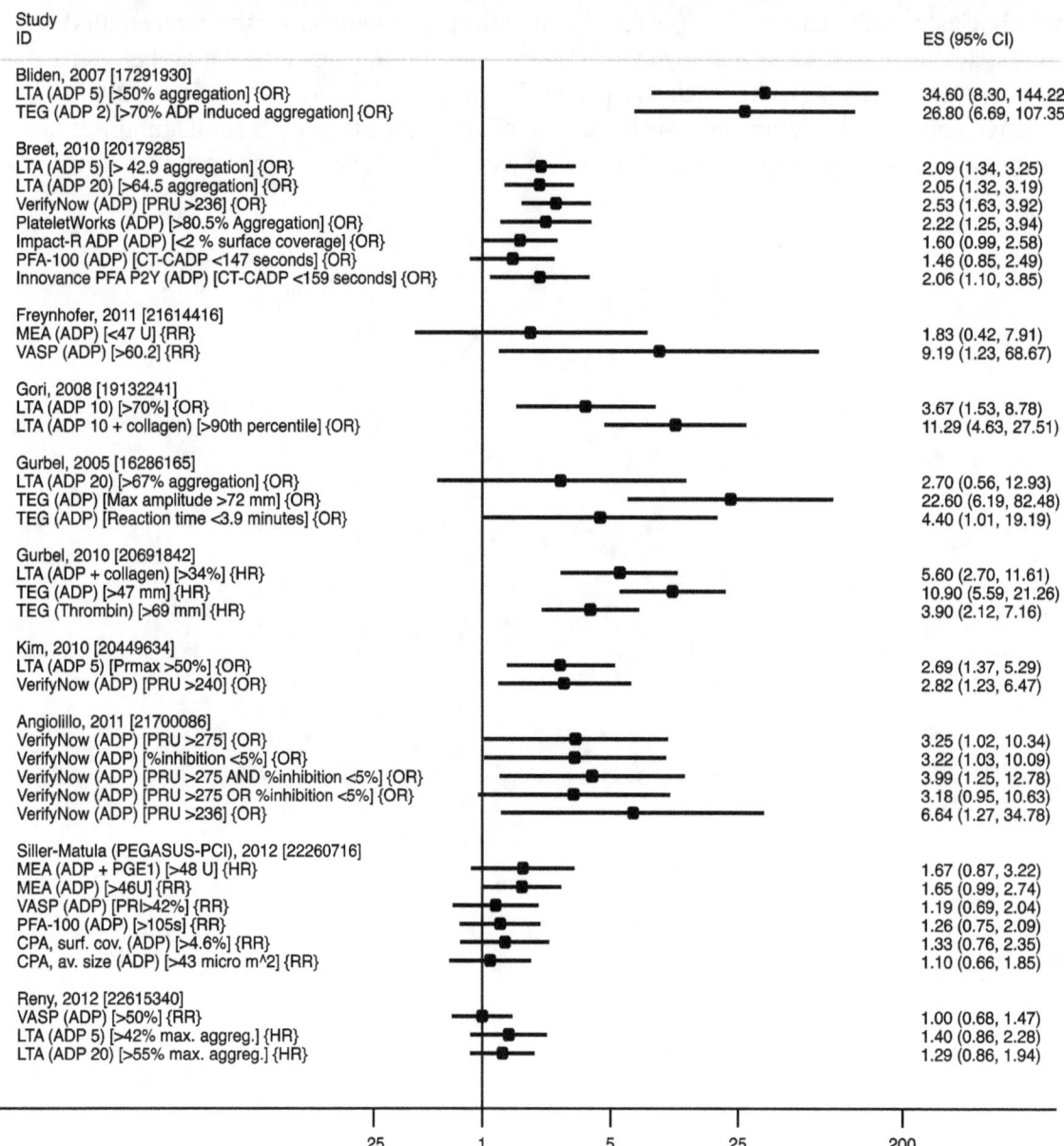

Study ID — ES (95% CI)

Bliden, 2007 [17291930]
LTA (ADP 5) [>50% aggregation] {OR} — 34.60 (8.30, 144.22)
TEG (ADP 2) [>70% ADP induced aggregation] {OR} — 26.80 (6.69, 107.35)

Breet, 2010 [20179285]
LTA (ADP 5) [> 42.9 aggregation] {OR} — 2.09 (1.34, 3.25)
LTA (ADP 20) [>64.5 aggregation] {OR} — 2.05 (1.32, 3.19)
VerifyNow (ADP) [PRU >236] {OR} — 2.53 (1.63, 3.92)
PlateletWorks (ADP) [>80.5% Aggregation] {OR} — 2.22 (1.25, 3.94)
Impact-R ADP (ADP) [<2 % surface coverage] {OR} — 1.60 (0.99, 2.58)
PFA-100 (ADP) [CT-CADP <147 seconds] {OR} — 1.46 (0.85, 2.49)
Innovance PFA P2Y (ADP) [CT-CADP <159 seconds] {OR} — 2.06 (1.10, 3.85)

Freynhofer, 2011 [21614416]
MEA (ADP) [<47 U] {RR} — 1.83 (0.42, 7.91)
VASP (ADP) [>60.2] {RR} — 9.19 (1.23, 68.67)

Gori, 2008 [19132241]
LTA (ADP 10) [>70%] {OR} — 3.67 (1.53, 8.78)
LTA (ADP 10 + collagen) [>90th percentile] {OR} — 11.29 (4.63, 27.51)

Gurbel, 2005 [16286165]
LTA (ADP 20) [>67% aggregation] {OR} — 2.70 (0.56, 12.93)
TEG (ADP) [Max amplitude >72 mm] {OR} — 22.60 (6.19, 82.48)
TEG (ADP) [Reaction time <3.9 minutes] {OR} — 4.40 (1.01, 19.19)

Gurbel, 2010 [20691842]
LTA (ADP + collagen) [>34%] {HR} — 5.60 (2.70, 11.61)
TEG (ADP) [>47 mm] {HR} — 10.90 (5.59, 21.26)
TEG (Thrombin) [>69 mm] {HR} — 3.90 (2.12, 7.16)

Kim, 2010 [20449634]
LTA (ADP 5) [Prmax >50%] {OR} — 2.69 (1.37, 5.29)
VerifyNow (ADP) [PRU >240] {OR} — 2.82 (1.23, 6.47)

Angiolillo, 2011 [21700086]
VerifyNow (ADP) [PRU >275] {OR} — 3.25 (1.02, 10.34)
VerifyNow (ADP) [%inhibition <5%] {OR} — 3.22 (1.03, 10.09)
VerifyNow (ADP) [PRU >275 AND %inhibition <5%] {OR} — 3.99 (1.25, 12.78)
VerifyNow (ADP) [PRU >275 OR %inhibition <5%] {OR} — 3.18 (0.95, 10.63)
VerifyNow (ADP) [PRU >236] {OR} — 6.64 (1.27, 34.78)

Siller-Matula (PEGASUS-PCI), 2012 [22260716]
MEA (ADP + PGE1) [>48 U] {HR} — 1.67 (0.87, 3.22)
MEA (ADP) [>46U] {RR} — 1.65 (0.99, 2.74)
VASP (ADP) [PRI>42%] {RR} — 1.19 (0.69, 2.04)
PFA-100 (ADP) [>105s] {RR} — 1.26 (0.75, 2.09)
CPA, surf. cov. (ADP) [>4.6%] {RR} — 1.33 (0.76, 2.35)
CPA, av. size (ADP) [>43 micro m^2] {RR} — 1.10 (0.66, 1.85)

Reny, 2012 [22615340]
VASP (ADP) [>50%] {RR} — 1.00 (0.68, 1.47)
LTA (ADP 5) [>42% max. aggreg.] {HR} — 1.40 (0.86, 2.28)
LTA (ADP 20) [>55% max. aggreg.] {HR} — 1.29 (0.86, 1.94)

.25   1   5   25   200

Abbreviations: ADP = adenosine diphosphate; CI = confidence interval; CT = closure time; EPI = epinephrine; LTA = light-transmission aggregometry; max = maximum; MEA = Multiplate analyzer; PFA = Platelet Function Analyzer; PRU = platelet reactivity units; RR = relative risk; TEG = thromboelastography; U = units; VASP = vasodilator-stimulated phosphoprotein. RRs compare event rates among patients with high versus low platelet reactivity (as defined by each study, for each test employed). Solid squares (and horizontal lines) indicate the RR of acute coronary syndromes (and the corresponding 95% CI) for individual studies. The vertical line indicates an RR of 1.

Stent Thrombosis

Four studies reported comparative information regarding the ability of assays for measuring platelet reactivity to predict stent thrombosis for patients undergoing PCI with stent implantation (Figure 33).[82,140,154,183] LTA was used in three studies and the VerifyNow P2Y12 assay and the

PFA-100 assays were each used in two studies; other tests are shown in the figure. Overall, point estimates for the predictive ability of alternative test methods were variable (within each study); however, CIs were extremely wide (and overlapping), suggesting that there is substantial uncertainty regarding the relative predictive ability of the compared tests for stent thrombosis and that there is insufficient evidence on comparative test performance for this outcome.

Figure 33. Comparative studies assessing the predictive ability of platelet-reactivity assays for stent thrombosis

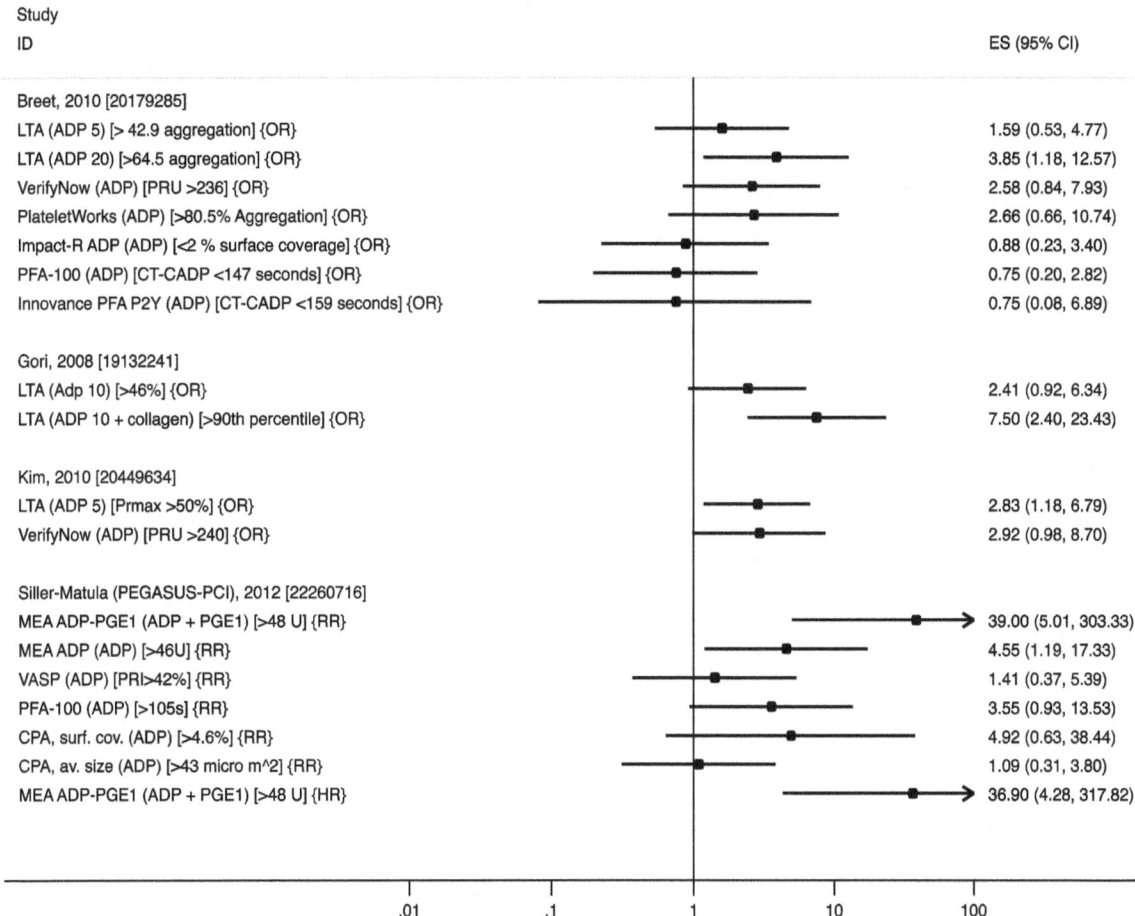

Abbreviations: ADP = adenosine diphosphate; CI = confidence interval; CT = closure time; EPI = epinephrine; LTA = light-transmission aggregometry; max = maximum; PFA = Platelet Function Analyzer; PRU = platelet reactivity units; RR = relative risk; U = units.

RRs compare event rates among patients with high versus low platelet reactivity (as defined by each study, for each test employed). The solid squares (and horizontal lines) indicate the RR of stent thrombosis (and the corresponding 95% CI) for individual studies. The vertical line indicates an RR of 1.

Comparisons Between Genetic Testing for CYP2C19 Variants and Phenotypic Testing for Platelet Reactivity

Only four studies[82,88,95,111] provided extractable information regarding the relative prognostic ability of genetic testing for CYP2C19 loss-of-function variants and phenotypic testing of platelet reactivity for MACE (4 studies) or stent thrombosis (3 studies). These studies have been considered with regards to the individual tests they evaluated in the preceding sections of the report (Key Question 1b or 2b, as applicable). Data that would allow us to formally compare the tests while accounting for the within-person correlation induced by applying multiple tests to the same patient were not reported. Below, for each outcome and each study separately, we have plotted the prognostic sensitivity and prognostic specificity of the tests in the receiver operating characteristic space. Given that these studies represent a very small subset of the studies reporting information on genetic or phenotypic testing, no firm conclusions can be drawn from their results.

MACE

Four studies reported information on the prognostic value of genetic and phenotypic tests for MACE.[82,88,95,111] Test performance was generally limited, however the paucity of the data does not allow firm conclusions. The specific tests compared are described in the legend of Figure 34.

Figure 34. Comparative studies assessing the predictive ability of genetic testing for CYP2C19 variants and platelet-reactivity assays for MACE

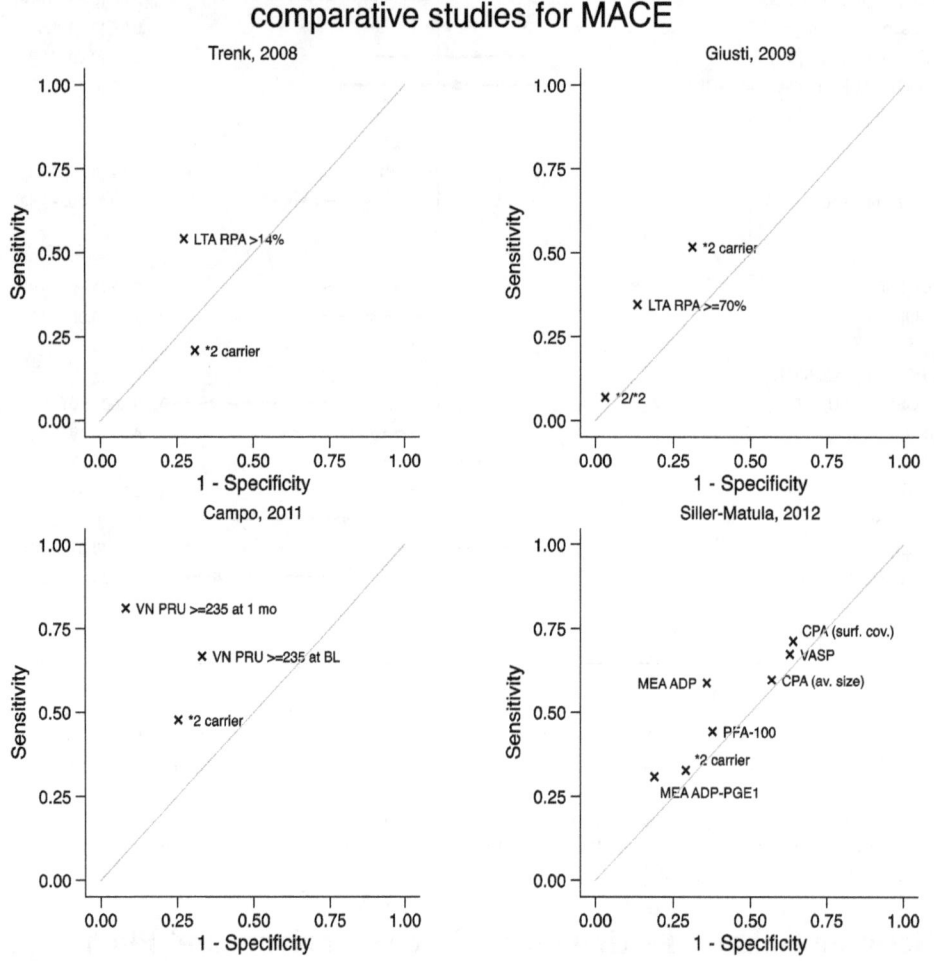

Abbreviations: *2/*2 denotes homozygote for the CYP2C19 *2 allele; *2 carrier denotes the combination of *2/*2 and *2/*1 individuals; av. size = average size; ADP = adenosine diphosphate; BL = baseline; CPA = cone and plate analyzer; LTA = light transmission aggregometry; MACE = major adverse cardiovascular event; MEA = Multiplate analyzer; mo = month; PFA = platelet function analyzer; PGE1 = prostaglandin E1; PRU = platelet reactivity unit; RPA = residual platelet aggregation; surf. cov. = surface coverage; VASP = vasodilator-stimulated phosphoprotein phosphorylation; VN = VerifyNow P2Y12 assay. Details regarding the study designs, populations, and outcomes are presented in Appendix E.

116

Stent Thrombosis

Three studies reported information on the prognostic value of genetic and phenotypic tests for stent thrombosis.[82,88,95] Test performance was generally limited, however the paucity of the data does not allow firm conclusions. The specific tests compared are described in the legend of Figure 35.

Figure 35. Comparative studies assessing the predictive ability of genetic testing for CYP2C19 variants and platelet-reactivity assays for stent thrombosis

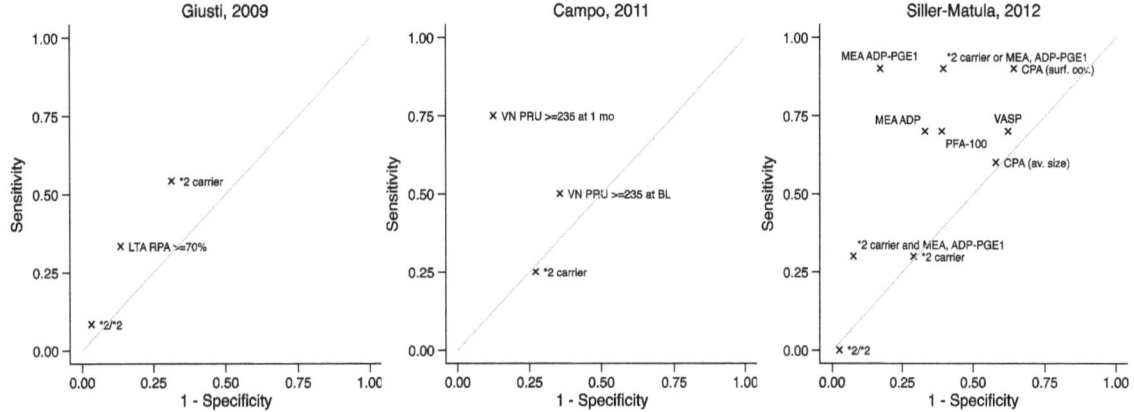

Abbreviations: *2/*2 denotes homozygote for the CYP2C19 *2 allele; *2 carrier denotes the combination of *2/*2 and *2/*1 individuals; av. size = average size; ADP = adenosine diphosphate; BL = baseline; CPA = cone and plate analyzer; LTA = light transmission aggregometry; MACE = major adverse cardiovascular event; MEA = Multiplate analyzer; mo = month; PFA = platelet function analyzer; PGE1 = prostaglandin E1; PRU = platelet reactivity unit; RPA = residual platelet aggregation; surf. cov. = surface coverage; VASP = vasodilator-stimulated phosphoprotein phosphorylation; VN = VerifyNow P2Y12 assay. Details regarding the study designs, populations, and outcomes are presented in Appendix E.

Risk of Bias for Studies Reviewed for Key Question 2b

The detailed assessment of 11 risk-of-bias items for studies evaluating the predictive ability of phenotypic testing regarding clinical outcomes or platelet reactivity (during followup) is presented in Appendix E. Briefly, all studies used a longitudinal design (not case–control; per our inclusion criteria) and no studies had substantial loss-to-followup. Inappropriate exclusions were uncommon however information on blinding was often not reported (particularly for the index test) or not used. Using the arbitrary cutoffs based on the number of adequately addressed risk of bias items 35 studies were rated as quality "A," 80 studies were rated as quality "B," and 12 were rated as quality "C."

Assessing Small-Study Effects

For the two assays (VerifyNow P2Y12 and VASP) and for outcomes for which we performed meta-analyses of predictive value we assessed differences between more precise (larger) and less precise (smaller) studies using the Egger regression-based test for small study effects. Table 10 summarizes our key findings.

Table 10. Small study effects in meta-analyses of the value of platelet reactivity for predicting clinical outcomes among clopidogrel-treated patients with ischemic heart disease

Assay	Outcome	P-Value for Small-Study Effects
VerifyNow P2Y12	All-cause mortality	0.147
	Cardiovascular mortality	0.383
	MACE	**0.001**
	Stent thrombosis	**0.048**
	Bleeding events (all severity levels)	0.764
	Bleeding events (major)	0.611
VASP assay	MACE	0.230
	Cardiovascular mortality	0.113
	Stent thrombosis	0.769
	Acute coronary syndromes	0.311

Abbreviations: MACE = major adverse cardiovascular events, VASP = vasodilator-stimulated phosphoprotein. Significant p-values are in bold type.

Statistically significant "small study effects" were identified among studies of the VerifyNow P2Y12 assay included in meta-analyses of MACE and stent thrombosis. Again, we caution that these statistically significant results should not be overinterpreted as proof for the presence of publication bias given both the statistical properties of the Egger test and the fact that alternative causes (true heterogeneity between smaller and larger studies, chance, or other biases) can also produce significant results. Nonetheless, these results suggest that selective publication of more extreme results in smaller studies may have affected the available data and limits somewhat the strength of the conclusions that can be drawn (e.g., it contributed to our decision to grade the strength of evidence on MACE as moderate, rather than high).

Key Question 2c. What is the impact of modifying factors on the association between phenotypic test results and clinical outcomes?

We reviewed studies to identify any evidence that patient- or system-level factors or test characteristics could modify the predictive ability of phenotypic testing for platelet reactivity. Evidence of effect modification by person-level characteristics (e.g., age, sex, disease severity) is best obtained from comparisons within a given study (i.e., among subgroups of the patient population that were selected using the same criteria and managed in a similar way). Additional evidence on effect modification can be derived from exploratory comparisons across studies, by assessing study-level characteristics (e.g., the setting of care or study design characteristics) or characteristics of the overall patient population (e.g., populations selected on the basis of ancestry).[f] In the following sections we discuss each of these sources of information regarding effect modification separately.

---

[f]We refer to the information obtained from cross-study comparisons as "exploratory" because comparisons for a given characteristic across studies may be confounded (by other study features). Our ability to statistically "control" for such differences is typically limited by the relatively small number of available studies available for meta-analysis.

Effect Modification Within Studies

In total, seven studies reported information on effect modification of the predictive effect of platelet reactivity. All studies reported information on clinical outcomes. Relevant results have been summarized in Table 11; however, we caution that because only a small subset of the eligible studies provided adequate information to statistically assess effect modification, selective reporting is highly likely.

Studies assessed the following factors as potential modifiers: IIb/IIIa inhibitor as an adjunct treatment for PCI (two studies), diabetes mellitus (three studies), and chronic kidney disease (one study). Two studies used the VASP assay to assess platelet reactivity, three used the VerifyNow P2Y12 assay (one of which also used VerifyNow ASA[g]), one used LTA (with ADP as the agonist), and one used the Multiplate analyzer. Statistically significant interaction effects were reported only in two studies. The first study[227] assessed whether the predictive value of the VASP assay is different among patients with coronary artery disease who have coexisting chronic kidney disease versus those who do not. The study found statistically significant interaction effects for several clinical outcomes (all-cause mortality, cardiac death, and a composite outcome of all-cause mortality, myocardial infarction, or target-lesion revascularization), in all cases suggesting that the prognostic effect of high on-clopidogrel platelet reactivity was stronger among patients with chronic kidney disease. The second study assessed whether the prognostic effect of the VerifyNow P2Y12 assay is different among patients with high ($\geq$3 mg/L) versus low (<3 mg/L) CRP levels. The study reported a statistically significant interaction effect, suggesting that high on-clopidogrel platelet reactivity was associated with increased risk for the primary outcome (MACE, defined as all-cause death, nonfatal MI, stent thrombosis, and stroke) compared to low reactivity among patients with diabetes but not among non-diabetic patients.

---

[g]This assay uses arachidonic acid as the agonist, to measure "aspirin resistance."

Table 11. Studies reporting information on effect modification

Author Year Country PMID Study name (when available)	Patient Population	Antiplatelet Regimen	Platelet Reactivity Measurement Method (agonist) [assay and manufacturer] Threshold Definition	Effect Modifier	Summary of Findings*
Bliden[137] 2007 US 17291930 NR	Patients on clopidogrel-based therapy for ≥1 mo undergoing scheduled PCI	Aspirin ≥81 mg/d for ≥7 d before PCI; clopidogrel 75 mg/d for ≥1 mo	LTA (ADP 5 μmol/L) [Chronolog Lumi-Aggregometer; Model 490-4D; Chronolog, Havertown, PA] ≥50% on-clopidogrel reactivity [based on prior literature]	IIb/IIIa inhibitor treatment (used vs. not)	Predictive effect of on-treatment reactivity stratified by IIb/IIIa inhibitor treatment for the composite outcome of death, MI, TVR, stroke, non-TVR, or rehospitalization for ischemia [calculated values] IIb/IIIa inhibitor used: high reactivity vs. normal reactivity OR=29.33 (95% CI, 2.40 to 357.85) IIb/IIIa inhibitor not used: high reactivity vs. normal reactivity OR=32.67 (95% CI, 7.12 to 149.79) P for interaction=0.94 [chi-square test for heterogeneity]

120

Table 11. Studies reporting information on effect modification (continued)

Author Year Country PMID Study name (when available)	Patient Population	Antiplatelet Regimen	Platelet Reactivity Measurement Method (agonist) [assay and manufacturer] Threshold Definition	Effect Modifier	Summary of Findings*
Campo[187] 2010 Multinational 20951320 3T/2R ancillary study	Patients undergoing PCI were screened for aspirin and clopidogrel responsiveness (poor-responders were randomized to tirofiban or placebo); the current study reported on long term outcomes regardless of baseline response status	Aspirin 100 mg/d indefinitely; clopidogrel 75 mg/d for ≥1 mo for patients with stable CAD receiving BMS, or for ≥1 yr for patients with UA or receiving DES	VerifyNow Aspirin (AA agonist) for aspirin responsiveness; VerifyNow P2Y12 (ADP agonist) for clopidogrel responsiveness [Accumetrics, San Diego, CA] For VerifyNow Aspirin ARU ≤550 and VerifyNow P2Y12 % platelet inhibition ≥40% were considered indicative of full response to aspirin and clopidogrel, respectively [cutoff values were those used in the 3T/2R study]	IIb/IIIa inhibitor treatment (used vs. not); in poor responders at baseline, use of IIb/IIIa inhibitor was randomized; the choice was "operator's choice" in responders	Predictive effect of "nonresponder status" stratified by IIb/IIIa inhibitor treatment [calculated values]. Periprocedural ischemic events (up to 3 d post-PCI). *IIb/IIIa inhibitor used:* high reactivity vs. normal reactivity OR=1.63 (95% CI, 0.54 to 4.92).*IIb/IIIa inhibitor not used:* high reactivity vs. normal reactivity OR=2.76 (95% CI, 1.42 to 5.36).P for interaction =0.42 [chi-square test for heterogeneity] Periprocedural MI (up to 3 d post -PCI). *IIb/IIIa inhibitor used:* high reactivity vs. normal reactivity OR=4.20 (95% CI, 1.77 to 9.93) *IIb/IIIa inhibitor not used:* high reactivity vs. normal reactivity OR=7.72 (95% CI, 4.60 to 13.04). P for interaction=0.22 [chi-square test for heterogeneity]. Death, MI, or stroke (3 d–1 yr post-PCI). *IIb/IIIa inhibitor used:* high reactivity vs. normal reactivity OR=2.97 (95% CI, 0.95 to 9.28) *IIb/IIIa inhibitor not used:* high reactivity vs. normal reactivity OR=3.59 (95% CI, 1.74 to 7.39) P for interaction=0.78 [chi-square test for heterogeneity]

Table 11. Studies reporting information on effect modification (continued)

Author Year Country PMID Study name (when available)	Patient Population	Antiplatelet Regimen	Platelet Reactivity Measurement Method (agonist) [assay and manufacturer] Threshold Definition	Effect Modifier	Summary of Findings*
El Ghannudi[224] 2011 France 21524751 NR	Patients undergoing PCI with stent placement for ACS or stable CAD	Clopidogrel (various loading doses); all patients were on aspirin treatment	VASP assay (ADP ± PGE1) [Diagnostica Stago (Biocytex), Asnieres, France] using flow cytometry

Poor response was defined as VASP PRI>61% [based on prior literature] | Diabetes mellitus (yes vs. no) | Results from univariate analyses (platelet reactivity was not a significant predictor of outcomes in nondiabetic patients and adjusted results were NR)
Diabetic patients
HR for PRI >61% vs. ≤61% for CV death=5.798 (95% CI, 1.25 to 26.86)
HR for PRI >61% vs. ≤61% for all-cause mortality=3.84 (95% CI, 1.04 to 14.23)
HR for PRI >61% vs. ≤61% for MACE=2.01 (95% CI, 0.96 to 4.23)
Non-diabetic patients
HR for PRI >61% vs. ≤61% for CV death=1.74 (95% CI, 0.43 to 7.00)
HR for PRI >61% vs. ≤61% for all-cause mortality=1.53 (95% CI, 0.47 to 5.04)
HR for PRI >61% vs. ≤61% for MACE=1.06 (95% CI, 0.55 to 2.03)

Interaction p-value [diabetic vs. nondiabetic] for CV death=0.26; for all-cause mortality=0.31; for MACE=0.20 [calculated values, chi-square test for heterogeneity] |

122

Table 11. Studies reporting information on effect modification (continued)

Author Year Country PMID Study name (when available)	Patient Population	Antiplatelet Regimen	Platelet Reactivity Measurement Method (agonist) [assay and manufacturer] Threshold Definition	Effect Modifier	Summary of Findings*
Mangiacapra[196] 2010 Multinational 20723634 NR	Patients undergoing elective PCI with stent implantation for stable angina or NSTE ACS	Pre-PCI: clopidogrel loading dose 600 mg or on-clopidogrel chronic treatment (75 mg/d for ≥5 d); post-PCI: clopidogrel maintenance (75 mg/d for ≥1 mo after BMS implantation or 12 mo after DES implantation or patients with ACS) All patients received aspirin (100 mg/d) pre-PCI and continued with the same maintenance dose indefinitely	VerifyNow P2Y12 (ADP) [Accumetrics, San Diego, CA] High platelet reactivity was defined as VerifyNow PRU >240 [based on prior literature]	Diabetes mellitus (yes vs. no)	Effect of high vs. low platelet reactivity, stratified by diabetes status (calculated values) on periprocedural MI *Diabetic patients:* OR=5.89 (95% CI, 1.46 to 23.81) *Nondiabetic patients,* OR=1.82 (95% CI, 0.44 to 7.65) Interaction p-value [diabetic vs. nondiabetic]=0.25 [chi-square test for heterogeneity]
Morel[227] 2011 France 21251579 NR	Patients undergoing PCI for stable CAD or ACS	Clopidogrel loading dose (300 or 600 mg); all patients received aspirin	VASP assay (ADP ± PGE1) [Biocytex, Diagnostica Stago, Asnieres, France] using flow cytometry Poor response was defined as VASP PRI >61% [based on prior work from the same authors]	CKD (present vs. not)	Effect of nonresponse to clopidogrel (vs. response), stratified by CKD status (calculated values) *Patients with CKD* All-cause mortality, OR=12.145 (95% CI, 2.604 to 56.647) Cardiac death, OR=10.923 (95% CI, 2.325 t0 51.314) STE MI, OR=1.449 (95% CI, 0.197 to 10.637) NSTE MI, OR=2.219 (95% CI, 0.357 to 13.780) TVR, OR=1.157 (95% CI, 0.295 to 4.538) Definite stent thrombosis, OR=1.440 (95% CI, 0.088 to 23.567) Probable stent thrombosis, OR=6.128 (95% CI, 0.664 to 56.528) Definite/probable stent thrombosis, OR=3.859 (95% CI, 0.718 to 20.730) Possible stent thrombosis, OR=17.387 (95% CI, 0.939 to 321.819) All types of stent thrombosis, OR=8.659 (95% CI, 1.808

Table 11. Studies reporting information on effect modification (continued)

Author Year Country PMID Study name (when available)	Patient Population	Antiplatelet Regimen	Platelet Reactivity Measurement Method (agonist) [assay and manufacturer] Threshold Definition	Effect Modifier	Summary of Findings*
					to 41.457) MACE, OR=3.556 (95% CI, 1.433 to 8.822) *Patients without CKD* All-cause mortality, OR=0.648 (95% CI, 0.164 to 2.557) Cardiac death, OR=0.762 (95% CI, 0.138 to 4.228) STE MI, OR=0.507 (95% CI, 0.052 to 4.930) NSTE MI, OR=1.242 (95% CI, 0.476 to 3.241) TVR, OR=1.146 (95% CI, 0.552 to 2.382) Definite stent thrombosis, OR=2.079 (95% CI, 0.457 to 9.456) Probable stent thrombosis, OR=0.764 (95% CI, 0.069 to 8.523) Definite/probable stent thrombosis, OR=1.556 (95% CI, 0.441 to 5.490) Possible stent thrombosis, OR=0.507 (95% CI, 0.021 to 12.559) All types of stent thrombosis, OR=1.289 (95% CI, 0.385 to 4.321) MACE, OR=1.026 (95% CI, 0.538 to 1.956) Interaction p-values [chi-square tests for heterogeneity], by outcome (CKD vs. no CKD) All-cause mortality, p=0.005; cardiac death, p=0.023; STE MI, p=0.495; NSTE MI, p=0.581; TVR, p=0.990; definite stent thrombosis, p=0.821; probable stent thrombosis, p=0.213; definite/probable stent thrombosis, p=0.396; possible stent thrombosis, p=0.107; all types of stent thrombosis, p=0.057; MACE, p=0.029

124

Table 11. Studies reporting information on effect modification (continued)

Author Year Country PMID Study name (when available)	Patient Population	Antiplatelet Regimen	Platelet Reactivity Measurement Method (agonist) [assay and manufacturer] Threshold Definition	Effect Modifier	Summary of Findings*
Park[211] 2011 S. Korea 22152948 NR	Patients who had undergone PCI with DES implantation for stable angina or ischemia, or NSTE-MI	Aspirin loading (200 mg) followed by maintenance therapy (100–200 mg); clopidogrel "optimal treatment" (defined as maintenance therapy with 75 mg/d for ≥5 d or a loading dose of 300 or 600 mg ≥12 h pre-PCI)	VerifyNow P2Y12 (ADP) [Accumetrics, San Diego, CA] Poor response was defined as PRU >235 or %inhibition <15% [cutoffs were chosen to be "similar" to previous studies]	CRP levels (≥3 mg/L vs. <3 mg/L)	Among patients with elevated CRP levels, high on-clopidogrel platelet reactivity was associated with increased risk for the primary outcome (MACE, defined as all-cause death, nonfatal MI, stent thrombosis, and stroke) compared to low reactivity; "these findings were not observed in patients with non-elevated CRP"; interaction p-value=0.02.
Siller-Matula[244] 2012 Austria 22305813 NR	Patients undergoing PCI with stent implantation	Loading with clopidogrel (600 mg) + aspirin (100 mg); maintenance with clopidogrel (75 mg/d) + aspirin (100 mg/d)	Multiplate analyzer (ADP) [Verum Diagnostica GmbH, Munich, Germany] Poor response was defined as reactivity ≥48U [chosen on the basis of data, to maximize the sum of sensitivity and specificity]	Diabetes (present vs. not)	For MACE (stent thrombosis, acute coronary syndrome, death, stroke, or repeat revascularization by PCI or CABG): prognostic ability of high on-clopidogrel platelet reactivity among patients with diabetes: OR=2.18 (95% CI, 1.20 to 3.95); p=0.04. Prognostic ability of high on-clopidogrel platelet reactivity among patients without diabetes: OR=1.86 (95% CI, 1.03 to 3.37); p=0.048. Interaction p=0.923

Abbreviations: ADP = adenosine diphosphate; ARU = aspirin reactivity units; BMS = bare metal stent; CAD = coronary artery disease; CI = confidence interval; CKD = chronic kidney disease; CV = cardiovascular; d = days, DES = drug eluting stent; HR = hazard ratio, LTA = light-transmission aggregometry, MACE = major adverse cardiovascular events; MI = myocardial infarction; mo=months, NR = not reported; NSTE = non–ST-elevation; OR = odds ratio; PCI = percutaneous coronary intervention; PGE1 = prostaglandin E1, PRI = platelet reactivity index, PRU = platelet reactivity units, STE = ST-elevation; TVR = target-vessel revascularization; UA = unstable angina, VASP = vasodilator-stimulated phosphoprotein; yr = years.

*The description "calculated values" indicates that the results are based on statistical procedures we conducted in cases where studies provided sufficient statistics for the assessment of effect modification but did not assess its statistical significance.

†Information from the randomized comparison has been reviewed in the section of this report relevant to Key Question 3.

3T/2R = Tailoring Treatment with Tirofiban in patients showing Resistance to aspirin and/or Resistance to clopidogrel; AA = arachidonic acid; ACS = acute coronary syndromes;

125

Effect Modification Across Studies

On the basis of our protocol and the availability of data from studies considered eligible for Key Question 2b, we assessed the following characteristics as potential modifiers of the predictive effect of platelet reactivity by performing comparisons across studies using subgroup analysis: disease subtype (acute coronary syndromes vs. mixed coronary artery disease populations), setting of care (PCI vs. other), duration of followup (≤30 days vs. >30 days); and year when enrollment was started (continuous variable). For setting of care (PCI versus not) there was no variability across studies (all were conducted in the setting of interventional procedures); as such no meta-analysis was performed. Meta-regressions were performed only for one outcome (MACE) reported in more than 10 studies and for high versus low reactivity measured with the VerifyNow assay (all other assays had less than 10 studies considered sufficiently similar for meta-analysis for all outcomes assessed). Table 12 summarizes the findings of our meta-regression analyses.

Table 12. Meta-regression results for study-level effect modifiers of the predictive value of phenotypic testing for platelet reactivity using the VerifyNow P2Y12 assays in patients with ischemic heart disease: major adverse cardiovascular events

Effect Modifier	Groups Compared	No. of Studies	RR (95% CI) Within Subgroup	rRR (95% CI); P-Value
All studies	NA	13	2.48 (1.86 to 3.32)	NA
ACS vs. ischemic heart disease	Other ischemic heart disease or mixed	8	2.10 (1.55 to 2.86)	1.86 (0.99 to 3.52); 0.055
	ACS	5	3.68 (2.26 to 6.00)	
Duration of followup	>30 d	11	2.29 (1.72 to 3.05)	2.63 (0.83 to 8.32); 0.101
	≤30 d	2	6.03 (2.13 to 17.10)	
Enrollment start year	(continuous variable)	12	NA	1.06 (0.82 to 1.38); 0.649

Abbreviations: ACS = acute coronary syndromes; CI = confidence interval; d = days; NA = not applicable; RR = relative risk; rRR = relative RR (between groups).
Results across all studies are provided for comparison. One study did not report the year of start of enrollment.

Taken together, analyses of effect modification within-studies and across studies did not provide sufficient evidence that any factor substantially modifies the predictive effect of platelet reactivity.

Key Questions 3a and 3b Regarding Alternative Testing Strategies

The overarching question of the impact of testing (genetic or phenotypic) on outcomes can be answered by comparative studies of alternative test-and treat strategies. Direct comparisons of testing strategies, particularly those in which assignment to a specific test-based strategy is random, are generally very rare. However, other study designs can provide information on the clinical utility of the tests of interest to this review. We grouped the studies we identified for this Key Question into three categories:

1. *Randomized trials of test-and-treat strategies*: These studies randomize patients to alternative management strategies, at least one of which is based on a test of interest. Patients are then followed up for intermediate or clinical outcomes. Random treatment assignment provides an unconfounded estimate of the effect of test-based management compared to alternative therapeutic strategies on outcomes.

2. *Randomized treatment trials that evaluate treatment-effect modification:* These are randomized studies in which patients in all groups undergo the test of interest at baseline. Treatment assignment is based on randomization and thus is independent of test results. Because these studies include both test-positive and test-negative patients in each treatment arm, they can be used to assess test result × treatment interactions. The presence of an interaction effect indicates that the relative treatment benefits (or harms) differ by test status; the results can also be used to infer whether improved outcomes should be expected if treatment choice were guided by test results.
3. *Randomized trials with test-based selection:* These studies select patients on the basis of baseline test results and then randomize them into non–test-based treatment groups. When properly randomized and conducted, these studies can provide unconfounded estimates of the treatment effect conditional on a particular test result but do not provide information on whether the treatment effect is modified by the test results.

Key Question 3 focused on efficacy outcomes (platelet reactivity as an intermediate marker of response and patient-relevant clinical outcomes). Information on harms is summarized later in the Results section, under Key Question 4. In the following sections, we discuss studies belonging to each of three designs—studies of test-and-treat strategies, studies of treatment-effect modification, and studies with test-based selection—separately for genetic testing (CYP2C19 variants) and for phenotypic testing (platelet reactivity). Table 13 summarizes the number of studies and outcomes assessed for each of the designs we reviewed for Key Question 3.

Table 13. Number of studies relevant to Key Question 3a or 3b and outcomes assessed, by study design and test used

Study Design	Genetic Testing for CYP2C19 Variants	Phenotypic Testing for Platelet Reactivity
***Comparative studies of test-and-treat strategies* (testing vs. no testing or comparisons between alternative test-and-treat strategies)**	1 RCT (clinical and intermediate outcomes)	6 RCTs + 1 NRCS (4 for clinical outcomes; 3 both for clinical and intermediate outcomes)
***RCTs of treatment-effect modification by test results* (difference in treatment effects across levels of the biomarkers)**	12 (5 for clinical outcomes; 6 for intermediate outcomes; 1 for both)	3 (1 for clinical outcomes; 2 for intermediate outcomes)
***RCTs with test-based selection* (comparison of treatments among patients selected on the basis of biomarker level)**	1 (clinical and intermediate outcomes)	14 (4 for clinical outcomes only; 4 for intermediate outcomes only; 6 for both)

Abbreviations: NRCS = nonrandomized comparative study; RCT = randomized controlled trial.

Key Question 3a. What is the comparative effectiveness of genetic testing for CYP2C19 variants and phenotypic testing for platelet reactivity for therapeutic decisionmaking?

Genetic Testing for CYP2C19 Variants

Study of Test-and-Treat Strategies
We identified a single-center, "pilot study" (as described by the authors) comparing a strategy of testing for CYP2C19 variants versus no testing strategy to guide treatment decisionmaking in a predominantly white population (95 percent). Table 14 summarizes

information on the comparators and patient population of the study; Table 15 summarizes information on the design of the trial; and Table 16 summarizes test-related information. Of note, the trial used a point-of-care genotyping assay (Spartan RX CYP2C19) to obtain genotyping results for the CYP2C19 *2 allele rapidly (within ~1 hour after sampling).

Table 14. Descriptive characteristics of studies of test-and-treat strategies using genetic testing of CYP2C19 variants

Author Year Country PMID Study Name (if available)	Selected Population	Total N Enrolled Male (%) Age* Dyslipidemia (%) Current smokers (%) HTN (%) Diabetes (%)	Initial and Compared Treatment Strategies
Roberts[86] 2012 Canada 22464343 RAPID-GENE	Adult patients undergoing PCI for the treatment of NSTE-ACS or stable CAD; patients who had been administered antiplatelet treatment other than aspirin + clopidogrel, or anticoagulation, were excluded	N=200 (187 with complete followup) 146 (78%) 60 (9) 152 (81%) 58 (31%) 119 (64%) 39 (21%)	All patients were treated with a loading dose of clopidogrel (600 mg) ≥24 h pre-PCI; adjuvant pharmacotherapy during PCI was restricted to bivalirudin. Patients were then randomized to 1 of 2 treatment strategies: *CYP2C19 genotyping-guided treatment:* Genotyping was performed for identifying *2 carrier status at the time of randomization. Carriers of the *2 allele (i.e., *2/*1 and *2/*2) were given prasugrel 10 mg/d, with the first dose immediately after PCI. Non-carriers received clopidogrel 75 mg/d. *Control treatment:* maintenance clopidogrel (75 mg/d)

Abbreviations: ACS = acute coronary syndrome; CAD = coronary artery disease; d = day; HTN = hypertension; NSTE = non-ST elevation; PCI = percutaneous coronary intervention.
*Mean (standard deviation), unless otherwise stated.

Table 15. Study design characteristics of studies of test-and-treat strategies using genetic testing of CYP2C19 variants

Author Year Country PMID Study Name (if available)	Enrollment period	Randomization Procedure	Blinding	Number of Participating Centers	Followup Duration	Setting	Target Enrollment from a priori power analysis	Procedure for Multiple Comparisons	Funding
Roberts[86] 2012 Canada 22464343 RAPID-GENE	August 2012 – July 2011	Randomization sequence was computer generated and blocked in randomly selected block sizes of 4 and 6; patients were allocated to trial groups using opaque, serially numbered, sealed envelopes.	Interventional cardiologists and data analysts were masked to genetic carrier status and subsequent treatment for the duration of the study. Patients were not masked to treatment allocation.	Single center	For pharmacodynamics outcomes 7 d; for clinical outcomes 30 d	Cardiology institute of university hospital	Targeted 200; enrolled 200; analyzed 187 [powered to detect a difference in the treatment effect among *2 carriers]	Not used	Industry only (manufacturer of genotyping assay)

Abbreviation: d = days.

129

Table 16. Test information in studies of test-and-treat strategies using genetic testing of CYP2C19 variants

Author Year Country PMID Study Name (if available)	Assay for Genetic Testing (Manufacturer)	Test Time Point Interval Between Sampling and Genotyping Results Interval Between Collection and DNA Extraction	N Tested Test Success Rate (%)	Alleles Genotyped	Genotype Grouping	Rationale for Grouping Alleles
Roberts[86] 2012 Canada 22464343 RAPID-GENE	Spartan RX CYP2C19 point-of-care testing device; please see the section on Key Question 1a for additional information on analytic validity from this trial (Spartan Biosciences, Ottawa, ON, Canada)	All patients were tested "at the time of randomization" Acquisition of samples and initiation of analysis = 8 min; *2 genotyping results within 60 min of activation	200 patients were tested Results were obtained from all patients; erroneous results (as compared to sequencing) were obtained in 1 patient (misclassified as carrier)	*2 [rs4244285]	Carriers=*2/*2 or *2/*1 or *3/*3 Non-carriers=*1/*1	Unclear

Abbreviation: min = minutes.

130

Clinical Outcomes

The study reported monitoring the following clinical outcomes: a composite outcome of cardiovascular death, non-fatal myocardial infarction, readmission to hospital, and stent thrombosis. Twenty-three of 91 patients (25 percent) assigned to the rapid genotyping group were CYP2C19 *2 carriers (4 were homozygotes); 23 of 96 (24 percent) in the standard therapy group were CYP2C19 *2 carriers (3 were homozygotes). No clinical adverse ischemic outcomes were observed in either group, at 7 or 30 days of followup.

Intermediate Outcome: Platelet Reactivity During Followup

Intermediate outcomes were assessed with the VerifyNow P2Y12 assay (Accumetrics, San Diego, CA). The primary study endpoint was the proportion of CYP2C19*2 carriers with a P2Y12 reactivity value of more than 234 units (PRU) after 1 week of dual antiplatelet therapy. The cut-off for high reactivity was derived from previous published studies. All patients underwent platelet-function testing immediately after PCI and at 7 days after randomization. Table 17 summarizes the key findings regarding intermediate outcomes.

Table 17. Summary of intermediate outcomes in studies of test-and-treat strategies using genetic testing of CYP2C19 variants

Author Year Country PMID Study Name (if available)	Treatment Groups (sample size)	Followup Duration	Summary of Findings
Roberts[86] 2012 Canada 22464343 RAPID-GENE	*CYP2C19 genotyping-guided treatment:* prasugrel for *2 carriers; clopidogrel for non-carriers (102 randomized; 91 included in analyses; 23 of whom were *2 carriers) *Control treatment:* clopidogrel (98 randomized; 96 included in analyses; 23 of whom were *2 carriers)	1 wk after randomization	*Among *2 carriers only* Proportion with high on-treatment platelet reactivity (PRU >234) = 0% in the genotyping-guided group vs. 30% in the control treatment group (p=0.009) Proportion with high on-treatment platelet reactivity (PRU >208) = 1% in the genotyping-guided group vs. 48% in the control treatment group (p=0.002) Change in PRU from baseline to d 7 among *2 carriers in the genotyping-guided group=-123.09 (SD=77.2) vs. -8.48 (SD=74.0) in the control treatment group (p<0.001) Platelet inhibition = 73.3% (SD=20.3) in the genotyping-guided group vs. 27.0% (SD=13.4) in the control treatment group (p<0.001) *In the whole trial population* Proportion with high on-treatment platelet reactivity (PRU >234) = 10% in the genotyping-guided group vs. 17% in the control treatment group (p=0.067) Proportion with high on-treatment platelet reactivity (PRU >208) = 15% in the genotyping-guided group vs. 31% in the control treatment group (p<0.001) Platelet inhibition = 56.5% (SD=24.5) in the genotyping-guided group vs. 43.9% (SD=22.9) in the control treatment group (p<0.001)

Abbreviations: PRU = platelet reactivity unit; SD = standard deviation; wk = week.

Assessment of Risk of Bias of the Study

A detailed assessment of risk of bias for this trial is presented in Appendix F. Briefly, this was a well-conducted, single-center, pilot study that was based on an a priori power analysis and met its accrual target. Although approximately 6.5 percent of enrolled patients were excluded from the analyses, the reasons for exclusion do not appear to have introduced bias. The procedure for generating the randomized sequence was appropriate for obtaining random allocation of participants. Interventional cardiologists and data analysts were masked to genotype information and treatment assignment; however, patients were not masked to treatment allocation. Statistical analyses were preplanned and results (summarized above) were reported in adequate detail, for all pre-specified outcomes (both primary and secondary).

Randomized Trials Reporting Information on Treatment-Effect Modification by CYP2C19 Genotype Status

We identified 12 studies (reported in 13 publications) describing randomized controlled trials that provide information on effect modification by CYP2C19 variants. Six studies (reported in seven publications)[h] provided information on clinical outcomes, five on intermediate outcomes (platelet reactivity during followup), and one on both types of outcome.

Information on the genetic assays used, the specific variants genotyped, and the grouping of genotypes for analysis is presented Table 18 for all studies of treatment-effect modification by CYP2C19 variants. In most cases, authors claimed to have based the classification of genotypes on prior published literature; however, studies genotyped different variants, resulting in heterogeneous exposure groupings.

---

[h]Three publications reported information on a single population each, and one publication reported information on two independent populations.

Table 18. Test information for studies of treatment-effect modification by CYP2C19 genotype status

Author Year Country PMID Study Name (if available)	Assay for Genetic Testing (Manufacturer)	Test Time Point		N Tested Test Success Rate (%)	Alleles Genotyped	Genotype Grouping	Rationale for Grouping Alleles
		Interval Between Sampling and Genotyping Results	Interval Between Collection and DNA Extraction				
Pare[109] 2010 Multinational 20979470 ACTIVE A	TaqMan assays [no additional information provided]	NR NR NR		Not estimable (data presented only on the successfully genotyped patients)	*2 [rs4244285]; *3 [rs4986893]; *4 [rs12248560]	Poor metabolizers=*2/*2 or *2/*3 or *3/*3 Intermediate metabolizers=*2/*1 or *3/*1 Extensive metabolizers=*1/*1 Ultra metabolizers=*17/*1 or *17/*17 Unknown metabolizers=*2/*17 or *3/*17	Based on prior literature; however, results from an alternative classification were presented as Appendix material
Pare[109] 2010 Multinational 20979470 CURE	TaqMan assays [no additional information provided]	NR NR NR		Not estimable (data presented only on the successfully genotyped patients)	*2 [rs4244285]; *3 [rs4986893]; *4 [rs12248560]	Poor metabolizers=*2/*2 or *2/*3 or *3/*3 Intermediate metabolizers=*2/*1 or *3/*1 Extensive metabolizers=*1/*1 Ultra metabolizers=*17/*1 or *17/*17 Unknown=*2/*17 or 3/*17	Based on prior literature; however, results from an alternative classification were presented as Appendix material

Table 18. Test information for studies of treatment-effect modification by CYP2C19 genotype status (continued)

Author Year Country PMID Study Name (if available)	Assay for Genetic Testing (Manufacturer)	Test Time Point / Interval Between Sampling and Genotyping Results / Interval Between Collection and DNA Extraction	N Tested / Test Success Rate (%)	Alleles Genotyped	Genotype Grouping	Rationale for Grouping Alleles
Mega[99,258] 2009 Multinational 19106084 19414633 TRITON-TIMI 38	98% of the genotyping procedures were performed with the Targeted Human DMET 1.0 Assay [Affymetrix, no additional details provided]; for the *17 allele and for no-call samples on the DMET chip (2% of samples) genotyping was performed with bi-directional sequencing or exon-specific PCR	NR NR NR	Not estimable (data presented only on the successfully genotyped patients)	*1A, *2A, *3, *4, *5A, *6, *7, *8, *9, *10, *12, *13, *14	Noncarriers=*1A/*1A Carriers=*1/*2A, *1A/*3, *1A/*4, *1A/*8, *2A/*2A, *2A/*3, *2A/*4, *2A/*5A, *2A/*8 Unknown=*1A/*9, *1A/*10, *2A/*17, *6/*17	Based on prior literature
Mega[259] 2010 Multinational 20801494 TRITON-TIMI 38	Detailed information not provided in the paper however the study by Mega et al. 2009[99] (see above row) was cited for the genotyping methods and grouping of genotypes.	NR NR NR	Not estimable (data presented only on the successfully genotyped patients)	For CYP2C19: as above In addition, genotyping was performed for ABCB1 C3435T (rs1045642) and results by combining both tests were reported	For CYP2C19: as above For ABCB1 C3435T: TT carriers vs. CC or CT carriers† Combined results were presented by grouping patients with CYP2C19 reduced-function alleles and ABCB1 TT carriers vs. CYP2C19 loss-of-function allele noncarriers and ABCB1 CC/CT carriers†	Based on prior literature

134

Table 18. Test information for studies of treatment-effect modification by CYP2C19 genotype status (continued)

Author Year Country PMID Study Name (if available)	Assay for Genetic Testing (Manufacturer)	Test Time Point Interval Between Sampling and Genotyping Results Interval Between Collection and DNA Extraction	N Tested Test Success Rate (%)	Alleles Genotyped	Genotype Grouping	Rationale for Grouping Alleles
Kim[260] 2011 S. Korea 21511217 ACCELAMI2C19	Single base primer extension assay (SNaPshot kit, Applied Biosystems, Foster City, CA) on the ABI 3100 genetic analyzer (Applied Biosystems, Foster City, CA)	NR NR NR	140 MI patients were identified; CYP2C19 genotype could be determined in 126 (88.6%)	*2 [rs4244285]; *3 [rs4986893]	Carriers=*2/*1 or *3/*1 or *3/*3 Noncarriers=*1/*1	Not explicitly reported
Wallentin[104] 2010 Multinational 20801498 PLATO	TaqMan assays [Applied Biosystems, Life Technologies, Pleasanton CA]	Blood samples were obtained "as close to [time of] randomization as possible" NR NR	10,285 98.8–99.5%	CYP2C19*1–*8, *17 In addition, genotyping was performed for ABCB1 C3435T (rs1045642) and results by combining both tests were reported	For CYP2C19: Any LOF allele (*2–*8) No LOF allele (*1 or *17) For major bleeding only: Any LOF allele (*2–*8) but no GOF allele (not *17) No LOF or GOF allele (*1) Any GOF allele (*17) For ABCB1 C3435T:† High expression (C/C) Intermediate expression (C/T) Low expression (T/T) Combined results were presented by grouping patients with any CYP2C19 loss-of-function allele and ABCB1 TT carriers vs. all other patients	Based on prior literature

135

Table 18. Test information for studies of treatment-effect modification by CYP2C19 genotype status (continued)

Author Year Country PMID Study Name (if available)	Assay for Genetic Testing (Manufacturer)	Test Time Point / Interval Between Sampling and Genotyping Results / Interval Between Collection and DNA Extraction	N Tested	Test Success Rate (%)	Alleles Genotyped	Genotype Grouping	Rationale for Grouping Alleles
Varenhorst[261] 2009 Sweden 19429918 TABR	Targeted Human DMET 1.0 Assay (Affymetrix, Santa Clara, CA) for all alleles except *17; *17 was genotyped using PCR-RFLP methods	NR NR NR	For CYP2C19 variants: 98 (100% success rate)		*1A, *2A, *3, *4, *5A, *6, *7, *8, *9, *10, *12, *13, *14, *17	Extensive metabolizers=*17/*17, *1A/*17, *1A/*1A Reduced metabolizers=*1A/*2A, *1A/*8, *2A/*2A Uncertain functional status=*2A/*17	Based on prior literature
Tantry[262] 2010 USA and UK 21079055 ONSET/OFFSET and RESPOND Genotype Studies	TaqMan Assay (Life Technologies, Pleasanton, CA)	NR NR NR	NR (results reported only on successfully genotyped individuals)		*2 [rs4244285]; *3 [rs4986893]; *4 [rs28399504]; *5 [rs56337013]; *6 [rs72558184]; *7 [rs72558186]; *8 [rs41291556]; *17 [rs12248560]	3 genotype grouping schemes were used: *Grouping 1* Ultra metabolizers=*17/*17 or *17/*1 Extensive metabolizers=*1/*1 Intermediate metabolizers=*2-*8/*1 or *2-*8/*17 Poor metabolizers=*2-*8/*2-*8 *Grouping 2* Loss-of-function carriers=*2-*8/*1 or *2-*8/*17 or *2-*8/*2-*8 Loss-of-function noncarriers=*1/*1 or *17/*17 or *17/*1 *Grouping 3* Gain-of-function carriers=*17/*17 or *17/*1 Extensive metabolizers=*1/*1 Loss-of-function carriers=*2-*8/*1 or *2-*8/*17 or *2-*8/*2-*8 Results were also presented separately for the observed diplotypes.	Not explicitly reported

136

Table 18. Test information for studies of treatment-effect modification by CYP2C19 genotype status (continued)

Author Year Country PMID Study Name (if available)	Assay for Genetic Testing (Manufacturer)	Test Time Point; Interval Between Sampling and Genotyping Results; Interval Between Collection and DNA Extraction	N Tested; Test Success Rate (%)	Alleles Genotyped	Genotype Grouping	Rationale for Grouping Alleles
Hwang[263] 2010 S. Korea 20823393 ACCEL-RESISTANCE, DM, and COMPLEX trials	Single base primer extension assay (SNaPshot kit, Applied Biosystems, Foster City, CA) on the ABI 3100 genetic analyzer (Applied Biosystems, Foster City, CA)	NR NR NR	140 patients undergoing PCI in the 3 RCTs were identified; CYP2C19 genotype could be determined in 114 (76%)	*2 [rs4244285]; *3 [rs4986893]	Carriers=*2/*1 or *3/*1 or *3/*3 Noncarriers=*1/*1	Not explicitly reported (however the authors cite a previous study from the same center)
Gladding[191] 2008 New Zealand 19463375 PRINC	TaqMan assay (Applied Biosystems, Foster City, CA) on ABI PRISM 7000 Sequence Detection System (Applied Biosystems, Foster City, CA)	NR NR NR	60 patients participating in the PRINC study; analyses relevant to this KQ only included 43 patients (the genotyping success rate was not estimable)	*2 [rs4244285]; *4 [rs28399504]; *17 [rs12248560]; results on the *17 variant allele were not reported in analyses relevant to this KQ	Carriers=*2/*2 or *2/*4 or *4/*4 or *2/*1 or *4/*1 Noncarriers=*1/*1	Not explicitly reported (results relevant to this KQ were not reported for all genotyped alleles)
Park[264] 2011 S. Korea 21345843 CILON-T	TaqMan fluorogenic 5' nuclease assay (ABI, Foster City, CA) for *2 and *3 SNaPshot multiplex kit (ABI PRISM) for *17	NR NR NR	483 (successful in 474/483=98.1%) [in 5 patients, the DNA amount was not enough to carry out the genotyping of all 3 SNPs, and genotyping of *2 failed in 3 patients and of *3 in 1 patient]	CYP2C19*2 [rs4244285]; *3 [rs4986893]; *17 [rs12248560]	Carriers of CYP2C19 LOF allele (*2 or *3 with any other allele) Noncarriers (*1/*1, *17/*17, or *1/*17)	NR

137

Table 18. Test information for studies of treatment-effect modification by CYP2C19 genotype status (continued)

Author Year Country PMID Study Name (if available)	Assay for Genetic Testing (Manufacturer)	Test Time Point / Interval Between Sampling and Genotyping Results / Interval Between Collection and DNA Extraction	N Tested / Test Success Rate (%)	Alleles Genotyped	Genotype Grouping	Rationale for Grouping Alleles
Bhatt[85] 2012 Multinational 22450429 CHARISMA	PCR-RFLP for *2 and *17 [no additional details reported]; TaqMan allelic discrimination assay for *3	NR NR NR	4924 samples were collected; 4862 had adequate DNA for analysis of which 4819 had "defined ancestry;" 4537 patients comprised the study population in main analysi	CYP2C19*2 [rs4244285]; *3 [rs4986893]; *17 [rs12248560 and rs11188072]	Poor metabolizers=*2/*2 or *2/*3 or *3/*3 Intermediate metabolizers=*2/*1 or *3/*1 Extensive metabolizers=*1/*1 Ultra metabolizers=*17/*1 or *17/*17 Unknown metabolizers=*2/*17 or *3/*17	NR; results are presented for alternative classifications
Collet[265] 2011 France 21511218 CLOVIS-2	TaqMan Validated SNP assays (900HT sequence Detection System; Applied Biosystems, Courtaboeuf, France)	NR NR NR	43 heterozygous carriers were matched 1:1 with 43 wild-type homozygous patients; 8 homozygous carriers were matched 1:2 ratio with 16 wild-type homozygous patients (110 randomized patients); 106 patients completed both periods of the crossover study	*2, *3, *4, *5, *6 No *3, *5, or *6 alleles were detected in the sample	Carriers=*2/*1 or *2/*2 Noncarriers=*1/*1	NR

Abbreviations: CURE = Clopidogrel in Unstable Angina to Prevent Recurrent Events; DM = diabetes mellitus; DMET = Drug Metabolizing Enzyme and Transporter; KQ = Key Question; NR = not reported; ONSET/OFFSET and RESPOND; PCI = percutaneous coronary intervention; PCR = polymerase chain reaction; PLATO = Platelet Inhibition and Patient Outcomes; PRINC = Plavix Response in Coronary Intervention; RCT = randomized controlled trial; RFLP = restriction fragment length polymorphism; TRITON-TIMI 38 = Trial to Assess Improvement in Therapeutic Outcomes by Optimizing Platelet Inhibition With Prasugrel–Thrombolysis in Myocardial Infarction 38; UK = United Kingdom.
†ABCB1 is a gene that encodes a protein involved in the intestinal absorption of clopidogrel.[266]

Clinical Outcomes

Of the six studies (reported in seven publications) providing clinical outcome information, five[85,99,104,109,258] were large (>1000 participants), multicenter, randomized trials of clopidogrel-based treatment versus alternative treatments (three compared aspirin plus clopidogrel vs. aspirin monotherapy, one compared aspirin plus clopidogrel vs. aspirin plus prasugrel, and one compared aspirin plus clopidogrel vs. aspirin plus ticagrelor); each of these had at least one outcome event. The sixth study[260] was a small (126 patients) short-duration (30 days) trial comparing dual-antiplatelet therapy (aspirin plus clopidogrel) versus triple antiplatelet therapy (aspirin, clopidogrel, and cilostazol) for patients with myocardial infarction treated with "uneventful PCI." Because of the short followup period and small sample size, no clinical events were observed in this study.

Of the five larger studies, one included patients with non–ST-elevation acute coronary syndromes (the CURE [Clopidogrel in Unstable Angina to Prevent Recurrent Events] trial), one involved patients with ST-elevation or non–ST-elevation acute coronary syndromes (the PLATO [Platelet inhibition and patient Outcomes] trial), one included those with moderate-to-high-risk acute coronary syndromes who were undergoing PCI (TRITON-TIMI 38 [Trial to Assess Improvement in Therapeutic Outcomes by Optimizing Platelet Inhibition with Prasugrel–Thrombolysis in Myocardial Infarction 38]), one included a mixed population of patients with manifest thrombotic disease (coronary, cerebrovascular, and peripheral artery disease) along with individuals at high risk for developing atherothrombotic disease (CHARISMA [Clopidogrel for High Atherothrombotic Risk and Ischemic Stabilization, Management and Avoidance] trial), and one enrolled patients with atrial fibrillation who were not candidates for vitamin K antagonist therapy (ACTIVE A).

CURE, CHARISMA, and ACTIVE A compared aspirin plus clopidogrel (at standard doses) with aspirin monotherapy; TRITON-TIMI 38 compared aspirin plus clopidogrel versus aspirin plus prasugrel; and the PLATO trial compared aspirin plus clopidogrel versus aspirin plus ticagrelor. All trials were designed and powered to detect the main effect of antiplatelet therapies but were not specifically powered to detect heterogeneity of treatment effects and included only a subsample of the overall study population in the genetic substudy. Furthermore, these studies were conducted in predominantly or exclusively white populations (>90 percent in all cases), who have a relatively low prevalence of CYP2C19 loss-of-function alleles, possibly limiting the applicability of the findings to non-white individuals. Perhaps more importantly, the relatively low prevalence of loss-of-function alleles in white populations limits the studies' power to detect associations of small or moderate magnitude, particularly under a recessive genetic model.

The genetic substudy of the CURE trial (of patients with non–ST-elevation acute coronary syndromes) reported treatment-effect estimates (for dual-antiplatelet therapy vs. aspirin monotherapy) among poor, intermediate, extensive, and ultra-metabolizers, as well as patients with genotypes of unknown functional status.[109] (See Table 13 for definitions of genotype groups as implemented in the study.) Detailed results from time-to-event analyses for the two primary composite outcomes assessed in the study (cardiovascular death, nonfatal myocardial infarction, or stroke; and cardiovascular death, nonfatal myocardial infarction, stroke, recurrent ischemia, or hospitalization for unstable angina) are presented in Table 14. Overall, there was no statistically significant heterogeneity of treatment effects across genotype groups (p=0.12 and p=0.29 for the first and second composite outcomes, respectively) when patients were grouped into five genotype-defined categories (poor, intermediate, extensive, ultra, or unknown status). However, an analysis assessing effect modification between gain-of-function carrier status under a dominant model (i.e., one or two *17 alleles vs. none) and treatment (clopidogrel plus aspirin vs. aspirin monotherapy) produced a statistically significant result, such that *17 carriers had a larger reduction in cardiovascular events with clopidogrel, as compared with placebo, than did non-carriers (p=0.02 and p=0.03 for the first and second composite outcomes, respectively).

The genetic substudy of TRITON-TIMI 38 enrolled patients with moderate-to-high–risk acute coronary syndromes who underwent PCI.[99] The substudy reported treatment-effect estimates (for clopidogrel plus aspirin vs. prasugrel plus aspirin) among carriers and noncarriers of reduced-function CY2C19 alleles (see Table 13 for definitions of genotype groups as implemented in the study). Detailed results on the study's primary efficacy endpoint (a composite of cardiovascular death, myocardial infarction, or stroke) at 15 months of followup are presented in Table 14. The study reported that there was statistically significant treatment-effect heterogeneity among genotype groups (p=0.046). Using the events reported in the study, we calculated that the odds ratio for the primary efficacy outcome among carriers of reduced-function alleles was 1.45 (95% CI 0.91, 2.31), compared with 0.81 (95% CI 0.60, 1.10) among noncarriers (p=0.04 for the difference between estimates). These results suggest that there was statistically significant treatment-effect heterogeneity between carriers and noncarriers in this study. The combined grouping of CYP2C19 and ABCB1[i] genotypes was a statistically significant predictor of outcomes among patients receiving clopidogrel-based therapy (p=0.0018) but not among patients receiving prasugrel-based therapy (p=0.485). The study did not report results of a test of interaction between treatment and genotype groups defined jointly by CYP2C19 and ABCB1 status.

The genetic substudy of the PLATO trial enrolled patients with acute coronary syndromes.[118] The substudy reported treatment-effect estimates (for clopidogrel plus aspirin vs. ticagrelor plus aspirin) among carriers and noncarriers of loss-of-function CY2C19 alleles (see Table 18 for definitions of genotype groups as implemented in the study). Detailed results on the study's primary efficacy endpoint (a composite of cardiovascular death, myocardial infarction, or stroke) at 12 months of followup are presented in Table 19; there was no statistically significant treatment-effect heterogeneity between carriers of any loss-of-function allele and those without a loss-of-function allele (p=0.46). Neither were the results statistically significant for subcomponents of the primary outcome (cardiovascular death or myocardial infarction; interaction p=0.30). For definite stent thrombosis, the study did not provide an interaction p-value (because the number of events was too low); however, the treatment effect was similar in both genotype groups (same direction and magnitude; assuming normality for the log hazard ratio of each group defined by genotype, we calculated a z-score p-value of 0.76 for the relative hazard ratio). In addition, the combined grouping of CYP2C19 and ABCB1 genotypes did not yield a statistically significant interaction for the primary outcome between treatment group and genotype group (p=0.13).

The genetic substudy of the CHARISMA trial enrolled patients with known atherothrombotic disease (including coronary, cerebrovascular, and peripheral artery disease), along with individuals at high risk for developing atherothrombotic disease.[85] Patients were randomized to receive clopidogrel plus aspirin or aspirin plus placebo. Results from time-to-event analyses were reported for the treatment effect among poor, intermediate, extensive, and ultra-metabolizers, as well as patients with genotypes of unknown functional status (see Table 18 for definitions of genotype groups as implemented in the study). Detailed results regarding the

---

[i] ABCB1 is a gene that encodes a protein involved in the intestinal absorption of clopidogrel.[266]

primary composite outcome of myocardial infarction (non-fatal or fatal), stroke (non-fatal or fatal), or cardiovascular death are presented in Table 19. Overall, there was no significant heterogeneity of treatment effects across genotype groups (p=0.21). Similar results were obtained for the secondary outcome (p=0.55; for the composite outcome of myocardial infarction (non-fatal or fatal), stroke (non-fatal or fatal), cardiovascular death, hospitalization for unstable angina, transient ischemic attack, or revascularization procedure).

Finally, the genetic substudy of the ACTIVE A trial enrolled patients with atrial fibrillation and at least one additional risk factor for stroke who were not considered appropriate candidates for vitamin K–antagonist therapy. Patients were randomized to aspirin monotherapy or dual-antiplatelet therapy with aspirin and clopidogrel. Results from time-to-event analyses were reported for the treatment effect among poor, intermediate, extensive, and ultra-metabolizers, as well as patients with genotypes of unknown functional status (see Table 18 for definitions of genotype groups as implemented in the study). Detailed results regarding the composite outcome of any major vascular event (stroke, systemic embolism outside the central nervous system, myocardial infarction, or death from vascular causes) are presented in Table 19. Overall, there was no significant heterogeneity of treatment effects across genotype groups (p=0.32).

Table 19. Clinical outcomes in studies of treatment-effect modification by CYP2C19 genotype status

Author Year Country PMID Study name (if available)	Outcome Definition (timing)	Subgroup defined by genotype	Treatment group	Number with outcome/total number within phenotype-treatment group	Comparison between treatments, within genotype groups ES (95% CI); p-value [statistical test]	Comparison of treatment effects across genotype groups
Pare[109]* 2010 Multinational 20979470 CURE	First primary composite outcome=CV death, nonfatal MI, or stroke	Poor metabolizers	Dual antiplatelet therapy	4/61	HR=0.44 (95% CI, 0.12 to 1.61) [Cox proportional hazards model; adjusted for age, sex, ancestry]	p=0.12
			Aspirin monotherapy	6/55		
		Intermediate metabolizers	Dual antiplatelet therapy	37/437	HR=0.72 (95% CI, 0.48 to 1.10) [Cox proportional hazards model; adjusted for age, sex, ancestry]	
			Aspirin monotherapy	54/442		
		Extensive metabolizers	Dual antiplatelet therapy	112/1033	HR=0.92 (95% CI, 0.71 to 1.19) [Cox proportional hazards model; adjusted for age, sex, ancestry]	
			Aspirin monotherapy	121/987		
		Ultra metabolizers	Dual antiplatelet therapy	66/847	HR=0.53 (95% CI, 0.39 to 0.72) [Cox proportional hazards model; adjusted for age, sex, ancestry]	
			Aspirin monotherapy	112/826		
		Unknown metabolizers	Dual antiplatelet therapy	11/152	HR=0.69 (95% CI, 0.33 to 1.47) [Cox proportional hazards model; adjusted for age, sex, ancestry]	
			Aspirin monotherapy	18/176		

142

Table 19. Clinical outcomes in studies of treatment-effect modification by CYP2C19 genotype status (continued)

Author Year Country PMID Study name (if available)	Outcome Definition (timing)	Subgroup defined by genotype	Treatment group	Number with outcome/total number within phenotype-treatment group	Comparison between treatments, within genotype groups ES (95% CI); p-value [statistical test]	Comparison of treatment effects across genotype groups
	Second primary composite outcome=CV death, nonfatal MI, or stroke, recurrent ischemia, or hospitalization for UA	Poor metabolizers	Dual antiplatelet therapy	13/61	HR=0.93 (95% CI, 0.41 to 2.11) [Cox proportional hazards model; adjusted for age, sex, ancestry]	p=0.29
			Aspirin monotherapy	11/55		
		Intermediate metabolizers	Dual antiplatelet therapy	70/437	HR=0.87 (95% CI, 0.63 to 1.19) [Cox proportional hazards model; adjusted for age, sex, ancestry]	
			Aspirin monotherapy	84/442		
		Extensive metabolizers	Dual antiplatelet therapy	193/1033	HR=0.90 (95% CI, 0.74 to 1.10) [Cox proportional hazards model; adjusted for age, sex, ancestry]	
			Aspirin monotherapy	206/987		
		Ultra metabolizers	Dual antiplatelet therapy	123/847	HR=0.68 (95% CI, 0.53 to 0.85) [Cox proportional hazards model; adjusted for age, sex, ancestry]	
			Aspirin monotherapy	167/826		
		Unknown metabolizers	Dual antiplatelet therapy	19/152	HR=0.63 (95% CI, 0.36 to 1.11) [Cox proportional hazards model; adjusted for age, sex, ancestry]	
			Aspirin monotherapy	34/176		

143

Table 19. Clinical outcomes in studies of treatment-effect modification by CYP2C19 genotype status (continued)

Author Year Country PMID Study name (if available)	Outcome Definition (timing)	Subgroup defined by genotype	Treatment group	Number with outcome/total number within phenotype-treatment group	Comparison between treatments, within genotype groups ES (95% CI); p-value [statistical test]	Comparison of treatment effects across genotype groups
Pare[109] 2010 Multinational 20979470 ACTIVE A	Primary efficacy outcome=any major vascular event (stroke, systemic embolism outside the CNS, MI, death from vascular causes)	Poor metabolizers	Dual antiplatelet therapy	1/9	HR=0.74 (95% CI, 0.05 to 12.04) [Cox proportional hazards model; adjusted for age, sex]	p=0.32
			Aspirin monotherapy	1/12		
		Intermediate metabolizers	Dual antiplatelet therapy	21/93	HR=0.85 (95% CI, 0.47 to 1.54) [Cox proportional hazards model; adjusted for age, sex]	
			Aspirin monotherapy	24/92		
		Extensive metabolizers	Dual antiplatelet therapy	34/199	HR=0.55 (95% CI, 0.36 to 0.83) [Cox proportional hazards model; adjusted for age, sex]	
			Aspirin monotherapy	68/235		
		Ultra metabolizers	Dual antiplatelet therapy	49/222	HR=0.97 (95% CI, 0.65 to 1.45) [Cox proportional hazards model; adjusted for age, sex]	
			Aspirin monotherapy	50/200		
		Unknown metabolizers	Dual antiplatelet therapy	7/37	HR=0.55 (95% CI, 0.21 to 1.47) [Cox proportional hazards model; adjusted for age, sex]	
			Aspirin monotherapy	10/35		

144

Table 19. Clinical outcomes in studies of treatment-effect modification by CYP2C19 genotype status (continued)

Author Year Country PMID Study name (if available)	Outcome Definition (timing)	Subgroup defined by genotype	Treatment group	Number with outcome/total number within phenotype-treatment group	Comparison between treatments, within genotype groups ES (95% CI); p-value [statistical test]	Comparison of treatment effects across genotype groups
Mega[99,258]† 2009 Multinational 19106084 19414633 TRITON-TIMI 38	Primary efficacy outcome=CV death, MI, or stroke; analysis for this outcome was performed base on intention-to-treat (as assigned)	Carriers of a reduced function allele	Clopidogrel + aspirin	46/395	OR=1.45 (95% CI, 0.91 to 2.31) [calculated values]	p=0.046 based on a test-for-interaction; p=0.04 [calculated from z-test between odds ratios]
			Prasugrel + aspirin	34/407		
		Noncarriers	Clopidogrel + aspirin	83/1064	OR=0.81 (95% CI, 0.60 to 1.10) [calculated values]	
			Prasugrel + aspirin	99/1048		

145

Table 19. Clinical outcomes in studies of treatment-effect modification by CYP2C19 genotype status (continued)

Author Year Country PMID Study name (if available)	Outcome Definition (timing)	Subgroup defined by genotype	Treatment group	Number with outcome/total number within phenotype-treatment group	Comparison between treatments, within genotype groups ES (95% CI); p-value [statistical test]	Comparison of treatment effects across genotype groups
Mega[99,258] 2010 Multinational 20801494 TRITON-TIMI 38	Primary efficacy outcome= CV death, MI, or stroke; analysis for this outcome was performed base on intention-to-treat (as assigned) at 15 mo	CYP2C19 reduced-function alleles and ABCB1 TT carriers‡	Clopidogrel + aspirin	17/125	OR for the treatment effect among CYP2C19 reduced-function allele noncarriers and ABCB1 CC/CT carriers‡=NR [not possible to calculate] OR for the treatment effect among CYP2C19 reduced-function allele carriers or ABCB1 TT carriers=NR [not possible to calculate]	p-value for the genotype effect across genotypes=0.0018 (clopidogrel-treated); 0.485 (prasugrel-treated)
			Prasugrel + aspirin	NR/110		
		CYP2C19 reduced-function allele noncarriers and ABCB1 TT carriers‡	Clopidogrel + aspirin	35/288		
			Prasugrel + aspirin	NR/278		
		CYP2C19 reduced-function alleles and ABCB1 CC/CT carriers‡	Clopidogrel + aspirin	29/268		
			Prasugrel + aspirin	NR/296		
		CYP2C19 reduced-function allele noncarriers and ABCB1 CC/CT carriers‡	Clopidogrel + aspirin	48/773		
			Prasugrel + aspirin	NR/767		

Table 19. Clinical outcomes in studies of treatment-effect modification by CYP2C19 genotype status (continued)

Author Year Country PMID Study name (if available)	Outcome Definition (timing)	Subgroup defined by genotype	Treatment group	Number with outcome/total number within phenotype-treatment group	Comparison between treatments, within genotype groups ES (95% CI); p-value [statistical test]	Comparison of treatment effects across genotype groups
Kim[260] 2011 S. Korea 21511217 ACCELAMI2C19	Major cardiovascular events=death, nonfatal MI, or urgent target vessel revascularization	Carriers	Triple therapy (adjunctive cilostazol)	0/39	OR not estimable	NA
			High-maintenance dose clopidogrel	0/38		
		Noncarriers	Triple therapy (adjunctive cilostazol)	0/25		
			High-maintenance dose clopidogrel	0/24		

147

Table 19. Clinical outcomes in studies of treatment-effect modification by CYP2C19 genotype status (continued)

Author Year Country PMID Study name (if available)	Outcome Definition (timing)	Subgroup defined by genotype	Treatment group	Number with outcome/total number within phenotype-treatment group	Comparison between treatments, within genotype groups ES (95% CI); p-value [statistical test]	Comparison of treatment effects across genotype groups
Wallentin[104] 2010 Multinational 20801498 PLATO	Primary composite outcome: CV death, MI, or stroke: 30 d	Any CYP2C19 LOF allele (*2–*8)	Ticagrelor + aspirin	NR/1384	HR=0.73 (95% CI, 0.52 to 1.03) [Cox regression with adjustment for ethnic group, sex, use of PPI, aspirin dose, smoking status, and diabetes]	0.20
			Clopidogrel+ aspirin	NR/1388		
		No CYP2C19 LOF allele (*1 or *17)	Ticagrelor + aspirin	NR/3554	HR=0.96 (95% CI, 0.76 to 1.22) [Cox regression with adjustment for ethnic group, sex, use of PPI, aspirin dose, smoking status, and diabetes]	
			Clopidogrel+ aspirin	NR/3516		
	Primary composite outcome: CV death, MI, or stroke: 12 mo	Any CYP2C19 LOF allele (*2–*8)	Ticagrelor + aspirin	115/1384	HR=0.77 (95% CI, 0.60 to 0.99) [Cox regression with adjustment for ethnic group, sex, use of PPI, aspirin dose, smoking status, and diabetes]	0.46
			Clopidogrel+ aspirin	149/1388		
		No CYP2C19 LOF allele (*1 or *17)	Ticagrelor + aspirin	296/3554	HR=0.86 (95% CI, 0.74 to 1.01) [Cox regression with adjustment for ethnic group, sex, use of PPI, aspirin dose, smoking status, and diabetes]	
			Clopidogrel+ aspirin	332/3515		
		Any CYP2C19 LOF allele (*2–*8) + ABCB1 C/C[a]	Ticagrelor + aspirin	NR/2253	HR=0.75 (95% CI, 0.62 to 0.91) [Cox regression with adjustment for ethnic group, sex, use of PPI, aspirin dose, smoking status, and diabetes]	0.13
			Clopidogrel+ aspirin	NR/2248		

148

Table 19. Clinical outcomes in studies of treatment-effect modification by CYP2C19 genotype status (continued)

Author Year Country PMID Study name (if available)	Outcome Definition (timing)	Subgroup defined by genotype	Treatment group	Number with outcome/total number within phenotype-treatment group	Comparison between treatments, within genotype groups ES (95% CI); p-value [statistical test]	Comparison of treatment effects across genotype groups
		No CYP2C19 LOF allele (*1 or *17) + ABCB1 C/T or T/T[a]	Ticagrelor + aspirin	NR/2710	HR=0.92 (95% CI, 0.77 to 1.11) [Cox regression with adjustment for ethnic group, sex, use of PPI, aspirin dose, smoking status, and diabetes]	
			Clopidogrel+ aspirin	NR/2698		
	CV death or MI	Any CYP2C19 LOF allele (*2–*8)	Ticagrelor + aspirin	102/1384	HR=0.73 (95% CI, 0.57 to 0.95) [Cox regression with adjustment for ethnic group, sex, use of PPI, aspirin dose, smoking status, and diabetes]	0.30
			Clopidogrel+ aspirin	138/1388		
		No CYP2C19 LOF allele (*1 or *17)	Ticagrelor + aspirin	273/3554	HR=0.86 (95% CI, 0.74 to 1.01) [Cox regression with adjustment for ethnic group, sex, use of PPI, aspirin dose, smoking status, and diabetes]	
			Clopidogrel+ aspirin	306/3516		
	Definite stent thrombosis (in patients who underwent stenting)	Any CYP2C19 LOF allele (*2–*8)	Ticagrelor + aspirin	15/943	HR=0.71 (95% CI, 0.36 to 1.37) [Cox regression with adjustment for ethnic group, sex, use of PPI, aspirin dose, smoking status, and diabetes]	NR (no. of events too low to calculate)
			Clopidogrel+ aspirin	21/934		
		No CYP2C19 LOF allele (*1 or *17)	Ticagrelor + aspirin	22/2341	HR=0.62 (95% CI, 0.36 to 1.05) [Cox regression with adjustment for ethnic group, sex, use of PPI, aspirin dose, smoking status, and diabetes]	
			Clopidogrel + aspirin	35/2300		

Table 19. Clinical outcomes in studies of treatment-effect modification by CYP2C19 genotype status (continued)

Author Year Country PMID Study name (if available)	Outcome Definition (timing)	Subgroup defined by genotype	Treatment group	Number with outcome/total number within phenotype-treatment group	Comparison between treatments, within genotype groups ES (95% CI); p-value [statistical test]	Comparison of treatment effects across genotype groups
Bhatt[85] 2012 Multinational 22450429 CHARISMA	Primary composite outcome: first occurrence of non-fatal or fatal MI, non-fatal or fatal stroke, or cardiovascular death	Poor metabolizers	Clopidogrel + aspirin	7/52	HR=1.86 (95% CI, 0.53 to 6.55) [Cox regression with adjustment for age, sex, inclusion criteria (symptomatic vs. asymptomatic), use of statins, use of calcium channel blockers, and cigarette usage]	0.621
			Aspirin + placebo	4/48		
		Intermediate metabolizers	Clopidogrel + aspirin	29/458	HR=1.31 (95% CI, 0.75 to 2.30) [Cox regression with adjustment for age, sex, inclusion criteria (symptomatic vs. asymptomatic), use of statins, use of calcium channel blockers, and cigarette usage]	
			Aspirin + placebo	21/445		
		Extensive metabolizers	Clopidogrel + aspirin	52/886	HR=1.16 (95% CI, 0.78 to 1.71) [Cox regression with adjustment for age, sex, inclusion criteria (symptomatic vs. asymptomatic), use of statins, use of calcium channel blockers, and cigarette usage]	
			Aspirin + placebo	49/920		
		Ultra metabolizers	Clopidogrel + aspirin	40/716	HR=0.82 (95% CI, 0.54 to 1.24) [Cox regression with adjustment for age, sex, inclusion criteria (symptomatic vs. asymptomatic), use of statins, use of calcium channel blockers, and cigarette usage]	
				48/715		
		Unknown metabolizers	Clopidogrel + aspirin	12/156	HR=1.30 (95% CI, 0.56 to 3.04) [Cox regression with adjustment for age, sex, inclusion criteria (symptomatic vs. asymptomatic), use of statins, use of calcium channel blockers, and cigarette usage]	
			Aspirin + placebo	10/145		

150

Table 19. Clinical outcomes in studies of treatment-effect modification by CYP2C19 genotype status (continued)

Author Year Country PMID Study name (if available)	Outcome Definition (timing)	Subgroup defined by genotype	Treatment group	Number with outcome/total number within phenotype-treatment group	Comparison between treatments, within genotype groups ES (95% CI); p-value [statistical test]	Comparison of treatment effects across genotype groups
	Secondary composite outcome: first occurrence of non-fatal or fatal MI, non-fatal or fatal stroke, cardiovascular death, hospitalization for unstable angina, TIA, or revascularization procedure	Poor metabolizers	Clopidogrel + aspirin	12/52	HR=1.04 (95% CI, 0.45 to 2.43) [Cox regression with adjustment for age, sex, inclusion criteria (symptomatic vs. asymptomatic), use of statins, use of calcium channel blockers, and cigarette usage]	0.895
			Aspirin + placebo	10/48		
		Intermediate metabolizers	Clopidogrel + aspirin	82/458	HR=1.09 (95% CI, 0.80 to 1.50) [Cox regression with adjustment for age, sex, inclusion criteria (symptomatic vs. asymptomatic), use of statins, use of calcium channel blockers, and cigarette usage]	
			Aspirin + placebo	73/445		
		Extensive metabolizers	Clopidogrel + aspirin	145/886	HR=0.95 (95% CI, 0.76 to 1.19) [Cox regression with adjustment for age, sex, inclusion criteria (symptomatic vs. asymptomatic), use of statins, use of calcium channel blockers, and cigarette usage]	
				161/920		
		Ultra metabolizers	Clopidogrel + aspirin	124/716	HR=1.01 (95% CI, 0.79 to 1.30) [Cox regression with adjustment for age, sex, inclusion criteria (symptomatic vs. asymptomatic), use of statins, use of calcium channel blockers, and cigarette usage]	
			Aspirin + placebo	121/715		

151

Table 19. Clinical outcomes in studies of treatment-effect modification by CYP2C19 genotype status (continued)

Author Year Country PMID Study name (if available)	Outcome Definition (timing)	Subgroup defined by genotype	Treatment group	Number with outcome/total number within phenotype-treatment group	Comparison between treatments, within genotype groups ES (95% CI); p-value [statistical test]	Comparison of treatment effects across genotype groups
		Unknown metabolizers	Clopidogrel + aspirin	23/156	HR=0.83 (95% CI, 0.47 to 1.45) [Cox regression with adjustment for age, sex, inclusion criteria (symptomatic vs. asymptomatic), use of statins, use of calcium channel blockers, and cigarette usage]	
			Aspirin + placebo	27/145		

Abbreviations: ACTIVE A Trial = Atrial Fibrillation Clopidogrel Trial with Irbesartan for Prevention of Vascular Events A trial; CABG = coronary artery bypass grafting; CHARISMA = Clopidogrel for High Atherothrombotic Risk and Ischemic Stabilization, Management, and Avoidance; CI = confidence interval; CNS = central nervous system; CURE Trial = Clopidogrel in Unstable Angina to Prevent Recurrent Events trial; CV = cardiovascular; d = day; ES = effect size; GOF = gain of function; HR = hazard ratio; LOF = loss of function; MI = myocardial infarction; mo = month; NA = not applicable; NR = not reported; OR = odds ratio; PLATO trial = PLATelet inhibition and patient Outcomes trial; PPI = proton-pump inhibitor; TIA = transient ischemic attack; TRITON TIMI 38 = Trial to Assess Improvement in Therapeutic Outcomes by Optimizing Platelet Inhibition with Prasugrel–Thrombolysis In Myocardial Infarction 38.

*The authors reported extensive subgroup and sensitivity analyses across different genotype groupings and after including or excluding subgroups of patients by race or ethnicity. The results relevant to treatment effect heterogeneity from these analyses are presented in the text of this section.

†Patients with genotypes of "unclear" functional significance were excluded.

‡ABCB1 is a gene that encodes a protein involved in the intestinal absorption of clopidogrel.[266]

152

Because of the large differences in included populations, treatments compared, and exposure and outcome definitions among studies reporting on treatment-effect modification by CYP2C19 variants on clinical outcomes, we did not perform a meta-analysis. Given that the drugs compared (clopidogrel, prasugrel, and ticagrelor) have different mechanisms of action, it is plausible that interaction effects could have different magnitudes or directions across studies. For purposes of illustration, we used the counts reported in the studies to compare the treatment effect among carriers of CYP2C19 loss-of-function alleles versus noncarriers. Figure 36 presents the results for the five studies in which at least one composite cardiovascular outcome occurred (see Table 14 for definitions of outcomes) and with the results stratified by genotype group, under two genetic models (dominant and recessive). The figure also demonstrates the relative treatment effect (i.e., the relative odds ratio) across the genotype groups—the equivalent of the genotype × treatment interaction. The relative treatment effect was statistically significant in only one study, and only under a dominant genetic model. In generally, effects were more imprecise under a recessive genetic model, due to the scarcity of homozygote individuals in the study populations.

Figure 36. Results from large randomized trials assessing effect modification by CYP2C19 variants on MACE

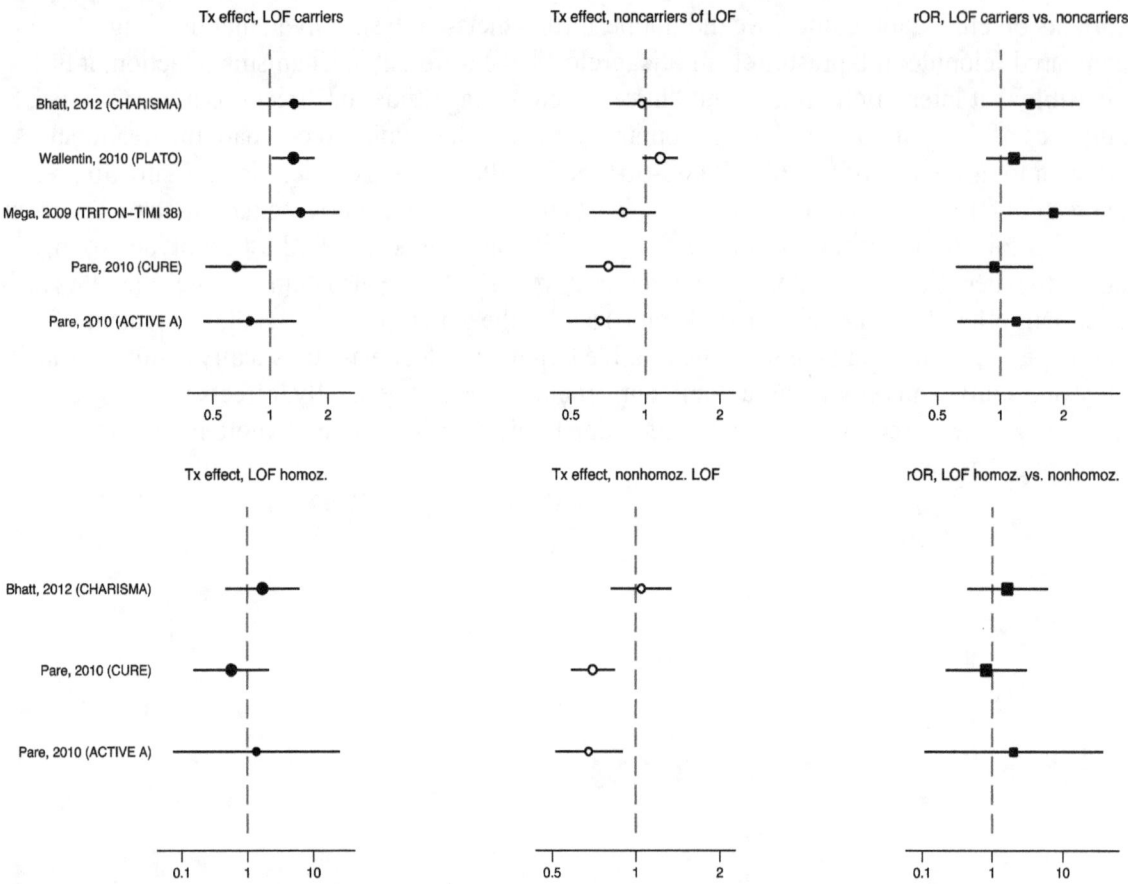

Abbreviations: ACTIVE A = Atrial Fibrillation Clopidogrel Trial with Irbesartan for Prevention of Vascular Events A; Clopidogrel for High Atherothrombotic Risk and Ischemic Stabilization, Management and Avoidance; CURE = Clopidogrel in Unstable Angina to Prevent Recurrent Events trial; homoz = homozygotes; PLATO = Platelet inhibition and patient Outcomes trial; TRITON-TIMI 38 = Trial to Assess Improvement in Therapeutic Outcomes by Optimizing Platelet Inhibition with Prasugrel–Thrombolysis in Myocardial Infarction; Tx = treatment.
The top set of panels presents forest plots of treatment effects (odds ratios) on major adverse cardiovascular events (MACE) among carriers of at least one loss-of-function (LOF) allele (top left panel); treatment effects among noncarriers of LOF alleles (top middle panel); and relative effects (relative odds ratios [rOR]) comparing the treatment effect among LOF carriers and LOF noncarriers (top right panel). The bottom set of panels presents forest plots of treatment effects on MACE among homozygotes for two LOF alleles (bottom left panel); treatment effects among non-homozygotes of LOF alleles (bottom middle panel); and relative effects (relative odds ratios [rOR]) comparing the treatment effect among homozygotes and non-homozygotes of LOF alleles (bottom right panel). Two studies did not provide adequate data for the comparisons of homozygotes and non-homozygotes. The CURE, CHARISMA, and ACTIVE A trials compared aspirin plus clopidogrel versus aspirin monotherapy; the TRITON-TIMI 38 trial compared aspirin plus clopidogrel versus aspirin plus prasugrel; the PLATO trial compared aspirin plus clopidogrel versus aspirin plus ticagrelor. Point estimates for treatment effects are shown as black circles (carriers) or white circles (noncarriers); point estimates for relative treatment effects are shown as black squares. For all symbols, size is inversely proportional to the standard error of each estimate. Horizontal lines denote 95% confidence intervals for all estimates. Vertical dashed lines denote no effect. Please see Tables 18 and 19 for full definitions of the genotype categories and outcomes reported by each study. References to individual studies are provided in Table 5.

Overall the available studies do not suggest that CYP2C19 genotype status is a strong modifier of the treatment effects evaluated in the studies. However, none of these studies were specifically designed to assess effect modification by genotype, they were conducted in heterogeneous populations and compared different pairs of treatments. Further, the studies

154

included only small subsets (in all cases <50 percent of the original trial populations) suggesting that selection bias may have affected their results. This was a concern particularly for the CHARISMA trial,85 where differences in baseline characteristics and outcome rates were observed between the patients included and those not included in the genetic substudy. Furthermore, details were not provided regarding the timing of obtaining samples for genetic analyses (but samples were generally not obtained at the trial baseline). In such cases, survivor bias (another form of selection bias) may also affect study results.

Intermediate Outcome: Platelet Reactivity During Followup

Seven studies assessing treatment-effect modification by CYP2C19 variants provided information on platelet reactivity during followup as an intermediate outcome (Table 20 and 21).[191,260-264] All seven were based on randomized trials comparing clopidogrel-based treatment to alternative therapies, had small to moderate sample sizes (range, 60 to 474 participants), and enrolled heterogeneous populations: two included patients with stable coronary artery disease, one included patients with myocardial infarction undergoing PCI, one included patients undergoing elective PCI, one enrolled patients with coronary artery disease receiving drug-eluting stents, one included "high-risk" patients undergoing PCI, and one included male patients who had experienced a myocardial infarction before age 45. All had short followup periods (<7 days to 6 weeks).

Table 20 describes the assays used, alleles genotyped, and genotype groupings used in the seven studies. Four of the six did not provide a rationale for the genotype grouping; one study used an enrichment design whereby patients with *2/*2 and *2/*1 genotype where matched to patients with *1/*1 genotype. The studies differed in the alleles genotyped and the genotype groupings used, leading to heterogeneity in the exposure definition. Platelet reactivity during followup was assessed by the VerifyNow P2Y12 assay in all seven studies, as well as by LTA in four studies and the VASP assay (with flow cytometry) in two studies. Key findings from these studies are summarized in Table 21. The overall results were variable and incomplete reporting sometimes precluded the quantitative assessment of test × treatment interactions. Because of the differences in designs, populations, treatments compared, and followup durations among the included studies, we did not perform a meta-analysis.

Table 20. Study characteristics in studies of treatment-effect modification by CYP2C19 genotype status with intermediate outcomes

Author Year Country PMID Study Name (if available)	Selection Criteria	Study Design	N Enrolled Male (%) Age* Dyslipidemia (%) Smokers (%) HTN (%) Diabetes (%) Race/Ethnicity (%)	Treatments Compared	Followup Duration
Varenhorst[261]† 2009 Sweden 19429918 TABR	Patients with stable coronary artery disease; patients were participants in a 2-center, double-blind, double-dummy RCT	Pre-specified genetic substudy of an RCT	98 89 (91%) 63.8 (6.0) NR 12 (12%) [unclear definition] NR 19 (19%) White=98 (100%)	All study subjects received aspirin 75 mg/d for 5–21 days prior to randomization and continued throughout the study. Following the open-label aspirin run-in period, subjects continuing to meet enrolment criteria were assigned to two groups: *Aspirin + prasugrel*: prasugrel loading dose 60 mg, followed by prasugrel 10 mg/d maintenance dose *Aspirin + clopidogrel*: clopidogrel 600 mg loading dose; clopidogrel 75 mg/d maintenance dose	30 d

156

Table 20. Study characteristics in studies of treatment-effect modification by CYP2C19 genotype status with intermediate outcomes (continued)

Author Year Country PMID Study Name (if available)	Selection Criteria	Study Design	N Enrolled Male (%) Age* Dyslipidemia (%) Smokers (%) HTN (%) Diabetes (%) Race/Ethnicity (%)	Treatments Compared	Followup Duration
Tantry‡[262] 2010 USA and UK 21079055 ONSET/OFFSET and RESPOND Genotype Studies	Patients with documented stable coronary artery disease; patients were participants in the double-blind, double-blind, parallel arm multicenter ONSET-OFFSET study or the double-blind, double-blind, crossover multicenter RESPOND study	Genetic substudies based on 2 RCTs [data from both were combined]	174 129 (74%) 63.9 (8.6) 164 (94%) 15 (9%) [current smokers] 137 (79%) 39 (22%) White=153 (88%); Black=15 (7%); other NR	In the ONSET/OFFSET trial: *Ticagrelor group*: ticagrelor (180 mg) loading dose; ticagrelor maintenance (90 mg) in the evening with a 12-hour interval between dosing, followed by ticagrelor maintenance 90 mg BID for 6 w *Clopidogrel group*: clopidogrel (600 mg) loading dose; clopidogrel maintenance (90 mg) in the evening with a 12-hour interval between dosing, followed by clopidogrel maintenance 75 mg/d for 6 w *Placebo group*: placebo (no treatment) loading dose; followed by placebo administration for 6 w In the RESPOND trial, previously identified responsive or nonresponsive to clopidogrel 300 mg loading dose (cut-off ≤10% absolute change of reactivity to LTA) patients were randomized into two groups for the first trial period: *Clopidogrel group*: 600 mg clopidogrel loading dose, followed by 75 mg/d maintenance dose for 2 w *Ticagrelor group*: 80 mg ticagrelor loading dose, followed by 90 mg BID maintenance dose Period 2 data for the RESPOND trial were not used in the pharmacodynamic investigation.	6 w for ONSET/OFFSET participants; 2 w for RESPOND participants

157

Table 20. Study characteristics in studies of treatment-effect modification by CYP2C19 genotype status with intermediate outcomes (continued)

Author Year Country PMID Study Name (if available)	Selection Criteria	Study Design	N Enrolled Male (%) Age* Dyslipidemia (%) Smokers (%) HTN (%) Diabetes (%) Race/Ethnicity (%)	Treatments Compared	Followup Duration
Kim[260] 2011 S. Korea 21511217 ACCELAMI2C19	Consecutive MI patients admitted to a single university hospital treated with "uneventful PCI"; patients were participants in the genetic expanded study of ACCEL-AMI	Genetic substudy of RCT	126 [with available genotyping information] 92 (73%) 61.7 (12.3) 35 (28%) 75 (60%) [current smokers] 59 (47%) 35 (28%) East Asian=126 (100%)	All patients received clopidogrel loading (600 mg) upon admission; followed by 75 mg/d maintenance dose. *High-maintenance dose clopidogrel:* clopidogrel 150 mg/d maintenance *Triple therapy (adjunctive cilostazol):* cilostazol 100 mg BID + clopidogrel 75/d maintenance All patients received aspirin 300 mg loading dose, followed by 200 mg/d maintenance dose for the duration of the study.	30 d

158

Table 20. Study characteristics in studies of treatment-effect modification by CYP2C19 genotype status with intermediate outcomes (continued)

Author Year Country PMID Study Name (if available)	Selection Criteria	Study Design	N Enrolled Male (%) Age* Dyslipidemia (%) Smokers (%) HTN (%) Diabetes (%) Race/Ethnicity (%)	Treatments Compared	Followup Duration
Hwang[263] 2010 S. Korea 20823393 ACCEL-RESISTANCE, DM, and COMPLEX trials (ACEL-POLYMORPHISM)§	High-risk patients undergoing PCI; patients were participants in the ACELL trials (patients in the RESISTANCE trial had HPPR; in the DM trial had diabetes mellitus; and in the COMPLEX trial had complex lesions for stent placement)§	Prespecified genetic substudy of 3 RCTs	114 [with available genotyping information] 88 (77%) 63.2 (9.5) 33 (29%) 51 (45%) [current smokers] 76 (67%) 37 (32%) East Asian=114 (100%)	All patients received clopidogrel loading dose of 300 mg upon ≥12 h before PCI or where on chronic clopidogrel treatment (75 mg/d for ≥7 d); followed by 75 mg/d maintenance dose. High-maintenance dose clopidogrel: clopidogrel 150 mg/d maintenance Triple therapy (adjunctive cilostazol): cilostazol 100 mg BID + clopidogrel 75/d maintenance All patients received aspirin 300 mg loading dose, followed by 200 mg/d maintenance dose for the duration of the study.	30 d

159

Table 20. Study characteristics in studies of treatment-effect modification by CYP2C19 genotype status with intermediate outcomes (continued)

Author Year Country PMID Study Name (if available)	Selection Criteria	Study Design	N Enrolled Male (%) Age* Dyslipidemia (%) Smokers (%) HTN (%) Diabetes (%) Race/ Ethnicity (%)	Treatments Compared	Followup Duration
Gladding[191]** 2008 New Zealand 19463375 PRINC	Patients undergoing elective PCI who were on aspirin treatment; patients were participants In the randomized PRINC trial	Genetic substudy of RCT	60 50 (83%) 68 (10) NR 6 (10%) [current smokers] 34 (57%) 11 (18%) White=57 (95%); others NR	The PRINC study design had 2 phases: a 2×2 factorial, randomized, placebo-controlled, double-blind study over the first 24 h, followed by a 1 w randomized, placebo-controlled, double-blind study. Patients were first randomized in a 2 × 2 manner to receive either 5 mg *verapamil or placebo at baseline and either placebo or 600 mg clopidogrel, 2 h from baseline.* All patients received 600 mg clopidogrel at the start of the PCI procedure, 10 min after administration of verapamil or placebo. The next day, patients were separately randomized to receive clopidogrel 75 or 150 mg once daily for 1 week, followed by 75 mg once daily thereafter.	7 d
Park[264] 2011 S. Korea 21345843 CILON-T	Patients undergoing implantation of drug-eluting stents; patients were participants in the CILON-T randomized trial	Genetic substudy of RCT	474 330 (70%) 63.3 (8.7) 220 (46%) 98 (21%) 322 (68%) 159 (34%) Korean = 474 (100%)	Patients who had not taken aspirin or clopidogrel before PCI were given a loading dose of aspirin (300 mg) and clopidogrel (300–600 mg) and then were randomized to: *Dual-antiplatelet therapy:* Aspirin (100 mg daily) and clopidogrel (75 mg daily) *Triple-antiplatelet therapy:* Aspirin (100 mg daily), clopidogrel (75 mg daily), and cilostazol (200 mg loading dose + 100 mg twice daily)	NR ("at discharge")

160

Table 20. Study characteristics in studies of treatment-effect modification by CYP2C19 genotype status with intermediate outcomes (continued)

Author Year Country PMID Study Name (if available)	Selection Criteria	Study Design	N Enrolled Male (%) Age* Dyslipidemia (%) Smokers (%) HTN (%) Diabetes (%) Race/Ethnicity (%)	Treatments Compared	Followup Duration
Collet[265] 2011 France 21511218 CLOVIS-2	Patients with MI before the age of 45, screened from the AFIJI multicenter registry. A total of 292 male patients were genotyped for CYP2C19*2. *2/*2 and *2/*1 patients were asked to participate in the trial. Age- and gender-matched CYP2C19 *1/*1 (noncarriers) from the AFIJI program were then recruited with a 1:1 ratio for each *2/*1 and a 2:1 ratio for each *2/*2 patient who was willing to participate.	Genetic substudy of crossover RCT	106 included in analyses 106 (100%) 40.1 (4.8) 73 (69%) NR 30 (28%) 16 (15%) European = 86 (81%): North African = 13 (12%); Black = 1 (1%); Asian = 6 (6%)	Patients were on maintenance aspirin (75 mg/d) and/or clopidogrel (75 mg/d) for ≥3 mo. They were randomized to an *open-label loading dose of 300 or 900 mg of clopidogrel* in a 2-period crossover fashion. Clopidogrel maintenance treatment (75 mg) was continued for ≥21 d before patients were crossed over to the alternate loading dose of clopidogrel. Measurements were obtained at baseline and 1, 2, 4, and 6 h post-loading in each study period.	At least 42 d (time on maintenance after each loading dose)

Abbreviations: AFIJI = Appraisal of risk Factors in young Ischemic patients Justifying aggressive Intervention; BID = twice daily; d = day; h = hours; NR = not reported; PCI = percutaneous coronary intervention; PRINC = Plavix Response in Coronary Intervention; RCT = randomized clinical trial; weeks
*Mean (standard deviation), unless otherwise stated.
†Some information extracted from Wallentin et al. 2008.[267]
‡Some information extracted from Gurbel et al. 2009[268] and Gurbel et al. 2010.[162]
§Although the HPPR study required presence of resistance to antiplatelet therapy, ascertained by reactivity testing, we included the study by Hwang et al. in this section (and not in

the section on studies randomizing patients after selection with reactivity testing) because the paper did not report separate results for patients in the ACCEL-RESISTANCE study, and such criteria were not used in the ACCEL-DM or ACCEL-COMPLEX trials.
**Some information extracted from Gladding et al. 2008.[269]

161

Table 21. Effect modification on the outcome of platelet reactivity in randomized trials stratifying patients by CYP2C19 genotype status

Author Year Country UID Study name (if available)	Treatment group	Subgroups defined by genotype	N	Assay (agonist) [manufacturer] for the assessment of platelet reactivity	Summary of results
Varenhorst[281] 2009 Sweden 19429918 TABR	Aspirin + prasugrel	Extensive metabolizers	35	VASP assay (ADP ±PGE1) [Biocytex, Marseille, France]	By PRI VASP: at 24 h, 14 d, and 29 d, the difference between extensive and reduced metabolizers was p<0.05 in clopidogrel treated patients but p=NS for prasugrel treated patients.
		Reduced metabolizers	15		
		Uncertain functional status	1		By PRU VerifyNow: at 24 h, 14 d, and 29 d, the difference between extensive and reduced metabolizers was p<0.05 in clopidogrel treated patients but p=NS for prasugrel treated patients.
	Aspirin + clopidogrel	Extensive metabolizers	37	VerifyNow P2Y12 (ADP) [Accumetrics, San Diego, CA]	Exact p-values were not reported; additional information provided only in graphical form (Figure 3 of the paper).
		Reduced metabolizers	9		
		Uncertain functional status	1		

162

Table 21. Effect modification on the outcome of platelet reactivity in randomized trials stratifying patients by CYP2C19 genotype status (continued)

Author Year Country UID Study name (if available)	Treatment group	Subgroups defined by genotype	N	Assay (agonist) [manufacturer] for the assessment of platelet reactivity	Summary of results
Tantry*[262] 2010 USA and UK 21079055 ONSET/OFFSET and RESPOND Genotype Studies	Ticagrelor group	Ultra metabolizers Extensive metabolizers Intermediate metabolizers Poor metabolizers	27 28 35 2	LTA (ADP 5 or 20 µmol/L) [Chronolog Optical Aggregometer, model 490-4D, no additional information provided]; VASP assay (ADP ±PGE1) [Biocytex, Marseille, France]; VerifyNow P2Y12 (ADP) [Accumetrics, San Diego, CA]	LTA (ADP 5 µM); p-value for the treatment effect within genotype group (ticagrelor vs. clopidogrel) Ultra metabolizers, p=0.0016 Extensive metabolizers, p=0.0004 Intermediate metabolizers, p<0.0001 Poor metabolizers, p=0.149
	Clopidogrel group	Ultra metabolizers Extensive metabolizers Intermediate metabolizers Poor metabolizers	28 31 20 3		LTA (ADP 20 µM); p-value for the treatment effect within genotype group (ticagrelor vs. clopidogrel) Ultra metabolizers, p=0.001 Extensive metabolizers, p=0.0001 Intermediate metabolizers, p<0.0001 Poor metabolizers, p=0.139

Table 21. Effect modification on the outcome of platelet reactivity in randomized trials stratifying patients by CYP2C19 genotype status (continued)

Author Year Country UID Study name (if available)	Treatment group	Subgroups defined by genotype	N	Assay (agonist) [manufacturer] for the assessment of platelet reactivity	Summary of results
	Ticagrelor group	LOF carriers LOF noncarriers GOF carriers	27 28 37		VerifyNow; p-value for the treatment effect within genotype group (ticagrelor vs. clopidogrel) Ultra metabolizers, p<0.0001 Extensive metabolizers, p<0.0001 Intermediate metabolizers, p<0.0001 Poor metabolizers, p=0.138
	Clopidogrel group	LOF carriers LOF noncarriers GOF carriers	28 31 23		VASP assay; p-value for the treatment effect within genotype group (ticagrelor vs. clopidogrel) Ultra metabolizers, p<0.0001 Extensive metabolizers, p<0.0001 Intermediate metabolizers, p<0.0001 Poor metabolizers, p=0.149 P-values from Wilcoxon rank-sum test. In all groups reactivity was lower in the ticagrelor group. Additional information provided only in graphical form (Figures 3-5). LTA (ADP 5 µM); p-value for the treatment effect within genotype group (ticagrelor vs. clopidogrel) Loss-of-function carriers, p<0.0001 Loss-of-function noncarriers, p<0.0001 Gain-of-function carriers, p=0.0016 LTA (ADP 20 µM); p-value for the treatment effect within genotype group (ticagrelor vs. clopidogrel) Loss-of-function carriers, p<0.0001 Loss-of-function noncarriers, p=0.0001 Gain-of-function carriers, p=0.001 VerifyNow; p-value for the treatment effect within genotype group (ticagrelor vs. clopidogrel) Loss-of-function carriers, p<0.0001 Loss-of-function noncarriers, p<0.0001 Gain-of-function carriers, p<0.0001

164

Table 21. Effect modification on the outcome of platelet reactivity in randomized trials stratifying patients by CYP2C19 genotype status (continued)

Author Year Country UID Study name (if available)	Treatment group	Subgroups defined by genotype	N	Assay (agonist) [manufacturer] for the assessment of platelet reactivity	Summary of results
					VASP assay; p-value for the treatment effect within genotype group (ticagrelor vs. clopidogrel) Loss-of-function carriers, p<0.0001 Loss-of-function noncarriers, p<0.0001 Gain-of-function carriers, p<0.0001 P-values from Wilcoxon rank-sum test. In all groups reactivity was lower in the ticagrelor group. Additional information provided only in graphical form (Figures 3-5).

Table 21. Effect modification on the outcome of platelet reactivity in randomized trials stratifying patients by CYP2C19 genotype status (continued)

Author Year Country UID Study name (if available)	Treatment group	Subgroups defined by genotype	N	Assay (agonist) [manufacturer] for the assessment of platelet reactivity	Summary of results
Kim†[250] 2011 S. Korea 21511217 ACCELAMI2C19	High-maintenance dose clopidogrel	Carriers Noncarriers	38 24	LTA (ADP 5 and 20 µmol/L) [AggRAM aggregometer, Helena Laboratories Corp., Beaumont, TX] VerifyNow P2Y12 (ADP) [Accumetrics, San Diego, CA]	*Maximal platelet aggregation by LTA 5 µmol/L at 30 d* *Carriers* Mean reactivity in high-maintenance dose clopidogrel group=37.6 (SD=16.0) Mean reactivity in triple therapy group=24.9 (SD=14.3) P-valuefor the treatment effect among carriers, <0.001 *Noncarriers* Mean reactivity in high-maintenance dose clopidogrel group=30.1 (SD=10.1) Mean reactivity in triple therapy group=28.2 (SD=11.5) P-value for the treatment effect among noncarriers=0.547
	Triple therapy (adjunctive cilostazol)	Carriers Noncarriers	25 39		*Maximal platelet aggregation by LTA 20 µmol/L at 30 d (mean reactivity)* *Carriers:* High-maintenance dose clopidogrel group, 52.3 (SD=17.5) Triple therapy group=35.0 (SD=19.3) P for the treatment effect among carriers <0.001 *Noncarriers* Mean reactivity in high-maintenance dose clopidogrel group=38.6 (SD=12.0) Mean reactivity in triple therapy group=37.5 (SD=13.2) P for the treatment effect among noncarriers=0.752 *Late platelet aggregation by LTA 5 µmol/L at 30 d* *Carriers* Mean reactivity in high-maintenance dose clopidogrel group=26.7 (SD=16.5) Mean reactivity in triple therapy group=15.2 (SD=12.4) P for the treatment effect among carriers=0.001 *Noncarriers* Mean reactivity in high-maintenance dose clopidogrel group=16.4 (SD=9.2) Mean reactivity in triple therapy group=13.6 (SD=11.7) P for the treatment effect among noncarriers=0.347

Table 21. Effect modification on the outcome of platelet reactivity in randomized trials stratifying patients by CYP2C19 genotype status (continued)

Author Year Country UID Study name (if available)	Treatment group	Subgroups defined by genotype	N	Assay (agonist) [manufacturer] for the assessment of platelet reactivity	Summary of results
					Late platelet aggregation by LTA 20 µmol/L at 30 d **Carriers** Mean reactivity in high-maintenance dose clopidogrel group=40.6 (SD=22.2) Mean reactivity in triple therapy group=23.5 (SD=19.2) P for the treatment effect among carriers=0.0001 **Noncarriers** Mean reactivity in high-maintenance dose clopidogrel group=21.8 (SD=14.8) Mean reactivity in triple therapy group=19.7 (SD=16.8) P for the treatment effect among noncarriers=0.649
					VerifyNow PRU at 30 d **Carriers** Mean reactivity in high-maintenance dose clopidogrel group=184.2 (SD=80.6) Mean reactivity in triple therapy group=171.9 (SD=86.3) P for the treatment effect among carriers=0.518 **Noncarriers** Mean reactivity in high-maintenance dose clopidogrel group=152.2 (SD=70.4) Mean reactivity in triple therapy group=136.6 (SD=70.0) P for the treatment effect among noncarriers=0.441
					VerifyNow %inhibition at 30 d **Carriers** Mean reactivity in high-maintenance dose clopidogrel group=40.3 (SD=23.5) Mean reactivity in triple therapy group=48.0 (SD=24.0) P for the treatment effect among carriers=0.157 **Noncarriers** Mean reactivity in high-maintenance dose clopidogrel group=54.7 (SD=22.3) Mean reactivity in triple therapy group=56.4 (SD=20.7) P for the treatment effect among noncarriers=0.783

167

Table 21. Effect modification on the outcome of platelet reactivity in randomized trials stratifying patients by CYP2C19 genotype status (continued)

Author Year Country UID Study name (if available)	Treatment group	Subgroups defined by genotype	N	Assay (agonist) [manufacturer] for the assessment of platelet reactivity	Summary of results
					HPR (cut-off >59% using LTA with ADP 20 μmol/L) at 30 d *Carriers* N (%) among high-maintenance dose clopidogrel group=17 (44.7%) N (%) among triple therapy group=6 (15.4%) P for the treatment effect among carriers=0.005 *Noncarriers* N (%) among high-maintenance dose clopidogrel group=2 (8.3%) N (%) among triple therapy group=0 (0%) P for the treatment effect among noncarriers=0.235

168

Table 21. Effect modification on the outcome of platelet reactivity in randomized trials stratifying patients by CYP2C19 genotype status (continued)

Author Year Country UID Study name (if available)	Treatment group	Subgroups defined by genotype	N	Assay (agonist) [manufacturer] for the assessment of platelet reactivity	Summary of results
Gladding[191] 2008 New Zealand 19463375 PRINC	1200 mg clopidogrel loading	Carriers Noncarriers	11 15	VerifyNow P2Y12 (ADP) [Accumetrics, San Diego, CA]	% inhibition (Mann–Whitney U test) among carriers at 4 h (600 mg vs. 1200 mg): median=14% vs. 37%; p=0.002 % inhibition (Mann–Whitney U test) among noncarriers at 4 h (600 mg vs. 1200 mg): median=35% vs. 43%; p=0.3
	600 mg clopidogrel loading	Carriers Noncarriers	8 9		% inhibition (Mann–Whitney U test) among carriers at 7 h (600 mg vs. 1200 mg): median=22% vs. 42%; p=0.09 % inhibition (Mann–Whitney U test) among noncarriers at 7 h (600 mg vs. 1200 mg): median=29% vs. 63%; p=0.05
	150 mg clopidogrel maintenance	Carriers Noncarriers	5 12		% inhibition (Mann–Whitney U test) among carriers at 7 d (150 mg vs. 75 mg): median=14% vs. 51%; p=0.042 % inhibition (Mann–Whitney U test) among noncarriers at 7 d (150 mg vs. 75 mg): median=32% vs. 51%; p=0.2
	75 mg clopidogrel maintenance	Carriers Noncarriers	9 6		
Hwang†[263] 2010 S. Korea 20823393 ACCEL-RESISTANCE, DM, and COMPLEX trials	High-maintenance dose clopidogrel	Carriers Noncarriers	43 22	LTA (ADP 5 and 20 μmol/L) [AggRAM aggregometer, Helena Laboratories Corp., Beaumont, TX] VerifyNow P2Y12 (ADP) [Accumetrics, San Diego, CA]	*Maximal platelet aggregation by LTA 5 μmol/L at 30 d* *Carriers* Mean reactivity in high-maintenance dose clopidogrel group=42.9 (SD=18.1) Mean reactivity in triple therapy group=28.4 (SD=13.9) P-value for the treatment effect among carriers<0.001 *Noncarriers* Mean reactivity in high-maintenance dose clopidogrel group=31.1 (SD=12.9) Mean reactivity in triple therapy group=26.7 (SD=15.2) P-value for the treatment effect among noncarriers=0.304

169

Table 21. Effect modification on the outcome of platelet reactivity in randomized trials stratifying patients by CYP2C19 genotype status (continued)

Author Year Country UID Study name (if available)	Treatment group	Subgroups defined by genotype	N	Assay (agonist) [manufacturer] for the assessment of platelet reactivity	Summary of results
	Triple therapy (adjunctive cilostazol)	Carriers Noncarriers	47 22		*Maximal platelet aggregation by LTA 20 μmol/L at 30 d* *Carriers* Mean reactivity in high-maintenance dose clopidogrel group=55.4 (SD=15.9) Mean reactivity in triple therapy group=40.5 (SD=16.7) P-value for the treatment effect among carriers<0.001 *Noncarriers* Mean reactivity in high-maintenance dose clopidogrel group=41.9 (SD=16.4) Mean reactivity in triple therapy group=36.0 (SD=19.2) P-value for the treatment effect among noncarriers=0.276 *Late platelet aggregation by LTA 5 μmol/L at 30 d* *Carriers* Mean reactivity in high-maintenance dose clopidogrel group=30.7 (SD=22.2) Mean reactivity in triple therapy group=16.7 (SD=11.5) P-value for the treatment effect among carriers<0.001 *Noncarriers* Mean reactivity in high-maintenance dose clopidogrel group=19.0 (SD=13.4) Mean reactivity in triple therapy group=14.9 (SD=13.4) P-value for the treatment effect among noncarriers=0.318 *Late platelet aggregation by LTA 20 μmol/L at 30 d* *Carriers* Mean reactivity in high-maintenance dose clopidogrel group=43.2 (SD=22.0) Mean reactivity in triple therapy group=26.4 (SD=17.4) P-value for the treatment effect among carriers<0.001 *Noncarriers* Mean reactivity in high-maintenance dose clopidogrel group=26.9 (SD=18.8) Mean reactivity in triple therapy group=21.2 (SD=19.0) P-value for the treatment effect among noncarriers=0.321

170

Table 21. Effect modification on the outcome of platelet reactivity in randomized trials stratifying patients by CYP2C19 genotype status (continued)

Author Year Country UID Study name (if available)	Treatment group	Subgroups defined by genotype	N	Assay (agonist) [manufacturer] for the assessment of platelet reactivity	Summary of results
					VerifyNow PRU at 30 d
					Carriers
					Mean reactivity in high-maintenance dose clopidogrel group=214.1 (SD=68.5)
					Mean reactivity in triple therapy group=191.6 (SD=78.4)
					P-value for the treatment effect among carriers=0.153
					Noncarriers
					Mean reactivity in high-maintenance dose clopidogrel group=149.7 (SD=65.4)
					Mean reactivity in triple therapy group=129.4 (SD=76.4)
					P-value for the treatment effect among noncarriers=0.348
					VerifyNow %inhibition at 30 d
					Carriers
					Mean reactivity in high-maintenance dose clopidogrel group=33.5 (SD=19.2)
					Mean reactivity in triple therapy group=45.8 (SD=21.2)
					P-value for the treatment effect among carriers=0.005
					Noncarriers
					Mean reactivity in high-maintenance dose clopidogrel group=65.2 (SD=12.8)
					Mean reactivity in triple therapy group=70.5 (SD=7.6)
					P-value for the treatment effect among noncarriers=0.317
					HPR (cut-off >50% using LTA with ADP 5 µmol/L) at 30 d
					Carriers
					N (%) among high-maintenance dose clopidogrel group=16 (37.2%)
					N (%) among triple therapy group=3 (6.4%)
					P-value for the treatment effect among carriers<0.001
					Noncarriers
					N (%) among high-maintenance dose clopidogrel group=3 (13.6%)
					N (%) among triple therapy group=1 (4.5%)
					P-value for the treatment effect among noncarriers=0.607

Table 21. Effect modification on the outcome of platelet reactivity in randomized trials stratifying patients by CYP2C19 genotype status (continued)

Author Year Country UID Study name (if available)	Treatment group	Subgroups defined by genotype	N	Assay (agonist) [manufacturer] for the assessment of platelet reactivity	Summary of results
Park[264] 2011 S. Korea 21345843 CILON-T	Dual-antiplatelet therapy:	LOF carriers Noncarriers	132 104	VerifyNow P2Y12 (ADP) [Accumetrics, San Diego, CA]	*Mean on-treatment platelet reactivity (in PRU)* Dual therapy, carrier (254±7) vs. noncarrier (208±7), p<0.001 Triple therapy, carrier (215±7) vs. noncarrier (199±9), p=0.167 Noncarrier, dual therapy (211±8) vs. triple therapy (196±9), p=0.242 Carrier, dual therapy (256±7) vs. triple therapy (213±6), p<0.001 *High on-treatment platelet reactivity (>240 PRU):* Dual therapy, carrier (60.8%) vs. noncarrier (36.5%), p<0.001 Triple therapy, carrier (43.7%) vs. noncarrier (33.3%), p=0.115 Noncarriers, triple therapy (33.3%) vs. dual therapy (36.5%), p=0.241 Carriers, triple therapy (43.7%) vs. dual therapy (60.8%), p<0.001 p=0.241 for proportion of high on-treatment platelet reactivity among triple therapy noncarrier, triple therapy carrier, and dual therapy noncarrier Multivariate analysis for independent predictors of high on-treatment platelet reactivity (adjusted for decade of age, sex, smoking, diabetes, CKD, and treatment group): *OR (95% CI) [p-value] vs. dual therapy, noncarrier:* Dual therapy, carrier 2.93 (1.64 to 5.21) [<0.001] Triple therapy, noncarrier 0.75 (0.39 to 1.44) [0.388] Triple therapy, carrier 1.19 (0.68 to 2.05) [0.545]
	Triple-antiplatelet therapy (adjunctive cilostazol)	LOF carriers Noncarriers	151 87		

172

Table 21. Effect modification on the outcome of platelet reactivity in randomized trials stratifying patients by CYP2C19 genotype status (continued)

Author Year Country UID Study name (if available)	Treatment group	Subgroups defined by genotype	N	Assay (agonist) [manufacturer] for the assessment of platelet reactivity	Summary of results
Collet[265] 2011 France 21511218 CLOVIS-2	*Clopidogrel loading dose of 300 or 900 mg (crossover RCT).* Clopidogrel maintenance treatment (75 mg) was continued for ≥21 days before patients were crossed over to the alternate loading dose group	*2/*2 *2/*1 1/1	7 41 58	LTA (ADP 20 μmol/L) [Model 490-4D, Chrono-Log Corporation, Kordia, Netherlands] VerifyNow P2Y12 (ADP) [Accumetrics, San Diego, CA]	There was a stepwise decrease of the relative reduction in residual platelet aggregation from wild-type/wild-type to *2/*2 patients, with a significant gene-dose effect following the 300 mg loading dose. The 300 mg loading dose resulted in a significant reduction in platelet aggregation in wild-type/wild-type and wild-type/*2 patients, but had no detectable effect on platelet activation in *2/*2 carriers (residual/maximal platelet aggregation[%]: 65.43 ±11.23 and 67.27 ±10.60 before vs. 60.10 ±28.75 and 66.97 ±23.91 after loading, respectively) The 900 mg loading dose blunted the effect of the CYP2C19*2 variant on relative reduction in residual platelet aggregation in wild-type/*2, which did not differ from wild-type/wild-type. The increased dose had little effect on *2/*2 carriers. The prevalence of high on-clopidogrel platelet reactivity (measured by LTA 20 μmol/L ADP with a cut-off of 64.5%) increased with the number of *2 alleles, although this effect was blunted after administration of the 900 mg loading dose in patients carrying a single *2 allele. High on-treatment reactivity was less frequent when measured by VerifyNow (PRU ≥235) with no significant gene-dose effect.

Abbreviations: ADP = adenosine diphosphate; CI = confidence interval; CKD = chronic kidney disease; d = day(s); GOF = gain-of-function; HPR = high platelet reactivity; LOF = loss-of-function; LTA = light-transmission aggregometry; PRINC = Plavix Response in Coronary Intervention; PRU = platelet reactivity units; RCT = randomized controlled trial; VASP = vasodilator-stimulated phosphoprotein.

*Results were extracted for the longest followup reported (2–6 weeks); results for each diplotype not presented.
†Results were extracted for the longest followup reported (30 d)

Assessment of Risk of Bias of Individual Studies

A detailed assessment of 17 risk-of-bias items for studies providing information on effect modification by CYP2C19 variants is presented in Appendix F (the table includes both studies reporting on clinical and those reporting on intermediate outcomes). Overall, the risk of bias of individual studies was variable. Generally, studies reporting on clinical outcomes (which were generally larger and had longer followup than those with platelet reactivity as an outcome) used robust methods for randomization and allocation concealment. However, these studies included only a small proportion of the patients enrolled in the corresponding parent trials (15 to 40 percent in trials reporting clinical followup of more than a month). In large RCTs providing information on treatment effect modification by genotype status, genetic analyses were not conducted at baseline, raising further concerns regarding selection bias. In contrast, in studies reporting information on laboratory outcomes (which tended to be smaller with short followup periods), 79 to 100 percent of the patients enrolled in the parent RCTs were also included in the genetic substudies. These smaller studies provided adequate descriptions of the methods used for generating the randomization sequence but did not provide sufficient information to assess methods of allocation concealment.

Study With Genetic Test–Based Selection of Patients

We identified a single multicenter trial (ELEVATE-TIMI 56) using genetic test-based selection of patients and then randomizing them to alternative antiplatelet treatments. The study enrolled 335 patients with known cardiovascular disease (57.1 percent with a history of myocardial infarction; 97.3 percent with a history of PCI) on maintenance clopidogrel therapy (75 mg daily). Table 22 presents the descriptive characteristics of the trial.

Table 22. Descriptive characteristics of the study with genetic test–based selection of patients

Author, Year Country PMID Study name	Selected Population	Study Design Treatment Strategies Compared	Assay [model, manufacturer]	Total N Enrolled Male (%) Age†, Dyslipidemia (%), Smokers (%), HTN (%), Diabetes (%)
Mega[87] 2011 USA 22088980 ELEVATE-TIMI 56	Patients receiving clopidogrel maintenance therapy (75 mg/d); eligible patients had to have an indication for clopidogrel therapy (either AMI or PCI, within ≥4 wk and ≤6 mo prior to enrollment)	Crossover RCT, double-blind (patients + outcome assessors) Patients on dual antiplatelet therapy (clopidogrel 75 mg/d + aspirin 81-325 mg/d) were genotyped for the presence of CYP2C19 *2 alleles and were then allocated to treatment on the basis of genotype: *Patients with at least one *2 allele* (carriers) were randomized to various sequences of receiving clopidogrel at doses of 75, 150, 225, and 300 mg/d. *Patients with no *2 alleles* (non-carriers) were randomized to doses of 75 or 150 mg (2 periods at each dose). All patients were asked to keep their aspirin dose stable during the study.	For selecting patients before randomization: pyrosequencing assay [Nanosphere Verigene 2C19/CBS nucleic acid research-use-only assay]	333 patients were genotyped and randomized to different dosing schemes 249 (75%) 60 (10) 315 (95%) NR 287 (86%) 118 (35%)

Abbreviations: d = day; HTN = hypertension; NR = not reported; PCI = percutaneous coronary intervention; RCT = randomized controlled trial; SD = standard deviation; wk = week.
The study reported results both regarding clinical outcomes and the intermediate outcome of platelet reactivity, which are summarized below.
†Mean (standard deviation), unless otherwise stated.

Clinical Outcomes

Table 23 summarizes information on clinical outcomes from the ELEVATE-TIMI 56 study.

Table 23. Key findings of studies with phenotypic test–based selection of patients and clinical outcomes

Author Year Country PMID Study Name	Treatment Groups (sample size)	Followup Duration	Summary of Findings
Mega[87] 2011 USA 22088980 ELEVATE-TIMI 56	*Patients with at least one *2 allele* (carriers = 86 patients) randomized to various sequences of receiving clopidogrel at doses of 75, 150, 225, and 300 mg/d (each for 14 d ±3 d) + aspirin *Patients with no *2 alleles* (non-carriers = 247) were randomized to doses of 75 or 150 mg (2 periods of 14 d ±3 d at each dose) + aspirin	~ 2 mo on treatment	There were no deaths or cerebrovascular events. Among CYP2C19*2 noncarriers, 2 patients had cardiac ischemic events while taking the 75 mg dose and 3 with the 150 mg dose. Among carriers of a CYP2C19*2 allele, 1 patient experienced a cardiac ischemic event while taking the 75 mg clopidogrel dose.

Abbreviations: mo = months.

Intermediate Outcome: Platelet Reactivity During Followup

Table 24 summarizes information on the intermediate outcome of platelet reactivity from the ELEVATE-TIMI 56 study.

Table 24. Key findings of the study with genetic test–based selection of patients and intermediate outcomes

Author Year Country PMID Study Name	Treatment Groups (sample size)	Followup Duration	Summary of Findings
Mega[87] 2011 USA 22088980 ELEVATE-TIMI 56	*Patients with at least one *2 allele* (carriers = 86 patients) randomized to various sequences of receiving clopidogrel at doses of 75, 150, 225, and 300 mg/d (each for 14 d ±3 d) + aspirin *Patients with no *2 alleles* (non-carriers = 247 patients) were randomized to doses of 75 or 150 mg (2 periods of 14 d ±3 d at each dose) + aspirin	~ 2 mo on treatment	Results were assessed with the VASP assay (primary analysis) and the VerifyNow assay (secondary analysis). When treated with a standard clopidogrel maintenance dose of 75 mg/d, both CYP2C19*2 heterozygotes and homozygotes had significantly higher on-treatment platelet reactivity than did noncarrier patients (p<0.001 for both pair-wise comparisons). Among CYP2C19*2 heterozygotes, higher clopidogrel maintenance doses (up to 300 mg) produced significant reductions in platelet reactivity (p<0.001 for trend). Each increase of 75 mg of the clopidogrel dose resulted in ~8% to 9% absolute reduction in VASP PRI. Pairwise comparisons between the higher daily doses of clopidogrel (150, 225, and 300 mg) and the 75 mg dose were all statistically significant (p<0.001). Results with the VerifyNow assay were similar to the VASP data across dose and genotype. Among CYP2C19*2 homozygotes, there was a trend toward less platelet reactivity with higher maintenance doses of clopidogrel; however, even with 300 mg daily of clopidogrel, these individuals had increased reactivity by VASP and VerifyNow. In CYP2C19*2 heterozygotes, 150 mg resulted in platelet reactivity that tended to be higher than that seen in noncarrier patients treated with 75 mg daily. The 225 mg dose resulted in platelet reactivity similar to that observed in response to standard clopidogrel dosing in noncarriers. The 300 mg dose resulted in superior reductions in platelet reactivity as compared with 75 mg dosing in noncarrier patients as measured both by VASP PRI and PRU (p<0.001 for both). For CYP2C19*2 homozygotes, even 300 mg daily of clopidogrel did not result in platelet reactivity levels similar to standard clopidogrel dosing in noncarriers.

Abbreviations: d = day; mo = month; PRI = platelet reactivity index; PRU = platelet reactivity unit.

Assessment of Risk of Bias of Individual Studies

A detailed assessment of 17 risk-of-bias items for the ELEVATE-TIMI 56 trial is presented in Appendix F. Overall, the trial was well conducted, with centralized randomization and blinding of both patients and outcome assessors (both for clinical and intermediate outcomes) to the treatments assessment. The sample size was based on a priori power analysis for platelet reactivity outcomes and the recruitment target was attained (333 patients randomized with a minimum of 254 required on the basis of the power calculation). There were minimal dropouts and losses to followup. However, the study was not powered for, and did not have adequate followup to provide robust evidence on, clinical outcomes.

Testing for Platelet Reactivity

Studies of Test-and-Treat Strategies

We identified seven studies directly comparing alternative test-and-treat strategies.[270-274] Six of the seven studies had a randomized design and one was a nonrandomized comparative study of test-and-treat strategies. Four compared VASP assay–guided therapy and non–test-guided therapy; two compared Multiplate analyzer-guided therapy and non–test-guided therapy (1 RCT and 1 nonrandomized comparative study); and one compared VerifyNow P2Y12–guided therapy versus non–test-guided therapy. The four studies evaluating the use of the VASP assay were of moderate size (the smallest enrolled 153 patients; the largest, 429 patients). The RCT evaluating the use of the Multiplate analyzer enrolled 192 patients and the nonrandomized comparative study evaluating the same assay enrolled 798 patients. The single study assessing VerifyNow was smaller (60 patients).

The six RCTs directly comparing alternative test-and-treat strategies assessed patients undergoing PCI; 4 enrolled patients with stable coronary artery disease or acute coronary syndromes and 1 enrolled exclusively patients undergoing elective stenting. The average patient age was equal to or older than 65 years in all RCTs. Patients had a relatively high burden of risk factors for cardiovascular disease. Four studies selected patients on the basis of a baseline assessment of platelet reactivity (enrolling only those with reactivity above a predetermined threshold); the fifth study included all patients, regardless of baseline reactivity.

The single nonrandomized comparative study also included patients undergoing PCI with stent implantation and did not use platelet reactivity as a selection criterion. Of note, the group receiving test-guided treatment was enrolled and followed up in a different research center than the group receiving non-test guided treatment (the Medical University of Vienna and the Kaiser Franz Josef Hospital, respectively). This renders the study results highly susceptible to confounding and selection bias. Our detailed assessment of the risk of bias of all seven studies comparing alternative test-and-treat strategies is presented at the end of this section.

The test-guided treatment groups in five studies (three using the VASP assay, one using the VerifyNow assay, and one using the Multiplate analyzer) employed repeat reactivity monitoring at multiple time points with modification of the administered clopidogrel dose on the basis of test results. The other two studies performed only a single assessment of platelet reactivity, with subsequent treatment modification in patients found to have reactivity values above a predefined threshold. Control groups were given clopidogrel-based therapy at standard doses.

Table 25 summarizes the selection criteria, population characteristics, and treatments compared in the five test-and-treat studies involving phenotypic testing.

The seven studies are relatively recent (with enrollment started between 2005 and 2009), and had relatively short followup durations (four had maximum followup of 30 days; two, 6 months; and one, a year). Four studies reported a prospective power calculation (and all had attained the enrollment goal). Table 26 summarizes the study design of included studies. Information on the assays used, test timing, and the number of patients screened for inclusion is presented in Table 27.

Table 25. Descriptive characteristics of studies of test-and-treat strategies using phenotypic testing of platelet reactivity

Author Year Country PMID Study Name (if available)	Selected Population	Total N Enrolled Male (%), Age,* Dyslipidemia (%), Current smokers (%), HTN (%), Diabetes (%)	Study design Initial and Compared Treatment Strategies
Wang[270] 2011 China 21538380	Patients with VASP PRI >50% 1 mo after undergoing PCI for refractory angina pectoris, silent ischemia on thallium scintigraphy, or NSTE ACS	N=306 214 (70%) 67 (11) 156 (51%) 118 (39%) 188 (61%) 132 (43%)	RCT All patients underwent angiography after a loading dose of aspirin (100 mg) and clopidogrel (300 mg); maintenance doses were 100 mg/d for aspirin and 75–375 mg/d for clopidogrel. One mo after PCI patients were randomized to 2 groups: *VASP-guided treatment:* VASP PRI was ascertained at 3, 6, 9, and 12 mo after the first analysis (1 mo post-PCI), when patients with PRI >50% received clopidogrel at a dose of 150 mg/d. At each subsequent monitoring visit the dose was increased by 75 mg/d if PRI remained >50% (for a maximum dose of 375 mg/d at 1 yr). If PRI was <25% at the 12-mp visit, the dose was decreased to 75mg/d. For PRI between 25% and 50%, the dose was not changed. *Control treatment:* A maintenance regimen of clopidogrel 75 mg/d was used.
Bonello[271] 2009 France 19101221	Patients with VASP PRI >50% undergoing nonemergent PCI for refractory angina pectoris under "optimal medical therapy," silent ischemia on thallium scintigraphy or NSTE ACS	N=429 345 (80%) 66 (11) 255 (59%) 238 (55%) 264 (62%) 155 (36%)	RCT All patients received a clopidogrel loading dose of 600 mg. Patients with PRI >50% afterward were randomized to 2 groups: *VASP-guided treatment:* Clopidogrel pretreatment was adjusted individually (pre-PCI) to obtain a VASP PRI <50% by prescribing up to 3 additional boluses of clopidogrel 600 mg 24 h after the previous dose; PRI was assessed 12 h after each administration until the value was <50%. If PRI remained >50% after the 3 additional loading doses, PCI was performed. *Control treatment:* PCI was carried out without an additional clopidogrel loading dose.

Table 25. Descriptive characteristics of studies of test-and-treat strategies using phenotypic testing of platelet reactivity (continued)

Author Year Country PMID Study Name (if available)	Selected Population	Total N Enrolled Male (%), Age*, Dyslipidemia (%), Current smokers (%), HTN (%), Diabetes (%)	Study design Initial and Compared Treatment Strategies
Bonello[272] 2008 France 18387444	Patients with VASP PRI >50% undergoing nonemergent PCI for refractory angina pectoris under "optimal medical therapy" or having silent ischemia on thallium scintigraphy or NSTE ACS	N=162 126 (78%) 66 (11) 86 (53%) 62 (38%) 98 (60%) 67 (41%)	RCT All patients received a clopidogrel loading dose of 600 mg. Patients with PRI >50% afterward were randomized to 2 groups: *VASP-guided treatment:* Clopidogrel pretreatment was adjusted individually (pre-PCI) to obtain a VASP PRI <50% by prescribing up to 3 additional boluses of clopidogrel 600 mg 24 h after the previous dose; PRI was assessed 12 h after each administration until the value was <50%. If PRI remained >50% after the 3 additional loading doses, PCI was performed. *Control treatment:* PCI was carried out without an additional clopidogrel loading dose.

Table 25. Descriptive characteristics of studies of test-and-treat strategies using phenotypic testing of platelet reactivity (continued)

Author Year Country PMID Study Name (if available)	Selected Population	Total N Enrolled Male (%), Age*, Dyslipidemia (%), Current smokers (%), HTN (%), Diabetes (%)	Study design Initial and Compared Treatment Strategies
Tousek[273] 2011 Czech Republic 21663983	Patients with VerifyNow PRU >240 undergoing PCI for stable angina, STE or NSTE MI, or UA	N=60 45 (75%) 66 (12) NR 22 (37%) 40 (67%) 18 (30%)	RCT All patients received a clopidogrel loading dose of 600 mg. Patients with VerifyNow PRU >240 afterward were randomized to 2 groups: *VerifyNow-guided treatment:* clopidogrel up-titration to 150 mg/d with further dose increases according to VerifyNow results every 7 days; the target PRU was <240 by 30 d. *Control treatment:* Standard clopidogrel maintenance dose of 75 mg/d.
Aleil[274] 2008 France 19463377 VASP-02	Patients undergoing elective PCI with coronary stenting	N=153 126 (82%) 64.9 (9.7) 100 (65%) 24 (16%) 97 (63%) 37 (24%)	RCT The day before PCI patients received clopidogrel (300 to 600 mg) loading dose and were then randomized into 2 groups (3:2 ratio): *VASP-guided treatment:* Clopidogrel maintenance dose of 75 mg/d for 2 wk. At 2 wk, VASP analysis was performed; patients with PRI ≥69% were administered a maintenance dose of 150 mg/d, and those with PRI <69% were kept on 75 mg/d, for an additional 2 wk. *Control treatment:* Clopidogrel maintenance dose of 150 mg/d for 4 wk.
Hazarbasanov[275] 2012 Bulgaria 22249353	Patients undergoing PCI	N=192 126 (66%) 64.5 (9.3) 129 (67%) 89 (46%) 170 (89%) 48 (25%)	RCT Patients with stable angina received clopidogrel loading (300 mg) 24 h before PCI. Patients presenting with ACS received clopidogrel loading (600 mg). Patients already on long-term clopidogrel therapy received an additional loading dose of 300 mg or 600 mg clopidogrel according to the clinical presentation. Patients were then randomized into 2 groups (1:1 ratio): *Multiplate analyzer-guided treatment:* patients with HPR received a 2nd loading dose of 600 mg clopidogrel and a doubled maintenance dose (150 mg/d) for 1 mo after PCI. Clopidogrel 75 mg/d was resumed after 30 d in all patients and continued for ≥3 mo post BMS placement or ≥12 mo post DES placement. *Control treatment:* clopidogrel 75 mg/d for ≥3 mo post BMS placement or ≥12 mo post DES placement.

Table 25. Descriptive characteristics of studies of test-and-treat strategies using phenotypic testing of platelet reactivity (continued)

Author Year Country PMID Study Name (if available)	Selected Population	Total N Enrolled Male (%), Age*, Dyslipidemia (%), Current smokers (%), HTN (%), Diabetes (%)	Study design Initial and Compared Treatment Strategies
Siller-Matula[276] 2012 Austria 22656044 MADONNA	Patients undergoing PCI with stent implantation for STEMI or NSTE-ACS	N=798 585 (73%) 65.0 (12.0) 608 (76%) 419 (53%) 676 (85%) 273 (34%)	NRCS The following treatment approaches were compared: *Multiplate analyzer-guided treatment:* patients received an initial loading dose of clopidogrel (600 mg) followed by measurement of on-treatment platelet reactivity (post PCI). Patients with high on-treatment platelet reactivity (≥50 U) were reloaded with clopidogrel (600 mg) and platelet reactivity was measured the day after re-loading. In case of high on-treatment platelet reactivity after a 2nd or 3rd clopidogrel loading, patients were re-loaded with clopidogrel 600 mg for the 4th time. After prasugrel became available, clopidogrel non-responders were loaded with prasugrel (in the absence of contraindications). For maintenance treatment, patients received the antiplatelet therapy matching with the last loading dose they received (clopidogrel responders received clopidogrel; clopidogrel non-responders - clopidogrel or prasugrel). Non-responders were hospitalized during the period of tailored antiplatelet therapy. *Control treatment:* a single clopidogrel loading dose (600 mg) followed by clopidogrel maintenance. All patients received 250 mg of acetylsalicylic acid intravenously during PCI followed by 100 mg per so a day. Patients were "matched" according to the indication for PCI (no details were reported on the matching methods). Patients in the non-guided group were included at the Medical University of Vienna whereas patients in the guided group at the Kaiser Franz Josef Hospital in Vienna.

Abbreviations: ACS = acute coronary syndrome; BMS = bare metal stent; d = day(s); DES = drug eluting stent; h = hours; HTN = hypertension; MI = myocardial infarction; mo = month; NR = not reported; NSTE = non-STEMI; PCI = percutaneous coronary intervention; PRI = platelet reactivity index; PRU = platelet reactivity units (arbitrary units); STE = ST-elevation; UA = unstable angina; VASP = vasodilator-stimulated phosphoprotein; wk = weeks.
*Age is given as mean years (standard deviation), unless otherwise stated.

Table 26. Study design characteristics of studies of test-and-treat strategies using phenotypic testing of platelet reactivity

Author Year Country PMID Study Name (if available)	Enroll-ment period	Random-ization procedure	Blinding	Number of partici-pating centers	Followup duration	Setting	Target enrollment from a priori power analysis	Proce-dure for multiple compar-isons	Funding
Wang[270] 2011 China 21538380	August 2008–October 2009	NR	Endpoints were recorded by an investigator who was not aware of treatment assignment or patient characteristics	Single center	1 yr	Cardiology department of university hospital	NR	Not used	Nonindustry only
Bonello[271] 2009 France 19101221	August 2007–March 2008	NR	Endpoints were recorded by an investigator who was not aware of treatment assignment or patient characteristics	Multicenter	30 d	4 cardiology centers	400 (429 actually enrolled)	Not used	NR
Bonello[272] 2008 France 18387444	March 2007–July 2007	NR	Endpoints were recorded by an investigator who was not aware of treatment assignment or patient characteristics	Multicenter	30 d	4 cardiology centers	160 (162 actually enrolled)	Not used	Nonindustry only
Tousek[273] 2011 Czech Republic 21663983	May 2009–July 2010	NR	NR	Single center	6 mo	Cardiology department of university hospital	NR	Not used	Nonindustry only
Aleil[274] 2008 France 19463377 VASP-02	April 2005–December 2007	Centralized randomization; no additional details reported	NR	Multicenter	30 d*	Multiple cardiology departments	NR	Not used	Partly industry; also assays provided by the manufacturer
Hazarbasanov[275] 2012 Bulgaria 22249353	May 2008–June 2009	NR	Open-label	Single center	6 mo	Cardiology department of university hospital	189 (192 actually enrolled)	Not used	Assays provided by the manufacturer

Table 26. Study design characteristics of studies of test-and-treat strategies using phenotypic testing of platelet reactivity (continued)

Author Year Country PMID Study Name (if available)	Enrollment period	Randomization procedure	Blinding	Number of participating centers	Followup duration	Setting	Target enrollment from a priori power analysis	Procedure for multiple comparisons	Funding
Siller-Matula[276] 2012 Austria 22656044 MADONNA	March 2007– November 2010	Not randomized	No blinding	2 centers; each center applied one of the compared approaches	30 d	The test-guided treatment group was treated in a university hospital; no details were provided for the center where the non-guided group was treated	351 patients per group (403 and 395 were actually enrolled)	Not used	NR

Abbreviations: d = days; mo = months; NR = not reported; yr = years.

*We extracted information at 30 d because this is the only time point when outcomes could have been affected by testing (in the VASP-guided group).

Table 27. Test information in studies of test-and-treat strategies using phenotypic testing of platelet reactivity

Author Year Country PMID Study Name (if available)	Platelet Reactivity Assay (Manufacturer)	Timing of Test Interval Between Sample Collection and Analysis Interval Between Sampling and Assay Results	N Tested; N Included Test Success Rate	Rationale for the Platelet Reactivity Threshold Chosen
Wang[270] 2011 China 21538380	VASP assay (VASP kit; Becton Dickinson, Franklin Lakes, NJ) using flow cytometry (Coulter EPICS XL cytometer, FACSCalibur, Becton Dickinson)	1 mo post-PCI for all patients; at 3, 6, 9, and 12 mo for patients in the VASP-guided treatment group NR NR	538 patients screened for inclusion; 306 had PRI >50% and fulfilled all other inclusion criteria NR	Not explicitly provided
Bonello[271] 2009 France 19101221	VASP assay (VASP kit; Diagnostica Stago, Asnieres, France) using flow cytometry (Coulter EPICS XL cytometer, Beckman Coulter Inc., Fullerton, CA)	≥6 h and within 24 h after the initial clopidogrel bolus; in the VASP-guided group, 12 h after each additional clopidogrel bolus NR NR	1122 patients screened for inclusion; 429 had PRI ≥50% and fulfilled all other inclusion criteria	Statement (in the introduction section) that measurements above the cut-off threshold are associated with higher risk of adverse cardiovascular outcomes; also, a previous randomized study from the same team of investigators.
Bonello[272] 2008 France 18387444	VASP assay (VASP kit; Diagnostica Stago, Asnieres, France) using flow cytometry (Coulter EPICS XL cytometer, Beckman Coulter Inc., Fullerton, CA)	24 h after the initial clopidogrel bolus; in the VASP-guided group, 12 h after each additional clopidogrel bolus NR NR	406 patients screened for inclusion; 162 had PRI ≥50% and fulfilled all other inclusion criteria	A previous study by the same team of investigators where a threshold of 50% could predict adverse cardiovascular outcomes with a sensitivity of 100%
Tousek[273] 2011 Czech Republic 21663983	VerifyNow P2Y12 assay (Accumetrics, San Diego, CA)	24-48 h after PCI (post–clopidogrel loading); in the VerifyNow-guided group, every 7 days thereafter for up to 30 d NR NR	378 patients screened for inclusion; 134 had PRU ≥240 and fulfilled all other inclusion criteria; and 60 patients were randomized	Not explicitly provided

184

Table 27. Test information in studies of test-and-treat strategies using phenotypic testing of platelet reactivity (continued)

Author Year Country PMID Study Name (if available)	Platelet Reactivity Assay (Manufacturer)	Timing of Test Interval Between Sample Collection and Analysis Interval Between Sampling and Assay Results	N Tested; N Included Test Success Rate	Rationale for the Platelet Reactivity Threshold Chosen
Aleil[274] 2008 France 19463377 VASP-02	VASP assay (VASP kit; Diagnostica Stago/Biocytex, Asnieres, France) using flow cytometry (FACS Calibur, Becton Dickinson, Plymouth, UK)	Before clopidogrel administration, 10-12 h post clopidogrel dosing, at 2 wk (to identify responders and switch nonresponders in the group originally assigned to 75 mg/d maintenance dose), and at 4 wk (to assess outcomes)	Inclusion was not based on baseline testing; 153 patients were included	Previous studies by the same team of investigators
Hazarbasanov[275] 2012 Bulgaria 22249353	Multiplate analyzer (ADP 6.4 µM) (Verum Diagnostica GmBH, Munich, Germany)	24 h after clopidogrel loading; in patients with high-platelet reactivity measurements were repeated 24 h after the second loading dose and at day 30 during the maintenance phase on 150 mg clopidogrel	Inclusion was not based on baseline testing; 192 patients were included	Consensus recommendations for the definition of high platelet reactivity
Siller-Matula[276] 2012 Austria 22656044 MADONNA	Multiplate analyzer (ADP 6.4 µM) (Verum Diagnostica GmBH, Munich, Germany)	Measurements were performed the day after PCI, ≥12 h post clopidogrel loading	Inclusion was not based on baseline testing; 798 patients were included	Previous published studies

Abbreviations: ADP = adenosine diphosphate; h = hour(s); mo = month(s); NR = not reported; PCI = percutaneous coronary intervention; VASP = vasodilator-stimulated phosphoprotein; PRU = platelet reactivity unit; wk = week(s).

Clinical Outcomes

All seven studies comparing alternative test-and-treat strategies reported information on cardiovascular mortality; six also reported on MACE (composite outcomes), five on stent thrombosis, three on acute coronary syndromes (myocardial infarction or unstable angina), three on myocardial infarction alone, two on all-cause mortality, and two on repeat revascularization. Overall, the studies had short followup durations and small to intermediate sample sizes; thus, the outcome rates were low and relative effect estimates (when possible to calculate) were often extreme (e.g., odds ratios <0.5) and had substantial uncertainty (wide CIs). Studies generally indicated that the groups with test-based monitoring had better outcomes (lower event rates) than the groups without test-based monitoring; however, the differences were often not statistically significant. For the outcome of cardiovascular mortality the study by Siller-Matula produced results in the opposite direction of all other studies (indicating worse outcomes with test-based treatment strategies). This may be attributable to potential confounding factors (because the Siller-Matula et al. study was not randomized) or may be a chance finding (confidence intervals were generally broad indicating substantial uncertainty around estimates of effect). Regardless of the reason for the observed inconsistency, it contributed to our decision to grade the strength of evidence for this outcome as insufficient. Detailed outcome information is summarized in Tables 28–33. To facilitate qualitative synthesis, we present forest plots of study estimates for outcomes assessed by at least six studies: cardiovascular mortality (Figure 37), stent thrombosis (Figure 38), and MACE (Figure 39). Meta-analyses were not performed owing to the differences in the populations included, interventions compared, and durations of followup used.

Table 28. Cardiovascular mortality in studies of test-and-treat strategies using phenotypic testing of platelet reactivity

Author Year Country PMID Study Name (if available)	Treatment Group Sample Size	No. with Outcome (%)	Time Point	Comparative Metric	95% CI	p-value [statistical test]
Wang[270] 2011 China 21538380	VASP-guided treatment N=150	6 (4.0%)	1 yr	OR=0.50 (calculated)	0.18 to 1.37 (calculated)	p=0.003* [unclear]
	Control N=156	12 (7.7%)				
Bonello[271] 2009 France 19101221	VASP-guided treatment N=215	0 (0%)	30 d	OR=0.11 (calculated)	0.01 to 2.03 (calculated)	p=0.06 [Fisher exact test]
	Control N=214	4 (1.8%)				
Bonello[272] 2008 France 18387444	VASP-guided treatment N=78	0 (0%)	30 d	OR=0.21 (calculated)	0.01 to 4.45 (calculated)	p=0.498 [Fisher exact test; calculated]
	Control N=84	2 (2.4%)				
Tousek[273] 2011 Czech Republic 21663983	VerifyNow-guided treatment N=30	0 (0%)	6 mo	Not defined	Not defined	NA
	Control N=30	0 (%)				
Aleil[274] 2008 France 19463377 VASP-02	VASP-guided treatment N=95 (93 included in analyses)	0 (0%)	30 d	Not defined	Not defined	NA
	Control N=58	0 (0%)				

Table 28. Cardiovascular mortality in studies of test-and-treat strategies using phenotypic testing of platelet reactivity (continued)

Author Year Country PMID Study Name (if available)	Treatment Group Sample Size	No. with Outcome (%)	Time Point	Comparative Metric	95% CI	p-value [statistical test]
Hazarbasanov[275] 2012 Bulgaria 22249353	Multiplate analyzer-guided treatment N=97	0 (0%)	6 mo	OR=0.136	0.007 to 2.660 (calculated)	p=0.12 [Fisher exact test]
	Control N=95	3 (3.2%)				
Siller-Matula[276] 2012 Austria 22656044 MADONNA	Multiplate analyzer-guided treatment N=403	8 (2%)	30 d	OR=1.58 (calculated)	0.51 to 4.87 (calculated)	p=0.422 [statistical test unclear]; p=0.58 (2-sided Fisher exact test; calculated)
	Control N=395	5 (1.3%)				

Abbreviations: CI = confidence interval; d = days; mo = months; NA = not applicable; NR = not reported; OR = odds ratio; VASP = vasodilator-stimulated phosphoprotein; yr = year.

"Calculated" indicates that the result was not reported by the article's authors; rather, we derived the result from reported raw data.

*Although p=0.003 was the reported p-value, recalculation using a chi-square test gives a p-value of 0.170 and recalculation using the Fisher exact test gives a p-value of 0.225. It is unclear how the reported p-value was calculated.

Figure 37. Cardiovascular mortality in studies of test-and-treat strategies using phenotypic testing for platelet reactivity

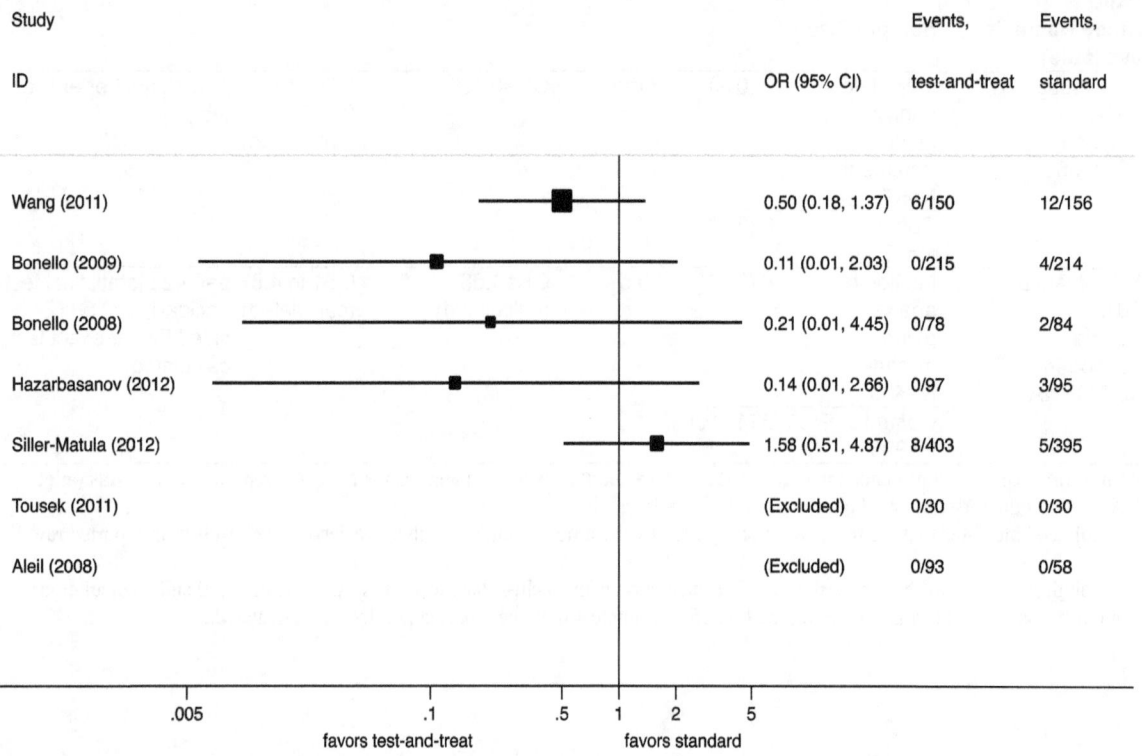

Abbreviations: CI = confidence interval; OR = odds ratio. See Table 25 for details on the strategies compared and the definitions of outcomes employed in each study.

Table 29. All-cause mortality in studies assessing test-and-treat strategies

Author Year Country PMID Study Name (if available)	Treatment Group Sample Size	No. with Outcome (%)	Time Point	Comparative Metric	95% CI	p-value [statistical test]
Wang[270] 2011 China 21538380	VASP-guided treatment N=150	NR	1 yr	NR	NR	p<0.01 [log-rank test
	Control N=156	NR				
Tousek[273] 2011 Czech Republic 21663983	VerifyNow-guided treatment N=30	0 (0%)	6 mo	Not defined	Not defined	NA
	Control N=30	0 (0%)				

Abbreviations: CI = confidence interval; mo = months; NA = not applicable; NR = not reported; VASP = vasodilator-stimulated phosphoprotein; yr = year.

Table 30. Stent thrombosis in studies of test-and-treat strategies using phenotypic testing of platelet reactivity

Author Year Country PMID Study Name (if available)	Treatment Group Sample Size	No. with Outcome (%)	Outcome Definition	Time Point	Comparative Metric	95% CI	p-value [statistical test]
Wang[270] 2011 China 21538380	VASP-guided treatment N=150	3 (2.0%)	Angiographically confirmed late ST	1 yr	OR=0.51 (calculated)	0.13 to 2.08 (calculated)	p=0.03* [unclear]
	Control N=156	6 (3.8%)					
Bonello[271] 2009 France 19101221	VASP-guided treatment N=215	1 (0.5%) [subacute thrombosis]	Early definite ST = total occlusion originating in or within 5 mm of the stent or visible thrombus within the stent or within 5 mm of the stent associated with ≥1 of the following signs present within 48 h: new onset of ischemic symptoms at rest; recent changes suggestive of acute ischemia on ECG at rest; typical increase and decrease in cardiac biomarkers according to Academic Research Consortium criteria	30 d	OR=0.10 (calculated)	0.01 to 0.75 (calculated)	p<0.01 for early definite stent thrombosis (p=0.25 for acute thrombosis; p=0.02 for subacute thrombosis) [Fisher exact test] p<0.01 [log-rank test]
	Control N=214	10 (4.7%) [8 subacute; 2 acute]					
Bonello[272] 2008 France 18387444	VASP-guided treatment N=78	0 (0%)	Early definite ST = angiographic confirmation of ST associated with at least 1 of the following signs present within 48 h: new onset of ischemic symptoms at rest; recent changes suggestive of acute ischemia on ECG at rest; typical increase and decrease in cardiac biomarkers according to Academic Research Consortium criteria	30 d	OR=0.11 (calculated)	0.01 to 2.15 (calculated)	p=0.121 [Fisher exact test; calculated]
	Control N=84	4 (4.8%) [3 subacute; 1 acute]					
Hazarbasanov[275] 2012 Bulgaria 22249353	Multiplate analyzer-guided treatment N=97	0 (0%)	Definite, probable, or possible ST according to Academic Research Consortium criteria	6 mo	OR=0.104 (calculated)	0.006 to 1.964 (calculated)	p=0.06 [Fisher exact test]
	Control N=95	4 (4.2%)					

Table 30. Stent thrombosis in studies of test-and-treat strategies using phenotypic testing of platelet reactivity (continued)

Author Year Country PMID Study Name (if available)	Treatment Group Sample Size	No. with Outcome (%)	Outcome Definition	Time Point	Comparative Metric	95% CI	p-value [statistical test]
Siller-Matula[276] 2012 Austria 22656044 MADONNA	Multiplate analyzer-guided treatment N=403	1 (<1%)	Definite and probable ST = ACS with either angiographic or pathological confirmation of thrombosis, or any unexplained death within 30 days or target vessel MI without angiographic confirmation of thrombosis or other identified culprit lesion, according to Academic Research Consortium criteria	30 d	OR=0.14 (calculated)	0.02 to 1.13 (calculated)	p=0.027 [statistical test unclear]; p=0.048 in multivariable adjusted Cox proportional hazards regression; p=0.04 [two-sided Fisher exact test; calculated]
	Control N=395	7 (1.8%)					

Abbreviations: ACS = acute coronary syndrome; CI = confidence interval; d = days; ECG = electrocardiogram; h = hour(s); OR = odds ratio; ST = stent thrombosis; VASP = vasodilator-stimulated phosphoprotein; yr = year.

"Calculated" indicates that the result was not reported by the article's authors; rather, we derived the result from reported raw data.

*Although p=0.03 was the reported p-value, recalculation using a chi-square test gives a p-value of 0.339 and recalculation using the Fisher exact test gives a p-value of 0.502. It is unclear how the reported p-value was calculated.

Figure 38. Stent thrombosis in studies of test-and-treat strategies using phenotypic testing for platelet reactivity

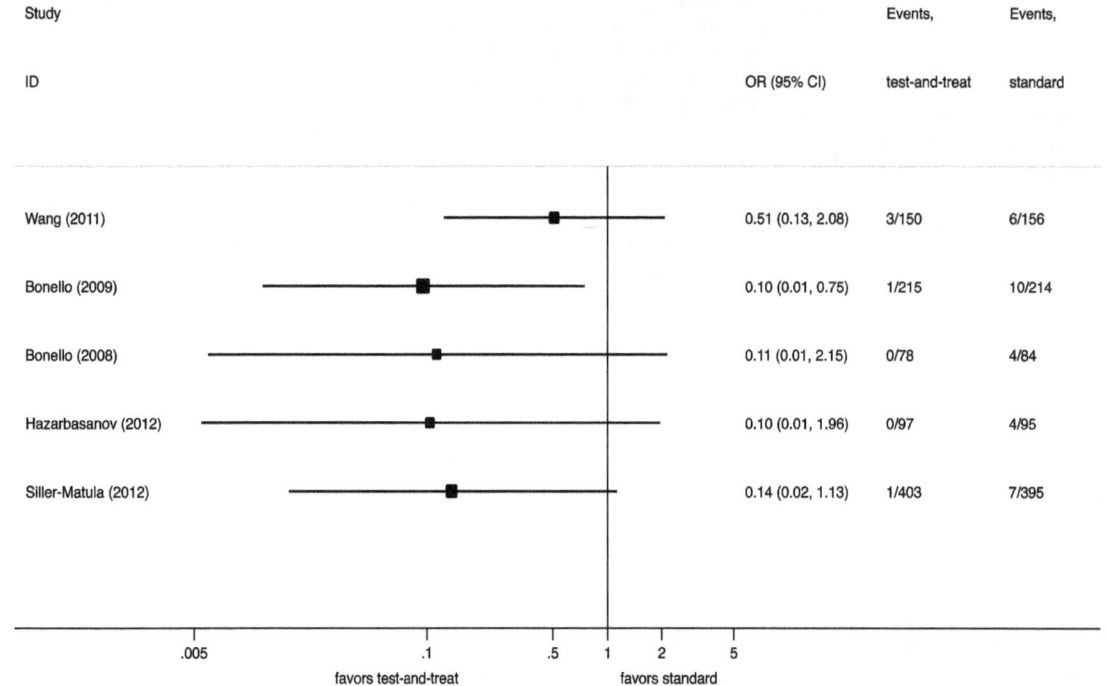

Stent thrombosis

Abbreviations: CI = confidence interval; OR = odds ratio. See Table 25 for details on the strategies compared and the definitions of outcomes employed in each study

190

Table 31. Major adverse cardiovascular events (composite) in studies of test-and-treat strategies using phenotypic testing of platelet reactivity

Author Year Country PMID Study Name (if available)	Treatment Group Sample Size	No. with Outcome (%)	Outcome Definition	Time Point	Comparative Metric	95% CI	p-value [statistical test]
Wang[270] 2011 China 21538380	VASP-guided treatment N=150	14 (9.3%)	Cardiovascular death, angiographically confirmed ST, recurrent ACS, or recurrent revascularization	1 yr	OR=0.43 (calculated)	0.22 to 0.85 (calculated)	p=0.008* [unclear]
	Control N=156	30 (19.2%)					
Bonello[271] 2009 France 19101221	VASP-guided treatment N=215	1 (0.5%)	Cardiovascular death, MI, or urgent repeat revascularization	30 d	OR=0.05 (calculated)	0.01 to 0.36 (calculated)	p<0.001 [Fisher exact test]
	Control N=214	19 (8.9%)					
Bonello[272] 2008 France 18387444	VASP-guided treatment N=78	0 (0%)	Cardiovascular death, angiographically confirmed ST, recurrent ACS, or repeat revascularization	30 d	OR=0.06 (calculated)	<0.01 to 1.01 (calculated)	p=0.007 [Fisher exact test] p<0.005 [log-rank p-value; log-rank statistic=7.75]
	Control N=84	8 (9.5%)					

191

Table 31. Major adverse cardiovascular events (composite) in studies of test-and-treat strategies using phenotypic testing of platelet reactivity (continued)

Author Year Country PMID Study Name (if available)	Treatment Group Sample Size	No. with Outcome (%)	Outcome Definition	Time Point	Comparative Metric	95% CI	p-value [statistical test]
Tousek[273] 2011 Czech Republic 21663983	VerifyNow-guided treatment N=30	1 (3.3%)	Death, MI, or stroke	6 mo	OR=0.48	0.04 to 5.6	p=0.55 [chi-square test]
	Control N=30	2 (6.7%)					
Aleil[274] 2008 France 19463377 VASP-02	VASP-guided treatment N=95 (93 included in analyses)	1 (1%) [patient was a nonresponder]	CV death, stroke, MI, documented ischemia requiring target-vessel revascularization, or "improvement" of medical treatment	30 d	OR=1.90 (calculated)	0.08 to 47.36 (calculated)	p>0.99 [Fisher exact test; calculated]
	Control N=58	0 (0%)					
Hazarbasanov[275] 2012 Bulgaria 22249353	Multiplate analyzer-guided treatment N=97	0 (0%)	CV death, MI, definite or probable stent thrombosis, or ischemic stroke	6 mo	OR=0.084 (calculated)	0.005 to 1.548	p=0.03 [Fisher exact test]
	Control N=95	5 (5.3%)					

Abbreviations: ACS = acute coronary syndrome; CI = confidence interval; CV cardiovascular; d = days; mo = months; MI = myocardial infarction; OR = odds ratio; ST = stent thrombosis; VASP = vasodilator-stimulated phosphoprotein; yr=year.

"Calculated" indicates that the result was not reported by the article's authors; rather, we derived the result from reported raw data.

*Although p=0.008 was the reported p-value, recalculation using a chi-square test gives a p-value of 0.014 and recalculation using the Fisher exact test gives a p-value of 0.015 (or 0.010 for a one-sided test). It is unclear how the reported p-value was calculated.

Figure 39. Major adverse cardiovascular events in studies of test-and-treat strategies using phenotypic testing of platelet reactivity

MACE

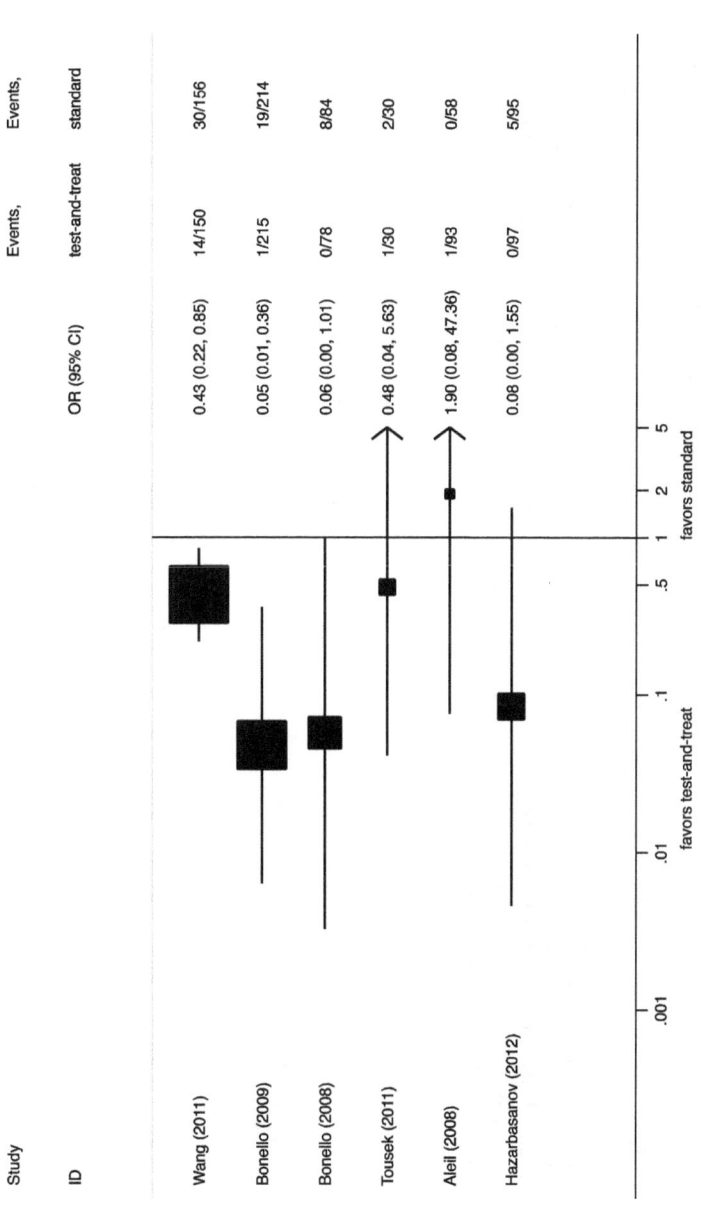

Study		Events,	Events,
ID	OR (95% CI)	test-and-treat	standard
Wang (2011)	0.43 (0.22, 0.85)	14/150	30/156
Bonello (2009)	0.05 (0.01, 0.36)	1/215	19/214
Bonello (2008)	0.06 (0.00, 1.01)	0/78	8/84
Tousek (2011)	0.48 (0.04, 5.63)	1/30	2/30
Aleil (2008)	1.90 (0.08, 47.36)	1/93	0/58
Hazarbasanov (2012)	0.08 (0.00, 1.55)	0/97	5/95

Abbreviations: CI = confidence interval; MACE = major adverse cardiovascular events; OR = odds ratio. See Table 25 for details on the strategies compared.

Table 32. Repeat revascularization in studies of test-and-treat strategies using phenotypic testing of platelet reactivity

Author Year Country PMID Study Name (if available)	Treatment Group Sample Size	No. with Outcome (%)	Outcome Definition	Time Point	Comparative Metric	95% CI	p-value [statistical test]
Wang[270] 2011 China 21538380	VASP-guided treatment N=150	3 (2.0%)	Recurrent revascularization by coronary angioplasty or CABG	1 yr	OR=0.33 (calculated)	0.09 to 1.26 (calculated)	p=0.027* [unclear]
	Control N=156	9 (5.8%)					
Bonello[271] 2009 France 19101221	VASP-guided treatment N=215	0 (0%)	Recurrent revascularization by urgent coronary angioplasty or CABG	30 d	OR=0.09 (calculated)	<0.01 to 1.61 (calculated)	p=0.06 [unclear]
	Control N=214	5 (2.3%)					

Abbreviations: CABG = coronary artery bypass grafting; CI = confidence interval; d = days; OR = odds ratio; VASP = vasodilator-stimulated phosphoprotein; yr = year.

"Calculated" indicates that the result was not reported by the article's authors; rather, we derived the result from reported raw data.

*Although p=0.027 was the reported p-value, recalculation using a chi-square test gives a p-value of 0.089 and recalculation using the Fisher exact test gives a p-value of 0.139. It is unclear how the reported p-value was calculated.

194

Table 33. Recurrent ACS in studies of test-and-treat strategies using phenotypic testing of platelet reactivity

Author Year Country PMID Study Name (if available)	Treatment Group Sample Size	No. with Outcome (%)	Outcome Definition	Time Point	Comparative Metric	95% CI	p-value [statistical test]
Wang[270] 2011 China 21538380	VASP-guided treatment N=150	2 (1.3%)	Recurrent ACS	1 yr	OR=0.69 (calculated)	0.11 to 4.18 (calculated)	p=0.1* [unclear]
	Control N=156	3 (2.1%)					
Bonello[271] 2009 France 19101221	VASP-guided treatment N=215	1 (0.5%)	MI	30 d	OR=0.10 (calculated)	0.01 to 0.75 (calculated)	p=0.01 [unclear]
	Control N=214	10 (4.8%)					
Bonello[272] 2008 France 18387444	VASP-guided treatment N=78	0 (0%)	Recurrent ACS	30 d	OR=0.21 (calculated)	0.01 to 4.45 (calculated)	p=0.498 [Fisher exact test; calculated]
	Control N=84	2 (2.4%)					
Tousek[273] 2011 Czech Republic 21663983	VerifyNow-guided treatment N=30	1 (3.3%)	MI	6 mo	OR=0.48	0.04 to 5.6	p=0.55 [unclear]
	Control N=30	2 (6.7%)					
Hazarbasanov[275] 2012 Bulgaria 22249353	Multiplate analyzer-guided treatment N=97	0 (0%)	MI	6 mo	OR=0.136	0.007 to 2.660 (calculated)	p=0.12 [Fisher exact test]
	Control N=95	3 (3.2%)					

195

Table 33. Recurrent ACS in studies of test-and-treat strategies using phenotypic testing of platelet reactivity (continued)

Author Year Country PMID Study Name (if available)	Treatment Group Sample Size	No. with Outcome (%)	Outcome Definition	Time Point	Comparative Metric	95% CI	p-value [statistical test]
Siller-Matula[276] 2012 Austria 22656044 MADONNA	Multiplate analyzer-guided treatment N=403	0 (0%)	ACS = MI or unstable angina	30 d	OR=0.05	0.003 to 0.78	p=0.001 [unclear statistical test]; p=0.001 [two-sided Fisher exact test; calculated]
	Control N=395	10 (2.5%)					

Abbreviations: ACS = acute coronary syndrome; CI = confidence interval; d = days; mo = months; MI = myocardial infarction; OR = odds ratio; VASP = vasodilator-stimulated phosphoprotein; yr = year.

"Calculated" indicates that the result was not reported by the article's authors; rather, we derived the result from reported raw data.

*Although p=0.1 was the reported p-value, recalculation using a chi-square test gives a p-value of 0.684 and recalculation using the Fisher exact test gives a p-value of 1.00. It is unclear how the reported p-value was calculated.

196

Intermediate Outcome: Platelet Reactivity During Followup

Four of the seven studies directly comparing alternative test-and-treat strategies reported information on platelet reactivity as an intermediate outcome (Appendix F). Although results generally indicated that platelet reactivity at the last followup assessment was lower in the groups that received test-based treatment than in those that received standard treatment, reporting was often incomplete and precluded statistical comparisons between groups. Furthermore, studies had short followup periods and it was unclear whether the observed differences in reactivity affected clinical outcomes.

Assessment of Risk of Bias of Individual Studies

A detailed assessment of 17 risk-of-bias items for studies comparing alternative test-and-treat strategies based on phenotypic testing for platelet reactivity is presented in Appendix F. Generally, the RCTs had moderate risk of bias. Because studies were prospectively conducted and because phenotypic testing is performed immediately after sample collection, the index test was assessed without knowledge of clinical or intermediate outcomes in all cases. However, information to judge whether outcomes were assessed without knowledge of the index-test result was often not reported. Subjects and personnel were not blinded and reporting was incomplete regarding the methods of generating the randomization sequence and concealing allocation. In one study[270] we observed substantial discrepancies between the statistical results provided by the authors and results from analyses that we performed using the reported event counts (despite using the same statistical procedures described in the paper's methods section). The single nonrandomized comparative study had high risk of bias because the two groups being compared (test-guided treatment and non-test guided treatment) were enrolled in different research institutions, increasing the probability that results were affected by confounding or selection bias.

One concern about test-and-treat studies conducted in the interventional setting pertains to delaying PCI until a particular level of reactivity is reached (particularly, in studies that perform repeat testing and modify treatment accordingly over the course of several weeks): the time to PCI tends to be longer in the experimental group than in the control group, although only one of the included studies provided relevant data (indicating that the time-to-PCI was indeed longer in patients assigned to test-based monitoring). This delay is potentially of concern because several studies have shown that delayed PCI may adversely impact clinical outcomes.

Studies of Treatment-Effect Modification by Baseline Platelet Reactivity

We identified three studies reporting information on effect modification by baseline platelet reactivity in patients randomized to alternative antiplatelet therapies.[242,277,278] Detailed information about the patient selection and patient characteristics is summarized in Table 34. Information about the assays used, test timing, and thresholds for platelet reactivity is presented in Table 35.

Table 34. Descriptive characteristics of the study of treatment-effect modification using phenotypic testing of platelet reactivity

Author Year Country PMID Study Name (if available)	Selection Criteria	Study Design	N Enrolled Male (%) Age* Dyslipidemia (%) Smokers (%) HTN (%) Diabetes (%)	Treatments Compared	Followup Duration
Montalescot[277] 2009 France 20062936 ACAPULCO	Patients with UA or NSTE MI who were to receive clopidogrel 900 mg loading dose	RCT comparing antiplatelet treatments in patients who were assed for platelet reactivity after a run-in period, before randomization	N=56 47 (84%) 61 (12) 9 (16%) 17 (30%) [current smokers] 37 (66%) 11 (20%)	Patients received clopidogrel 900 mg loading dose (single dose or cumulative dose when <900 mg had been previously admitted and aspirin (250-500 mg IV loading dose). They were then randomized to 2 groups: *Prasugrel +aspirin group*: prasugrel 10 mg maintenance dose + aspirin (maximum 100 mg/d) + placebo (instead of clopidogrel) *Clopidogrel + aspirin group*: clopidogrel 150 mg maintenance + aspirin (maximum 100 mg/d) + placebo (instead of prasugrel) After 2 wk patients were switched to the other group (crossover design) for another 2 wk.	Total study duration was 29 d; patients were on each treatment for 2 w (crossover design)
Capranzano[278] 2012 USA 22431415	Stable CAD patients on maintenance therapy with aspirin (81 mg/d) and clopidogrel (75 mg/d)	Crossover RCT comparing dual antiplatelet therapy (aspirin + clopidogrel) to triple therapy (aspirin + clopidogrel + cilostazol)	N=79 53 (67%) 60.8 (8.5) 77 (98%) 30 (38%) 72 (91%) 40 (51%)	Patients on aspirin + clopidogrel treatment and were randomized to receive *cilostazol (100 mg twice daily)* or *placebo* for 14 days. Patients then crossed over to the alternative treatment for an additional 4 days.	Total study duration was 28 d; patients were on each treatment for 2 w (crossover design)

198

Table 34. Descriptive characteristics of the study of treatment-effect modification using phenotypic testing of platelet reactivity (continued)

Author Year Country PMID Study Name (if available)	Selection Criteria	Study Design	N Enrolled Male (%) Age* Dyslipidemia (%) Smokers (%) HTN (%) Diabetes (%)	Treatments Compared	Followup Duration
Sibbing[242] Germany 2012 22682553 ISAR-REACT 4	Patients undergoing PCI for NSTE-MI	Parallel arm RCT comparing abciximab with heparin vs. bivalirudin antithrombotic treatment for PCI	N=564 438 (78%) 67.7 (10.8) 176 (31%) 124 (22%) 504 (89%) 176 (31%)	Patients received clopidogrel loading dose (600 mg) + aspirin (500 mg) pre-PCI; post-PCI treatment consisted of clopidogrel 2 × 75 mg/d for 3 days, followed by 75 mg/d for a recommended duration of 12 mo. Aspirin 2 × 100 mg/d indefinitely was also recommended. During PCI patients were randomized into 2 groups: *Abciximab + UFH:* bolus of 0.25 mg abciximab as well as a bolus dose of 70 units UFH per kilogram body weight, followed by a continuous infusion of abciximab 0.125 µg/kg body weight per minute for 12 h *Bivalirudin:* bolus bivalirudin 0.75 mg/kg, followed by a continuous infusion of 1.75 mg/kg per hour during PCI	30 d post randomization

Abbreviations: CAD = coronary artery disease; d = day(s); HTN = hypertension; MI = myocardial infarction; NSTE = non–ST-elevation; PCI = percutaneous coronary intervention; RCT = randomized controlled trial; UA = unstable angina; UFH = unfractionated heparin; wk = week(s).
*Mean (standard deviation), unless otherwise stated.

199

Table 35. Test information in the study of treatment-effect modification using phenotypic testing of platelet reactivity

Author Year Country PMID Study Name (if available)	Assay for Phenotypic Testing (agonist) [manufacturer]	Test Timepoint Interval Between Sampling and Genotyping Results Interval Between Collection and DNA extraction	N Tested Test Success Rate (%)	Threshold Used	Rationale for Threshold
Montalescot[277] 2009 France 20062936 ACAPULCO	LTA (ADP 5 and 20 µM) [Model 490-4D aggregometer, Chrono-Log Corporation, Kordia, Netherlands] VerifyNow P2Y12 (ADP) [Accumetrics, San Diego, CA] VASP assay (VASP kit; Biocytex, Marseilles, France) using flow cytometry (no additional details provided)	Pre-loading dose, 6-18 h after the 900 mg loading dose, and 16-28 h after the last maintenance dose at 2 w and 4 w	54 subjects received maintenance dose; 41 subjects completed the study; test success rate was not estimable	For maximal platelet reactivity by LTA ADP 20 µM: >50% For residual platelet aggregation by LTA ADP 5 µM: >14% For VASP PRI: ≥50% For VerifyNow PRU: ≥240 units	Based on prior literature (citations provided for each threshold)

Table 35. Test information in the study of treatment-effect modification using phenotypic testing of platelet reactivity (continued)

Author Year Country PMID Study Name (if available)	Assay for Phenotypic Testing (agonist) [manufacturer]	Test Timepoint Interval Between Sampling and Genotyping Results Interval Between Collection and DNA extraction	N Tested Test Success Rate (%)	Threshold Used	Rationale for Threshold
Capranzano[278] 2012 USA 22431415	*For assessing effect modification and outcomes:* VerifyNow P2Y12 (ADP) [Accumetrics, San Diego, CA] *For assessing outcomes only:* LTA (ADP 5 and 20 µM) [Model 490 aggregometer, Chrono-Log Corporation, Havertown, PA] VASP assay (VASP kit; Biocytex, Marseilles, France) using flow cytometry (no additional details provided)	Blood samples were collected 2–4 h after intake of antiplatelet medications at the following time-points: before randomization; 14 d after randomization; 14 d after crossover	Analyses were reported on 79 patients who completed the trial and had reactivity measurements; the parent trial enrolled 111 patients of whom 23.4% withdrew within 48-72 h due to adverse effects	For maximal platelet reactivity by LTA ADP 20 µM: >50% For residual platelet aggregation by LTA ADP 5 µM: >14% For VASP PRI: ≥50% For VerifyNow PRU: >240 units	Based on prior literature (citations provided for the threshold)

Table 35. Test information in the study of treatment-effect modification using phenotypic testing of platelet reactivity (continued)

Author Year Country PMID Study Name (if available)	Assay for Phenotypic Testing (agonist) [manufacturer]	Test Timepoint Interval Between Sampling and Genotyping Results Interval Between Collection and DNA extraction	N Tested Test Success Rate (%)	Threshold Used	Rationale for Threshold
Sibbing[242] Germany 2012 22682553 ISAR-REACT 4	Multiplate analyzer (ADP) [Verum Diagnostica, Munich, Germany]	Samples for the assessment of platelet reactivity were obtained before PCI and prior to the administration of study drug treatment	The platelet substudy was conducted in 2 centers enrolling 1195 (of the total 1721 included in the trial) of these 564 had platelet reactivity measurements available	≥468 AU × min	Based on prior literature and a consensus document (citations provided for the threshold)

Abbreviations: ADP = adenosine triphosphate; AU = arbitrary units; h = hours; LTA = light-transmission aggregometry; PRI = platelet reactivity index; PRU = platelet reactivity units; VASP = vasodilator-stimulated phosphoprotein; wk = week(s).

202

Clinical Outcomes

One study (based on the ISAR-REACT 4 trial) reported information on clinical outcomes. In the platelet reactivity sub-cohort of this trial, 205 patients (36 percent) had high on-clopidogrel platelet reactivity at the time of PCI (35.0 percent in the abciximab + heparin group vs. 37.6 percent in the bivalirudin group). A significant interaction was observed between study treatment arm and platelet aggregation regarding the combined efficacy endpoint (death, MI, or urgent target vessel revascularization; P for interaction = 0.037). Table 36 summarizes the findings for other clinical outcomes assessed in the study; significant effect modification was also observed for recurrent MI and a composite of recurrent myocardial infarction and death.

Table 36. Descriptive characteristics of the study of treatment-effect modification using phenotypic testing of platelet reactivity

Author, Year Country PMID Study name (if available)	Outcome	Abciximab + UFH (high platelet reactivity) N=96	Abciximab + UFH (normal platelet reactivity) N=178	Bivalirudin (normal platelet reactivity) N=109	Bivalirudin (High platelet reactivity) N=181	Interaction p-value
Sibbing[242] 2012	MACE = death, MI, or urgent TVR	9	12	24	9	p=0.037 [reported]; p=0.032 [calculated]
Germany	Death	1	3	1	1	p=0.586 [calculated]
22682553	Any recurrent MI	8	11	22	8	p=0.034 [calculated]
ISAR-REACT 4	Death or any recurrent MI	9	12	23	9	p=0.040 [calculated]
	Urgent TVR	0	1	2	0	p=0.246 [calculated]
	Definite stent thrombosis	0	1	1	0	p=0.364 [calculated]

Abbreviations: MACE = major adverse cardiovascular events; MI = myocardial infarction; TVR = target vessel revascularization; UFH = unfractionated heparin.
When needed, a continuity correction of 0.5 was used. P-values are calculated for a z-score comparison between log-odds ratios for the reactivity effect within each treatment group.

The remaining two studies did not report patient-relevant clinical outcomes stratified by platelet reactivity status at baseline. In one of them, one death (due to cancer) was observed and was not considered treatment related.

Intermediate Outcome: Platelet Reactivity During Followup

Two studies reported information on platelet reactivity during followup. The first[278] was a post-hoc evaluation based on a crossover RCT comparing triple therapy (aspirin, clopidogrel, and cilostazol) to double therapy (aspirin + clopidogrel + placebo) for patients with stable coronary artery disease. Among patients with high-platelet reactivity the mean change in platelet reactivity pre- and post-cilostazol (as assessed with the VerifyNow assay) was 53.4 platelet reactivity units (95% CI 24.7 to 82.1). Among patients with normal platelet reactivity the mean change in reactivity was 40.8 platelet reactivity units (95% CI 28.7 to 52.8). Based on these results we calculated that the p-value for interaction was 0.428 indicating that baseline platelet reactivity did not modify the effect of cilostazol on subsequent measurements.

The second study[277] reported the response rate among "poor responders" to the clopidogrel loading dose during prasugrel-based therapy and during clopidogrel-based therapy. Generally the response rates were higher during prasugrel therapy, regardless of the assay used to assess platelet reactivity. However, the study did not report the response status during followup for patients who were "responders" to the clopidogrel loading dose. Thus, the interaction between post–loading dose response to clopidogrel and treatment assignment could not be assessed.

Assessment of Risk of Bias

One study was considered to have a high risk of bias because outcome information was incompletely reported and information on the generation of the randomized sequence and allocation concealment was unclear. Another study was considered to have high risk of bias because it was a post hoc assessment based on a convenience sample enrolled in a crossover trial and because the parent trial had a large withdrawal rate (23 percent). The third study (the one reporting on clinical outcomes) had a moderate risk of bias. This study was based on a large randomized trial; however, only 564 (of a total of 1721) patients were included, representing a convenience sample of patients treated at centers where platelet reactivity testing was available. Furthermore, patients were included only if they attended the study locations at "core times" when the laboratory was operational. These aspects of the design render the study susceptible to selection bias; this concern was substantiated by the presence of differences in the distribution of several risk factors between patients included in the parent trial and those included in the platelet reactivity substudy.

Detailed information for each item considered in the risk-of-bias assessment is given in Appendix F.

Studies With Phenotypic Test–Based Selection of Patients

Fourteen studies met our inclusion criteria and reported information on the comparative effectiveness of treatments administered to patients selected on the basis of baseline platelet reactivity. The sample sizes ranged from 21 to more than 2000 participants and all 14 studies were relatively recent (published in 2008–2012). Eleven studies were performed mainly or exclusively in the PCI setting, two studies included patients with stable coronary artery disease (non-interventional setting), and one study enrolled patients on chronic hemodialysis receiving clopidogrel treatment. On-clopidogrel platelet reactivity was used as a selection criterion in all studies; it was assessed using the VerifyNow P2Y12 assay in nine studies, LTA in three studies, the VASP assay with flow cytometry in two studies; other assays in two studies (one study combined measurements from three assays to define high on-treatment reactivity). The treatment comparisons were between standard-dose clopidogrel-based therapy and high-dose clopidogrel in six studies, prasugrel in four studies, ticagrelor in two studies, and addition of a glycoprotein IIb/IIIa inhibitor in two studies.

Detailed information on patient selection, study design, patient characteristics, and assays used is summarized in Table 37.

Table 37. Descriptive characteristics of the studies with phenotypic test–based selection of patients

Author, Year Country PMID Study name (if available)	Selected Population	Study Design Treatment Strategies Compared	Assay (agonist) [model, manufacturer]	Total N Enrolled Male (%) Age* Dyslipidemia (%), Smokers (%), HTN (%), Diabetes (%)
Price[203] 2011 Multinational 21406646 GRAVITAS	Patients who had PCI with ≥1 drug-eluting stent for treating stable CAD or NSTE ACS; after protocol amendment, enrollment was expanded to include patients with STE MI. Patients on IIb/IIIa inhibitors were excluded. In patients with no prior exposure to clopidogrel, a dose of 600 mg had to have been administered ≤2 h post-PCI; patients already on clopidogrel must have received 75 mg/d for ≥7 d, or, if <7 d, a loading dose ≥300 mg when clopidogrel was started.	Double-blind, placebo-controlled RCT, multicenter Platelet reactivity was measured 12-24 h post-PCI. Patients with high-on treatment reactivity (PRU≥230) were randomized (central randomization, double-blind design) to two groups (standard- and high-dose clopidogrel). Also included a nonrandomized comparator arm of randomly selected patients among those without high on-clopidogrel reactivity (PRU <230); information on this group of patients has been summarized in the report section on Key Question 2b. *High-dose clopidogrel:* total 1st day day dose 600 mg, followed by 6-mo maintenance dose 150 mg/d *Standard-dose clopidogrel:* loading dose of placebo, followed by a dose of 75 mg/d + a placebo tablet Aspirin treatment (75-162 mg/d) was required for both groups.	For selecting patients and for assessing reactivity as an outcome: VerifyNow P2Y12 (ADP) [Accumetrics, San Diego, CA]	2214 (with PRU≥230) in the randomized groups; 586 (with PRU <230) in the randomly selected comparator group† 1441 (65%) 64.1 (10.5) 1934 (87%) 313 (14%) [current smokers] 1886 (85%) 1004 (45%)
Palmerini[228] 2010 Italy 19604542 DOUBLE	Patients with STE MI referred to a single center for PCI within 12 h of symptom onset	Randomized, single-center All patients received clopidogrel loading (300 mg); periprocedural abciximab and BMS were mandatory. Platelet reactivity was measured at baseline (after a loading dose of 300 mg and the first maintenance dose of 75 mg) and patients with PRI VASP <30% were excluded. Patients had been randomized before the first reactivity assessment into two groups (high- and standard-dose maintenance clopidogrel) *High-dose clopidogrel maintenance:* 150 mg/d for 1 mo *Standard-dose clopidogrel maintenance:* 75 mg/d for 1 mo All patients were on aspirin treatment (160 mg/d)	*For selecting patients:* Platelet VASP kit (ADP± PGE1) [Biocytex, Marseille, France] *For assessing reactivity as an outcome:* Platelet VASP kit (ADP± PGE1) [Biocytex, Marseille, France], LTA (NR) [Chronolog 700; no additional details provided], VerifyNow P2Y12 (ADP) [NR], whole blood impedance aggregometry (NR) [NR]	52 eligible (with VASP PRI ≥30%); 48 included in analyses (7.7% excluded) 43 (90%) 63 (12.2) 21 (44%) 32 (67%) [current or former smokers] 23 (48%) 8 (17%)

205

Table 37. Descriptive characteristics of the studies with phenotypic test–based selection of patients (continued)

Author, Year Country PMID Study name (if available)	Selected Population	Study Design Treatment Strategies Compared	Assay (agonist) [model, manufacturer]	Total N Enrolled Male (%), Age*, Dyslipidemia (%), Smokers (%), HTN (%), Diabetes (%)
Valgimigli[206] 2009 Multinational (Italy, Belgium, France, Spain) 19528337 3T/2R	Patients scheduled for coronary angiography, PCI, or both; presenting with stable or troponin-negative NSTE ACS were screened for inclusion; patients with evidence of myocardial damage or ongoing MI were excluded.	Patients were eligible for aspirin response evaluation (cut-off 550 units) if they were taking aspirin orally at doses of ≥80 mg/d for ≥5 days or received intravenous 500 mg aspirin ≥15 minutes before and did not receive clopidogrel or ticlopidine in the previous 7 days. Patients with aspirin poor responsiveness qualified for randomization before PCI only when clopidogrel screening requirements were met. Screening for clopidogrel response (cut-off: 40% inhibition) was undertaken in patients at steady state for aspirin provided ≥1 of the following requirements was fulfilled: the patient received a 600- or 300-mg loading dose ≥2 or 6 hours before, respectively, or the patient received a 75-mg maintenance clopidogrel dose for ≥7 consecutive days. Patients who were poor responders to both aspirin and clopidogrel followed the aspirin poor-responders randomization scheme. *IIb/IIIa inhibitor group:* tirofiban 50 mL diluted in 200 mL of 0.9% NaCl solution *Placebo group:* 50 mL of 0.9% NaCl was injected in 200 mL of 0.9% NaCl solution by an unblinded research study nurse (all other personnel were blinded to treatment assignment). Tirofiban was given as a bolus of 25 µg kg⁻¹ 3 min⁻¹, followed by an infusion of 0.15 µg kg⁻¹ min⁻¹ for 14 to 24 h. Intravenous aspirin at the time of PCI in patients at steady state for the treatment was allowed and left to the discretion of the treating physician. Anticoagulation during PCI was with heparin or bivalirudin. Rescue use of tirofiban was allowed (without unblinding).	VerifyNow P2Y12 (ADP) [Accumetrics, San Diego, CA] VerifyNow Aspirin (AA) [Accumetrics, San Diego, CA]	337 patients were poor responders to aspirin or clopidogrel; 174 were poor responders to clopidogrel alone; 26 were poor responders to both; 73 patients were excluded pre-randomization; 263 patients were randomized (147 were exclusively clopidogrel poor responders). For all randomized patients: 193 (73%) 68.2 (9.7) 141 (54%) 40 (15%) [current smokers] 188 (71%) 69 (26%)

206

Table 37. Descriptive characteristics of the studies with phenotypic test–based selection of patients (continued)

Author, Year Country PMID Study name (if available)	Selected Population	Study Design Treatment Strategies Compared	Assay (agonist) [model, manufacturer]	Total N Enrolled Male (%), Age,* Dyslipidemia (%), Smokers (%), HTN (%), Diabetes (%)
Cuisset[279] 2008 France 19463379	Patients with stable angina or a positive functional study with planned PCI with stent implantation of a de novo lesion in a native coronary artery; all patients were on chronic aspirin therapy (75 mg/d) and none were on clopidogrel	Blood samples were obtained ≥12 h after the loading dose of aspirin and clopidogrel; clopidogrel nonresponders (>70% on-clopidogrel reactivity used as the cut-off) were randomized to a IIb/IIIa inhibitor group or a conventional treatment group. Loading dose of clopidogrel (600 mg) and aspirin (250 mg) were administered the day before the procedure. Response was assessed ≥12 h after the loading dose of aspirin and clopidogrel; nonresponders were then randomized into the following groups: *IIb/IIIa inhibitor group:* systematic administration of abciximab to all patients. *Conventional treatment group:* use of IIb/IIIa agonists left at the discretion of physicians. Abciximab was administered with a 0.25 mg/kg of body weight bolus, followed by a 0.125 µg/kg/min [maximum, 10 µg/min] infusion for 12 h).Anticoagulation during the procedure was with heparin (50 U/kg in the IIb/IIIa group vs. 70 U/kg in the conventional treatment group). After discharge all patients received aspirin (75 mg) and clopidogrel (150 mg) maintenance doses for at least 1 mo.	LTA (ADP) [PAP4 aggregometer; Biodata Corporation; Wellcome, Paris, France]	149 nonresponders to clopidogrel 113 (76%) 65 (8.6) 111 (74%) 58 (39%) 93 (62%) 56 (38%)

207

Table 37. Descriptive characteristics of the studies with phenotypic test–based selection of patients (continued)

Author, Year Country PMID Study name (if available)	Selected Population	Study Design Treatment Strategies Compared	Assay (agonist) [model, manufacturer]	Total N Enrolled Male (%), Age* Dyslipidemia (%), Smokers (%), HTN (%), Diabetes (%)
Gurbel[162]‡ 2010 Multinational (N. America and Europe) 20194878 RESPOND	Patients with documented stable CAD who were on aspirin therapy (75-100 mg/d)	All patients received a loading dose of clopidogrel (300 mg) and response was assessed at 6-8 h post-loading. Nonresponse was defined as absolute change post-loading ≤10%; response status was confirmed 2-4 w before the first dose of study drug Both responders and nonresponders were randomized to 2 groups during period 1: *Clopidogrel:* clopidogrel 600 mg loading dose, followed by clopidogrel 75 mg/d maintenance for 14 d *Ticagrelor:* ticagrelor 180 mg loading dose, followed ticagrelor 90 mg BID maintenance dose In period 2, all nonresponders switched treatment, whereas half of the responders continued the same treatment, and the other half of the responders switched to the other treatment; both groups were treated for an additional 14 d. Patients continuing on the same treatments in both study periods did not receive loading doses of study drug during period 2. Switching patients received loading doses of the new drug. In addition to study drug, all patients received concomitant aspirin therapy (75 to 100 mg/d).	*For assigning patients to randomized groups:* LTA (ADP 20 μmol/L) [Chronolog Optical Aggregometer, model 490-4D; no other details] *For response assessment:* LTA (ADP 5 and 20 μmol/L, and collagen 2 μg/mL) [Chronolog Optical Aggregometer, model 490-4D; no other details], VerifyNow P2Y12 (ADP) [Accumetrics, San Diego, CA], Platelet VASP kit (ADP± PGE1) [Biocytex, Marseille, France], ADP-stimulated glycoprotein IIb/IIIa and P-selection expression by flow cytometry [no other details]	98 76 (78%) 65 (8) 92 (94%) 17 (17%) [current smokers] 79 (81%) 25 (26%)

Table 37. Descriptive characteristics of the studies with phenotypic test–based selection of patients (continued)

Author, Year Country PMID Study name (if available)	Selected Population	Study Design Treatment Strategies Compared	Assay (agonist) [model, manufacturer]	Total N Enrolled Male (%), Age,* Dyslipidemia (%), Smokers (%), HTN (%), Diabetes (%)
Alexopoulos[280] 2012 Greece 22789884	Consecutive patients with ACS undergoing PCI with stent implantation; patients receiving IIb/IIIa inhibitors were excluded	Single-blind, crossover RCT, single center At the time of PCI, clopidogrel-naive patients and those on clopidogrel 75 mg for <7 days without initial loading dose received a 600-mg clopidogrel. Patients on clopidogrel <7 days but with 300-mg loading or those on clopidogrel for >7 days did not receive any additional loading. All patients received an intra-arterial dose of 70 international units (IU)/kg heparin. After PCI, all patients received aspirin 100 mg/day indefinitely. Patients with HTPR were then randomized in a 1:1 ratio to *ticagrelor* 90 mg, 2 x daily or *prasugrel* 10 mg/d, until d 15 post-randomization. At 15 ±2 d platelet reactivity was assessed and patients crossed-over directly to the alternate therapy for an additional 15 days (no washout)	VerifyNow P2Y12 (ADP) [Accumetrics, San Diego, CA]	44 (with PRU ≥235) 37 (84%) 60 (9) 22 (50%) 28 (64%) 25 (57%) 10 (23%)
Gremmel[281] 2011 Austria 21546102	Patients undergoing angioplasty with stenting for CAD	With the exception of 2 patients (4.5%), who were already on continuous clopidogrel therapy, all patients received a loading dose of 300 (n = 33, 75%) or 600 mg (n = 9, 20.5%) clopidogrel prior to PCI. All patients received daily acetylsalicylic acid therapy (100 mg/d). Patients were then randomized into the following groups: *High maintenance dose group:* 100 mg aspirin and 150 mg clopidogrel per day for 3 mo post-PCI *Standard dose group:* aspirin 100 mg/d and clopidogrel 75 mg/d	VerifyNow P2Y12 (ADP) [Accumetrics, San Diego, CA], Platelet VASP (ADP± PGE1) [Diagnostica Stago, Biocytex, Marseille, France], Multiplate analyzer impedance aggregometry (ADP+PGE1) [Dynabyte, Munich, Germany]	44 patients (46 enrolled with 2 excluded due to non-adherence) with high reactivity on at least one of the 3 tests (PRU >235 or PRI >50% or AU ≥47) 30 (68) 68 (12) NR 18 (41%) NR 20 (45%)
Alexopoulos[282] 2011 Greece 21985070	Patients on regular maintenance hemodialysis (>6 mo)	Single-blind, crossover RCT, single center Hemodialysis patients who were receiving clopidogrel 75 mg/d maintenance treatment (>2 mo) underwent platelet reactivity testing. Those with high on-clopidogrel platelet reactivity were randomized in a 1:1 ratio to clopidogrel (150 mg/d) or prasugrel (10 mg/d), until d 15 post-randomization. At 15 ±2 d platelet reactivity was assessed again and patients crossed-over directly to the alternate therapy for an additional 15 d (no washout)	VerifyNow P2Y12 (ADP) [Accumetrics, San Diego, CA]	21 patients with PRU ≥ 235 14 (67%) 61.2 (12) 15 (71%) 5 (24%) 18 (86%) 10 (48%)

209

Table 37. Descriptive characteristics of the studies with phenotypic test–based selection of patients (continued)

Author, Year Country PMID Study name (if available)	Selected Population	Study Design Treatment Strategies Compared	Assay (agonist) [model, manufacturer]	Total N Enrolled Male (%), Age* Dyslipidemia (%), Smokers (%), HTN (%), Diabetes (%)
Alexopoulos[283] 2011 Greece 21982667	Consecutive patients on clopidogrel treatment (75/d) for >12 mo	Single-blind, crossover RCT, single center Patients had been receiving clopidogrel 75 mg/d for >12 mo when they underwent platelet reactivity testing. Those with high on-clopidogrel reactivity were randomized in a 1:1 ratio to clopidogrel (150 mg/d) or prasugrel (10 mg/d), until d 14 post-randomization. At 14 ±2 d platelet reactivity was assessed again and patients crossed-over directly to the alternate therapy for an additional 15 d (no washout)	VerifyNow P2Y12 (ADP) [Accumetrics, San Diego, CA]	31 patients with PRU ≥235 24 (86%) 69 (9) 27 (96%) 4 (14%) 24 (86%) 12 (43%)
Ari[216] 2012 Turkey EFFICIENT 21239075	Patients undergoing elective PCI	Non-blinded, active-control RCT, 2 centers Patients were taking aspirin (100 mg/d) for ≥ 5 d and clopidogrel (75 mg/d) for ≥ 3 d before intervention. Platelet reactivity was measured "just before" PCI. Patients with clopidogrel resistance (platelet inhibition <40%) were randomized to two treatment groups; patients with adequate response to clopidogrel (platelet inhibition ≥40%) were included as a non-randomize comparator arm treated with clopidogrel (75 mg/d); information on this group of patients is summarized in the report section on Key Question 2b. Randomized patients were assigned to the following two groups: *High-dose clopidogrel:* clopidogrel 150 mg/d for 1 mo + aspirin (100 mg/d) *Standard-dose clopidogrel:* clopidogrel 75 mg/d for 1 mo + aspirin (100 mg/d)	For selecting patients to randomize: VerifyNow P2Y12 (ADP) [Accumetrics, San Diego, CA] The VerifyNow Aspirin (AA) [Accumetrics, San Diego, CA] test was also used but not as a method for selecting patients	94 patients with platelet inhibition <40% included in the randomized comparison 72 (77%) 58 (10) NR 62 (66%) 47 (50%) 27 (29%)

210

Table 37. Descriptive characteristics of the studies with phenotypic test–based selection of patients (continued)

Author, Year Country PMID Study name (if available)	Selected Population	Study Design Treatment Strategies Compared	Assay (agonist) [model, manufacturer]	Total N Enrolled Male (%), Age,* Dyslipidemia (%), Smokers (%), HTN (%), Diabetes (%)
Trenk[284] 2012 Multinational (North America and Europe) 22520250 TRIGGER-PCI	Consecutive patients with stable CAD and clinical indications for PCI, who had undergone successful, elective coronary placement of at least 1 DES, were screened for inclusion. To be eligible for screening patients had to have been pre-treated with a loading dose of clopidogrel (600 mg) with aspirin (≥250 mg) within 24 h of the PCI; patients who had received IIb/IIIa inhibitors were excluded	Single-blind (assessors); placebo-controlled, multicenter Patients were pre-treated with a loading dose of clopidogrel (600 mg) + aspirin (≥250 mg) within 24 h of PCI. Reactivity testing was performed between 2-7 h after the first clopidogrel 75 mg maintenance dose the morning after PCI. Patients with high on-clopidogrel reactivity were randomized 1:1 to the following two groups: *Prasugrel + placebo*: prasugrel (60 mg) loading dose within 9 h after administration of the non-study-related clopidogrel maintenance dose (75 mg), followed by maintenance treatment of prasugrel 10 mg/d + placebo, starting the day after the loading dose of the study drug *Clopidogrel + placebo*: placebo loading dose within 9 h after administration of the non-study-related clopidogrel maintenance dose (75 mg), followed by maintenance treatment of clopidogrel (75 mg) + placebo, starting the day after the loading dose of the study drug	VerifyNow P2Y12 (ADP) [Accumetrics, San Diego, CA]	625 patients with PRU >208; 423 randomized for whom descriptive characteristics were reported (202 declined) 307 (73%) 66 (8) NR 61 (14%) 376 (89%) 177 (42%)

Table 37. Descriptive characteristics of the studies with phenotypic test–based selection of patients (continued)

Author, Year Country PMID Study name (if available)	Selected Population	Study Design Treatment Strategies Compared	Assay (agonist) [model, manufacturer]	Total N Enrolled Male (%), Age,* Dyslipidemia (%), Smokers (%), HTN (%), Diabetes (%)
Aradi[181] 2012 Hungary 21902692 DOSER	Clopidogrel-naïve patients with stable angina and significant de novo coronary stenosis amenable to ad hoc coronary stent implantation	Double-blind; placebo-controlled; single center. Immediately after coronary angiography and before PCI, patients received a clopidogrel loading dose (600 mg) + aspirin (300 mg). Use of glycoprotein IIb/IIIa inhibitors was prohibited. Reactivity assessment was performed 12-24 h after clopidogrel loading. Patients with high on-clopidogrel reactivity were randomized into 2 groups: *Standard dose clopidogrel:* clopidogrel maintenance at a dose of 75 mg/d for 1 mo *High-dose clopidogrel:* clopidogrel maintenance 150 mg/d for 1 mo. After 28 days, all patients returned to 75 mg maintenance dose of clopidogrel until 1 year. The study also included a non-randomized comparator arm consisting of all patients with normal platelet reactivity; information on this group of patients has been summarized in the report section on Key Question 2b.	For selecting patients to randomize: LTA (ADP) [CARAT TX4 four-channel light transmission aggregometer; Carat Diagnostics, Budapest, Hungary] For response assessment: LTA (ADP) [CARAT TX4 four-channel light transmission aggregometer; Carat Diagnostics, Budapest, Hungary]; Platelet VASP (ADP ± PGE1) [Biocytex, Marseilles, France],	74 patients with LTA maximal aggregation >= 46% were randomized 39 (53%) 62 (8) 41 (55%) 37 (50%; current + past) 63 (85%) 32 (43%)
Tang[247] 2012 China 22490487	Patients admitted for PCI who underwent successful coronary stenting	All patients received 300 mg of clopidogrel and aspirin at least 12 hours before the stenting. In the following three days after coronary stenting, patients received 100 mg of aspirin and 75 mg of clopidogrel per day. Three days after implantation of the stenting, peripheral venous blood samples for TEG were obtained. Patients with high-on treatment reactivity (to aspirin and clopidogrel) were randomized into 2 treatment groups: *Standard dual antiplatelet treatment:* aspirin 100 mg/d + clopidogrel (75 mg/d) *High dose dual antiplatelet therapy:* aspirin (200 mg/d) + clopidogrel (150 mg/d) The study also included a non-randomized comparator arm consisting of all patients with normal platelet reactivity; information on this group of patients has been summarized in the report section on Key Question 2b.	TEG analyzer (the device uses 4 channels: kaolin, activating agent A, arachidonic acid, and ADP) [Haemoscope Corporation, Niles, Illinois, USA]	60 patients had platelet inhibition <50% and were randomized 29 (48%) 63 (14) 13 (22%) 38 (63%; current) 31 (52%) 14 (23%)

212

Table 37. Descriptive characteristics of the studies with phenotypic test–based selection of patients (continued)

Author, Year Country PMID Study name (if available)	Selected Population	Study Design Treatment Strategies Compared	Assay (agonist) [model, manufacturer]	Total N Enrolled Male (%), Age,* Dyslipidemia (%), Smokers (%), HTN (%), Diabetes (%)
Alexopoulos[285] 2011 Greece 21511219	Consecutive patients undergoing PCI with stent implantation	Single-blind, crossover RCT, single center At the time of PCI, clopidogrel-naive patients and those on clopidogrel 75 mg for <7 days without initial loading dose received clopidogrel (600 mg). Patients on clopidogrel <7 days but with 300 mg loading or those on clopidogrel for >7 days did not receive any additional loading. All patients received an intra-arterial dose of 70 IU/kg heparin. After PCI, all patients received aspirin 325 mg/d for 1 mo followed by 100 mg/d indefinitely. Patients with HTPR were then randomized in a 1:1 ratio to prasugrel 10 mg/d or clopidogrel 150 mg/d, until d 30 post-randomization. At 30 ±2 d platelet reactivity was assessed and patients crossed-over directly to the alternate therapy for an additional 30 days (no washout)	VerifyNow P2Y12 (ADP) [Accumetrics, San Diego, CA]	71 patients with PRU ≥235 were randomized but 64 considered in analyses (2 dropouts for side effects; 5 for non-compliance) 57 (89%) 65 (11) 41 (64%) 30 (47%) 43 (67%) 23 (36%)

Abbreviations: AA = arachidonic acid; ACS = acute coronary syndrome; ADP = adenosine diphosphate; BMS = bare-metal stent; CAD = coronary artery disease; d = day; h = hour; HTN = hypertension; HTPR = high on-treatment platelet reactivity; IU = international units; LTA = light-transmission aggregometry; MI = myocardial infarction; mo = month; NR = not reported; NSTE = non–ST-elevation; PCI = percutaneous coronary intervention; PGE1 = prostaglandin E1; PMID = PubMed identification number; PRI = platelet reactivity index; PRU = platelet reactivity units; RCT = randomized controlled trial; SD = standard deviation; STE = ST-elevation; TEG = thromboelastography; VASP = vasodilator-stimulated phosphoprotein; w = week(s).

*Mean (standard deviation), unless otherwise stated.

†Patient characteristics extracted only for patients in the randomized groups (i.e., patients with PRU ≥ 230 randomly assigned to high- or low-dose clopidogrel strategies).

‡Despite including both responders and nonresponders, this study was categorized as a study of randomized treatment after test-based selection because patients were assigned to different treatments during the course of the study based on their original response status.

213

Clinical Outcomes

Clinical outcome comparisons between the randomized treatment groups were reported in 10 of the 14 studies. Only two trials (the GRAVITAS [Gauging Responsiveness with a VerifyNow Assay—Impact on Thrombosis and Safety] and the TRIGGER-PCI [Testing Platelet Reactivity In Patients Undergoing Elective Stent Placement on Clopidogrel to Guide Alternative Therapy With Prasugrel] trials) reported data from more than 100 randomized patients; we briefly discuss their key results here.

The GRAVITAS trial,[203] enrolling 2214 randomized patients—included patients who had undergone PCI for stable coronary artery disease or non–ST-elevation acute coronary syndrome and showed increased on-clopidogrel reactivity on the VerifyNow P2Y12 assay. The patients were randomized to high-dose clopidogrel or standard-dose clopidogrel, both in combination with aspirin. After 6 months of followup, there was no statistically significant difference between the randomized groups in the rate of cardiovascular death, nonfatal myocardial infarction, stent thrombosis, all-cause mortality, or composite cardiovascular outcomes (either cardiovascular death or nonfatal myocardial infarction, or cardiovascular death, nonfatal myocardial infarction, or stent thrombosis). The study also included followup information for a randomly selected group of patients with low platelet reactivity at baseline who were treated with standard-dose clopidogrel (see the Results section for Key Question 1b for details).

The TRIGGER-PCI study[284] compared prasugrel versus standard dose clopidogrel in 423 patients with high on-clopidogrel platelet reactivity (as measured by the VerifyNow P2Y12 assay). After 236 patients had completed the planned 6 month followup, a blinded interim review identified that a single primary endpoint event had been observed. Because of the very low event rate the trial was terminated early for futility. As such, for all outcomes, event rates were very low and differences in event rates between groups were not statistically significant.

The remaining 12 studies smaller sample sizes (ranging from 21 to 159 patients) and also had relatively short followup durations. Detailed information on clinical outcomes from all studies is presented in Table 38. Because the patient populations were heterogeneous, selected on the basis of different inclusion criteria, and assessed using different therapeutic regimens, we did not perform meta-analyses for any of the outcomes reported.

Table 38. Key findings of studies with phenotypic test–based selection of patients and clinical outcomes

Author Year Country PMID Study Name (if available)	Treatment Groups (sample size)	Followup Duration	Summary of Findings
Price[203] 2011 Multinational 21406646 GRAVITAS	*High-dose clopidogrel (n=1109)*: total first day dose 600 mg, followed by a maintenance dose of 150 mg/d for 6 mo *Standard-dose clopidogrel (n=1105)*: loading dose of placebo, followed by a dose of 75 mg/d + a placebo tablet	6 mo	Randomized comparison*: *CV death, nonfatal MI, or stent thrombosis*: HR=1.01 (95% CI, 0.58 to 1.76); p=0.97 CV death: HR=0.38 (95% CI, 0.10 to 1.43); p=0.14 Nonfatal MI: HR=1.12 (95% CI, 0.59 to 2.12); p=0.72 Stent thrombosis: HR=0.63 (95% CI, 0.21 to 1.93); p=0.42 CV death or nonfatal MI: HR=0.93 (95% CI, 0.53 to 1.64); p=0.80 All-cause death: HR=0.70 (95% CI, 0.27 to 1.85); p=0.48 Absolute difference in change of platelet reactivity from baseline at 30 d: -22% (95% CI, -26% to -18%); p<0.001 Absolute difference in change of platelet reactivity at 6 mo: -24% (95% CI, -28% to -20%); p<0.001

215

Table 38. Key findings of studies with phenotypic test–based selection of patients and clinical outcomes (continued)

Author Year Country PMID Study Name (if available)	Treatment Groups (sample size)	Followup Duration	Summary of Findings
Valgimigli[205]† 2009 Italy 19528337 3T/2R	*IIb/IIIa inhibitor group (n=68, clopidogrel-only nonresponders):* tirofiban 50 mL diluted in 200 mL of 0.9% NaCl solution *Placebo group (n=79, clopidogrel-only nonresponders):* 50 mL of 0.9% NaCl injected in 200 mL of 0.9% NaCl solution by an unblinded research study nurse (all other personnel were blinded to treatment assignment).	1 mo	Periprocedural MI (based on "the universal definition" of MI[285]) among clopidogrel-only nonresponders: 16.5% (11 events) in the tirofiban group vs. 30.8% in the placebo group (24 events); OR=0.44 (95% CI, 0.2 to 0.99); p=0.05 [calculated results] Periprocedural MI (based on "the universal definition" of MI[286]) among clopidogrel and aspirin nonresponders: 0% (0 events) in the tirofiban group vs. 25.0% in the placebo group [no effect size could be calculated] Among clopidogrel-only nonresponders no deaths were observed. No other outcome was reported separately for clopidogrel nonresponders. Among clopidogrel-only nonresponders a subgroup analysis by inhibition status (≥21% vs. <21%) on the effect of treatment on periprocedural MI was performed. The p-value for the interaction test was 0.35. The sample size of the compared groups was not extractable.

216

Table 38. Key findings of studies with phenotypic test–based selection of patients and clinical outcomes (continued)

Author Year Country PMID Study Name (if available)	Treatment Groups (sample size)	Followup Duration	Summary of Findings
Cuisset[279] 2008 France 19463379	IIb/IIIa inhibitor group (n=74): systematic administration of abciximab to all patients Conventional treatment group (n=75): use of IIb/IIIa agonists left at the discretion of physicians	1 mo	*Time-to-event analysis for CV-event free survival:* log-rank statistic=7.5; p=0.006 *Death from any cause, per procedural myonecrosis, acute or subacute definite or probable stent thrombosis and recurrent ACS:* 14 events in the IIb/IIIa inhibitor group vs. 30 events in the conventional treatment group; OR=0.35 (95% CI, 0.17 to 0.74); p=0.006 [calculated results] *Death:* 0 events in the IIb/IIIa inhibitor group vs. 1 event in the conventional treatment group; OR=0.33 (95% CI, 0.01 to 8.32); p=0.50 [calculated results] *Stent thrombosis:* 0 events in the IIb/IIIa inhibitor group vs. 1 events in the conventional treatment group; OR=0.33 (95% CI, 0.01 to 8.32); p=0.50 [calculated results] *Recurrent ACS:* 1 event in the IIb/IIIa inhibitor group vs. 2 events in the conventional treatment group; OR=0.50 (95% CI, 0.04 to 5.64); p=0.57 [calculated results] *Periprocedural myonecrosis:* 13 events in the IIb/IIIa inhibitor group vs. 26 events in the conventional treatment group; OR=0.40 (95% CI, 0.19 to 0.86); p=0.02 [calculated results]
Alexopoulos[280] 2012 Greece 22789884	Ticagrelor 90 mg, 2 x daily vs. prasugrel 10 mg/d (crossover RCT) Total N = 44 (43 completed the study)	1 mo (total duration)	No patient exhibited a major adverse cardiovascular event or a major bleeding event at either treatment group.
Gremmel[281] 2011 Austria 21546102	High-dose group: 100 mg aspirin and 150 mg clopidogrel per day for 3 mo post-PCI (N=21) Standard-dose group: aspirin 100 mg/d and clopidogrel 75 mg/d (N=23)	3 mo	One patient from each treatment group suffered stent thrombosis, and one patient from the standard treatment group exhibited an in-stent restenosis of the target lesion within the follow-up period of 3 months.

217

Table 38. Key findings of studies with phenotypic test–based selection of patients and clinical outcomes (continued)

Author Year Country PMID Study Name (if available)	Treatment Groups (sample size)	Followup Duration	Summary of Findings
Ari[216] 2012 Turkey EFFICIENT 21239075	*High-dose clopidogrel:* clopidogrel 150 mg/d for 1 mo + aspirin (100 mg/d) (N=47) *Standard-dose clopidogrel:* clopidogrel 75 mg/d for 1 mo + aspirin (100 mg/d) (N = 47)	6 mo	*MACE:* 2 events in the high-dose group vs. 8 in the standard-dose group; absolute risk difference = 12.7% (7.5 to 39.7); p=0.045

218

Table 38. Key findings of studies with phenotypic test–based selection of patients and clinical outcomes (continued)

Author Year Country PMID Study Name (if available)	Treatment Groups (sample size)	Followup Duration	Summary of Findings
Trenk[284] 2012 Multinational (North America and Europe) 22520250 TRIGGER-PCI	*Prasugrel + placebo:* prasugrel (60 mg) loading dose within 9 h after administration of the non-study-related clopidogrel maintenance dose (75 mg), followed by maintenance treatment of prasugrel 10 mg/d + placebo, starting the day after the loading dose of the study drug (N=212; 136 completed the study) *Clopidogrel + placebo:* placebo loading dose within 9 h after administration of the non-study-related clopidogrel maintenance dose (75 mg), followed by maintenance treatment of clopidogrel (75 mg) + placebo, starting the day after the loading dose of the study drug (N=211; 137 completed the study)	6 mo (early termination for futility)	*MACE (CV death or MI):* 0 events in the prasugrel-treated group vs. 1 event in the clopidogrel treated group; OR=0.33 (95% CI, 0.013 to 8.15); p=0.50 [calculated results] *CV death:* 0 events in the prasugrel-treated group vs. 0 events in the clopidogrel treated group; OR and p-value not estimable *MI:* 0 events in the prasugrel-treated group vs. 1 event in the clopidogrel treated group; OR=0.33 (95% CI, 0.013 to 8.15); p=0.50 [calculated results] *Definite or probable stent thrombosis:* 0 events in the prasugrel-treated group vs. 0 events in the clopidogrel treated group; OR and p-value not estimable *Urgent TVR:* 2 events in the prasugrel-treated group vs. 1 event in the clopidogrel treated group; OR=2.0 (95% CI, 0.18 to 22.23); p=0.57 [calculated results] *CV death, MI, or TVR:* 2 events in the prasugrel-treated group vs. 2 events in the clopidogrel treated group; OR=1.0 (95% CI, 0.14 to 7.13); p>0.99 [calculated results] *CV death, MI, stroke, or rehospitalization for cardiac ischemic events:* 2 events in the prasugrel-treated group vs. 6 events in the clopidogrel treated group; OR=0.33 (95% CI, 0.065, 1.63); p=0.17 [calculated results]; HR=0.40 (95% CI 0.09 to 2.69) *Non-CV death:* 0 events in the prasugrel-treated group vs. 1 event in the clopidogrel treated group; OR=0.33 (95% CI, 0.013 to 8.15); p=0.50 [calculated results]

219

Table 38. Key findings of studies with phenotypic test–based selection of patients and clinical outcomes (continued)

Author Year Country PMID Study Name (if available)	Treatment Groups (sample size)	Followup Duration	Summary of Findings
Aradi[181] 2012 Hungary 21902692 DOSER	*High-dose clopidogrel:* clopidogrel maintenance 150 mg/d for 1 mo After 28 days, all patients returned to 75 mg maintenance dose of clopidogrel until 1 year. (N=36) *Standard-dose clopidogrel:* clopidogrel maintenance at a dose of 75 mg/d for 1 mo (N=38)	12 mo	*CV death:* 0 events in the high-dose group vs. 1 event in the standard dose group; OR=0.34 (95% CI, 0.01 to 8.68); p=0.52 [calculated results]; p= 0.31 [log-rank test] *MI:* 0 events in the high-dose group vs. 3 events in the standard dose group; OR=0.14 (95% CI, 0.01 to 2.79); p=0.20 [calculated results]; p=0.08 [log-rank test] *TVR:* 1 event in the high-dose group vs. 5 events in the standard dose group; OR=0.19 (95% CI, 0.02 to 1.70); p=0.14 [calculated results]; p=0.09 [log-rank test] *CV death or MI:* 0 events in the high-dose group vs. 4 events in the standard dose group; OR=0.11 (95% CI, 0.01 to 2.02); p=0.14 [calculated results]; p=0.04 [log-rank test] *CV death, MI, or TVR:* 1 event in the high-dose group vs. 8 events in the standard dose group; OR=0.11 (95% CI, 0.01 to 0.91); p=0.04 [calculated results]; p=0.01 [log-rank test]
Tang[247] 2012 China 22490487	*High-dose dual antiplatelet therapy:* aspirin (200 mg/d) + clopidogrel (150 mg/d) (N=30) *Standard-dose dual antiplatelet treatment:* aspirin 100 mg/d + clopidogrel (75 mg/d) (N=30)	12 mo	Data extracted at 12 mo *CV death:* 0 events in the high-dose group vs. 1 events in the standard dose group; OR=0.32 (95% CI, 0.01 to 8.24); p=0.49 [calculated results] *Stent thrombosis:* 3 events in the high-dose group vs. 7 events in the standard dose group; OR=0.37 (95% CI, 0.09 to 1.58); p=0.18 [calculated results] *Recurrent unstable angina:* 7 events in the high-dose group vs. 13 events in the standard dose group; OR=0.40 (95% CI, 0.13 to 1.21); p=0.11 [calculated results] *MI:* 7 events in the high-dose group vs. 6 events in the standard dose group; OR=0.44 (95% CI, 0.10 to 1.97); p=0.29 [calculated results]
Alexopoulos[285] 2011 Greece 21511219	*Prasugrel* 10 mg/d or *clopidogrel* 150 mg/d (crossover RCT) Total N=71	2 mo	No deaths or strokes occurred in either treatment period.

Abbreviations: ACS = acute coronary syndrome; CI = confidence interval; CV = cardiovascular; d = day; HR = hazard ratio; LTA = light-transmission aggregometry; MACE = major adverse cardiovascular events; MI = myocardial infarction; mo = month; OR = odds ratio; PMID = PubMed identification number; PRI = platelet reactivity index; TIMI = Thrombolysis In Myocardial Infarction Study Group; TVR = target vessel revascularization.

*Detailed results on the comparison of patients with high versus low platelet reactivity receiving standard dose clopidogrel (i.e., the nonrandomized comparison) has been summarized in the results section on Key Question 2b.

†Outcome data were extracted only for patients with poor response to clopidogrel or clopidogrel and aspirin (i.e., we did not extract data on patients who were poor responders to aspirin alone).

Intermediate Outcome: Platelet Reactivity During Followup

Ten studies reported information on intermediate outcomes. Eight studies had a total duration of 3 months or less; five studies had a crossover design. The outcomes were assessed using different assays and were heterogeneously reported. The key findings are summarized in Table 39. Generally, patients on higher dose clopidogrel regimens or those receiving prasugrel showed greater responses in platelet reactivity compared to those receiving standard dose clopidogrel regimens.

Table 39. Key findings of studies with phenotypic test–based selection of patients and intermediate outcomes

Author Year Country PMID Study Name (if available)	Treatment Groups (sample size)	Followup Duration	Summary of Findings
Paltering[228] 2010 Italy 19604542 DOUBLE	*High-dose clopidogrel maintenance (n=24): 150 mg/d for 1 mo* *Standard-dose clopidogrel maintenance (n=24): 75 mg/d for 1 mo*	1 mo, assessments performed at 1 we	Mean change of PRI from baseline based on a random effects linear model in the high-dose group at 1 w: -27.8 (95% CI, -33.7 to -21.9); p=0.0001 Mean change of PRI from baseline based on a random effects linear model in the low-dose group at 1 w: -7.9 (95% CI, -14.1 to 1.8); p=0.11 Mean change of PRI from baseline based on a random effects linear model in the high-dose group at 30 d: -31.6 (95% CI, -37.6 to -25.7); p=0.0001 Mean change of PRI from baseline based on a random effects linear model in the low-dose group at 30 d: -18.7 (95% CI, -24.8 to -12.6); p=0.0001 Overall mean difference of PRI between groups (from the random effects linear model)=-15.4 (95% CI, -23.0 to -7.8); p=0.0001 Rate of poor response (defined as PRI>50%) in the high-dose group at 1 mo: 21% Rate of poor response (defined as PRI>50%) in the high-dose group at 1 mo: 71% (p=0.001 for the difference between groups) Mean difference between-groups by LTA (from the random effects linear model; unclear timepoint)=-13.1 (95% CI, -19.8 to -6.4); p=0.0001 Mean difference between-groups by VerifyNow (from the random effects linear model; unclear timepoint)=-57.1 (95% CI, -97.1 to -17.1); p=0.005 Mean difference between-groups by whole blood aggregometry (from the random effects linear model; unclear timepoint)=-1.3 (95% CI, -2.6 to -0.1); p=0.04 Adverse events (study-defined as such): 2 in the high dose group (1 epistaxis; 1 thrombocytopenia); 2 in the low-dose group (1 subacute stent thrombosis; 1 thrombocytopenia) Additional results are presented in Figures 1-3 of the paper.

Table 39. Key findings of studies with phenotypic test–based selection of patients and intermediate outcomes (continued)

Author Year Country PMID Study Name (if available)	Treatment Groups (sample size)	Followup Duration	Summary of Findings
Gurbel[162]* 2010 Multinational (N. America and Europe) 20194878 RESPOND	*Clopidogrel:* clopidogrel 600 mg loading dose, followed by clopidogrel 75 mg/d maintenance *Ticagrelor:* ticagrelor 180 mg loading dose, followed ticagrelor 90 mg BID maintenance dose Nonresponders=41 Responders=57 (crossover RCT)	1 mo	*NONRESPONDER COHORT* The proportion of patients who responded to ticagrelor was higher than those who responded to clopidogrel - using a cut-off of 10% absolute change; risk difference 0.25 (95% CI, 0.08 to 0.41); p=0.005 [McNemar test] - using a cut-off of 30% absolute change; risk difference 0.62 (95% CI, 0.42 to 0.79); p<0.001 [McNemar test] - using a cut-off of 50% absolute change; risk difference 0.13 (95% CI, 0.01 to 0.23); p=0.046[McNemar test] Inhibition of platelet aggregation (LTA ADP 20 μmol/L) was higher at all times with ticagrelor, compared to clopidogrel (P≤0.05); similar results were observed with LTA ADP 5 μmol/L and LTA collagen 2 μg/mL VerifyNow PRU was significantly lower with ticagrelor versus clopidogrel at all timepoints except the initial crossover-period (P≤0.05) During both treatment periods, VASP PRI was significantly lower in ticagrelor-treated patients. ADP-induced IIb/IIIa and P-selectin expression were lower at steady state in ticagrelor-treated patients. *RESPONDER COHORT* Platelet aggregation (LTA ADP 20 μmol/L) was lower after ticagrelor compared with clopidogrel therapy in period 1 and after crossing over in period 2. In patients who continued on the same therapy platelet aggregation was significantly lower at all timepoints after steady state with ticagrelor (p<0.05) Inhibition of platelet aggregation (LTA ADP 20 μmol/L) was higher after loading and maintenance ticagrelor therapy (p<0.05) except at period 2, day 15, 0 hours. Loading with ticagrelor after patients switched from clopidogrel was similar to the inhibition in patients treated with ticagrelor in period 1. In patients who did not switch, inhibition was greater with ticagrelor after steady state was reached (p<0.05). Similar results at steady state were obtained with LTA ADP 5 μmol/L and collagen 2 μg/mL (p<0.001). VerifyNow PRU was significantly lower with ticagrelor versus clopidogrel at all timepoints

223

Table 39. Key findings of studies with phenotypic test–based selection of patients and intermediate outcomes (continued)

Author Year Country PMID Study Name (if available)	Treatment Groups (sample size)	Followup Duration	Summary of Findings
			except the initial crossover-period up to 1 h (P≤0.05). Similar results were observed in patients who continued on the same therapy and those who switched.
			For comparisons at steady state VASP PRI was lower during ticagrelor treatment compared to clopidogrel. After treatments were switched, PRI was significantly lower with ticagrelor at all timepoints except on day 15 (in patients who crossed over; presumably due to carryover). PRI in patients who did not switch was lower during steady state ticagrelor therapy at "nearly all timepoints".
			ADP-induced IIb/IIIa and P-selectin expression were lower at steady state in ticagrelor-treated patients (p<0.001).
Alexopoulos[280] 2012 Greece 22789884	Ticagrelor 90 mg, 2 x daily vs. prasugrel 10 mg/d (crossover RCT) Total N = 44 (43 completed the study)	1 mo	Least squares mean difference = –68.3 PRU (95% CI, -88.6 to -48.1); p<0.001 [combined data throughout the study] Least squares mean difference = -56.7 PRU (95% CI, -83.3 to -30.2); p<0.001 [pre-crossover] Least squares mean difference = -79.3 PRU (95% CI, -110.6 to -48.0); p<0.001 [post-crossover]
Gremmel[281] 2011 Austria 21546102	High-dose group: 100 mg aspirin and 150 mg clopidogrel per day for 3 mo post-PCI (N=21) Standard-dose group: aspirin 100 mg/d and clopidogrel 75 mg/d (N=23)	3 mo	VerifyNow: high dose group mean = 190 ±78 PRU vs. standard dose mean = 262 ±74 PRU VASP assay: high dose group mean = 36.1 ±16.8 % vs. standard dose mean = 59.9 ±21.3 % Multiplate analyzer: high dose group mean = 26 ±16 AU vs. standard dose mean = 46 ±19 AU All p-values for the differences in means between treatment groups were p<0.003 [exact p-value not provided]
Alexopoulos[287] 2011 Greece 21985070	Clopidogrel 150 mg/d or prasugrel 10 mg/d (crossover RCT) Total N = 21	1 mo	Least squares mean difference = –123.2 PRU (95% CI, -157.8 to -88.7); p<0.001 [combined data throughout the study] High on-treatment platelet reactivity rates: prasugrel, n=4/21 (19%) vs. clopidogrel, n=18/21 (85.7%); p<0.001

Table 39. Key findings of studies with phenotypic test–based selection of patients and intermediate outcomes (continued)

Author Year Country PMID Study Name (if available)	Treatment Groups (sample size)	Followup Duration	Summary of Findings
Alexopoulos[283] 2011 Greece 21982667	*Clopidogrel* 150 mg/d or *prasugrel* 10 mg/d (crossover RCT) Total N = 28	1 mo	Least squares mean difference = –71.7 PRU (95% CI, -101.5 to -41.8); p<0.001 [combined data throughout the study]
			Least squares mean difference = -61.6 PRU (95% CI, -105.9 to -17.3); p=0.008 [pre-crossover]
			Least squares mean difference = -81.9 PRU (95% CI, -123.8 to -40.2); p<0.001 [post-crossover]
			High on-treatment platelet reactivity rates: prasugrel, n=3/26 (11.5%) vs. clopidogrel, n=12/26 (46.3%); p=0.003 [combined data throughout the study]
			High on-treatment platelet reactivity rates: prasugrel, n=2/13 (15.4%) vs. clopidogrel, n=8/15 (53.3%); p=0.06 [pre-crossover]
			High on-treatment platelet reactivity rates: prasugrel, n=1/14 (7.1%) vs. clopidogrel, n=4/12 (36.4%); p=0.1 [post-crossover]

225

Table 39. Key findings of studies with phenotypic test–based selection of patients and intermediate outcomes (continued)

Author Year Country PMID Study Name (if available)	Treatment Groups (sample size)	Followup Duration	Summary of Findings
Trenk[284] 2012 Multinational (North America and Europe) 22520250 TRIGGER-PCI	*Prasugrel + placebo:* prasugrel (60 mg) loading dose within 9 h after administration of the non-study-related clopidogrel maintenance dose (75 mg), followed by maintenance treatment of prasugrel 10 mg/d + placebo, starting the day after the loading dose of the study drug (N=212; 136 completed the study) *Clopidogrel + placebo:* placebo loading dose within 9 h after administration of the non-study-related clopidogrel maintenance dose (75 mg), followed by maintenance treatment of clopidogrel (75 mg) + placebo, starting the day after the loading dose of the study drug (N=211; 137 completed the study)	6 mo	After a median of 90 d median PRU on prasugrel was significantly lower than that on clopidogrel; p<0.001. The difference remained statistically significant at a median of 176 d. The between-treatment group difference in change for baseline was statistically significant at 90 d (p=0.001); the between-treatment group difference in change between 90 and 176 d was non-significant (p=0.338). 176 (94.1%) patients of the prasugrel group vs. 56 (29.6%) patients of the clopidogrel group had a PRU ≤208; p<0.001).
Aradi[181] 2012 Hungary 21902692 DOSER	*High-dose clopidogrel:* clopidogrel maintenance 150 mg/d for 1 mo After 28 days, all patients returned to 75 mg maintenance dose of clopidogrel until 1 year (N=36) *Standard dose clopidogrel:* clopidogrel maintenance at a dose of 75 mg/d for 1 mo (N=38)	1 mo (for reactivity measurements)	LTA maximal aggregation: high-dose clopidogrel group 33.8 ±15.1 vs. standard dose clopidogrel 37.0 ±13.5 LTA late aggregation: high-dose clopidogrel group 13.8 ±18.0 vs. standard dose clopidogrel 21.7 ±17.9 LTA disaggregation: high-dose clopidogrel group 64.9 ±31.2 vs. standard dose clopidogrel 49.9 ±32.1 LTA AUC: high-dose clopidogrel group 84.8 ±55.3 vs. standard dose clopidogrel 102.0 ±52.7 VASP PRI: high-dose clopidogrel group 37.2 ±17.1 vs. standard dose clopidogrel 60.8 ±17.2

Table 39. Key findings of studies with phenotypic test–based selection of patients and intermediate outcomes (continued)

Author Year Country PMID Study Name (if available)	Treatment Groups (sample size)	Followup Duration	Summary of Findings
Tang[247] 2012 China 22490487	*High dose dual antiplatelet therapy:* aspirin (200 mg/d) + clopidogrel (150 mg/d) (N=30) *Standard dual antiplatelet treatment:* aspirin 100 mg/d + clopidogrel (75 mg/d) (N=30)	12 mo	The inhibition rate of clopidogrel in the high dose group was 60.2% ±7.4, vs. 45.9% ±4.3 in the standard dose group; p<0.01. The difference remained statistically significant at 12 mo.
Alexopoulos[285] 2011 Greece 21511219	*Prasugrel 10 mg/d or clopidogrel* 150 mg/d (crossover RCT) Total N=71	2 mo	Least squares mean difference = –72.3 PRU (95% CI, -98.3 to -46.4); p<0.001 [combined data throughout the study] High on-treatment platelet reactivity was less frequent in the prasugrel group (4 of 53, 7.5%) compared to the clopidogrel group (19 of 53, 35.8%); p<0.001

Abbreviations: ADP = adenosine diphosphate; AUC = area under the curve; BID = twice daily; CI = confidence interval; d = day; LTA = light-transmission aggregometry; mo = month; PRI = platelet reactivity index; PRU = platelet reactivity units; RCT = randomized controlled trial; VASP = vasodilator-stimulated phosphoprotein; w = week(s).
*Despite including both responders and nonresponders, this study was categorized as a study of randomized treatment after test-based selection because patients were assigned to different treatments during the course of the study on the basis of their original response status.

227

Combined Genetic Testing for CYP2C19 Variants and Phenotypic Testing To Guide Antiplatelet Treatment

We identified four studies that provided information on treatment comparisons among patients selected on the basis of platelet reactivity and also provided information on the CYP2C19 genotype of participants.[285,287-289] The parent studies, their inclusion criteria, study designs, and outcomes are summarized in the immediately preceding section of this chapter. Briefly, two of these genetic sub-studies were conducted in the setting of small (21 and 64 patients) crossover RCTs of short duration (30 and 60 days),[287,288] one was based on a short-term parallel arm trial (2 weeks of followup),[283] and one study (GIFT [Genotype Information and Functional Testing]) was conducted in the setting of the large GRAVITAS trial with a followup of 6 months.[289] Analyses stratified by treatment and genotype status were not reported for clinical outcomes and all four studies reported results for the intermediate outcome of platelet reactivity. Studies did not report significant effect modification by genotype for this outcome (all analyses assumed a dominant model for loss-of-function alleles). However, analyses were inconclusive because studies were small and none had been prospectively powered specifically to assess effect modification by genotype.

Assessment of Risk of Bias of Individual Studies

A detailed assessment of 17 risk-of-bias items for studies comparing treatment effects in patients selected on the basis of phenotypic testing for platelet reactivity is presented in Appendix F. Overall, the risk of bias varied across the randomized studies. The large, multicenter GRAVITAS trial had low risk of bias, both regarding aspects related to the index test of interest as well as general aspects of randomized trial design (e.g., generation of the randomization sequence and allocation concealment).[203] The TRIGGER-PCI trial did not provide adequate information about the randomization procedure and allocation concealment or blinding of patients to treatment assignment; however outcomes assessors were blinded to treatment assignment.[284] Smaller studies (typically with short-term followup) were generally considered to have a higher risk of bias, owing to problems in the application of the tests of interest (e.g., an unclear rationale for the thresholds used) or incomplete reporting of outcomes. Furthermore, these studies often did not provide information sufficient to judge their risk of bias regarding general aspects of randomized trial design.

Key Question 3b. How do modifying factors affect the association of alternative test-and-treat strategies and patient outcomes?

Only four of the studies considered relevant to Key Question 3a provided information about the use of testing for clinical decisionmaking with data stratified by patient characteristics.

The first study reported results from the genetic substudy of the CURE trial comparing clopidogrel plus aspirin (dual-antiplatelet) and placebo plus aspirin in patients with non–ST-elevation myocardial infarction.[109] The study reported modification of the treatment effect by genotype status, stratified by ancestry. There was no significant interaction between genotype group and treatment (p=0.12 for the composite outcome of death from cardiovascular causes, nonfatal myocardial infarction, or stroke; p=0.28 for the composite outcome of death from cardiovascular causes, nonfatal myocardial infarction, stroke, recurrent ischemia, or hospitalization for unstable angina) among individuals of "European ancestry" and individuals of "Latin American ancestry" (p=0.81 and p=0.71, respectively, for the same outcomes).

The second study reported results from the genetic substudy of the CHARISMA trial, comparing clopidogrel plus aspirin versus placebo plus aspirin in patients with established atherothrombotic vascular disease (coronary, cerebrovascular, or peripheral artery disease).[85] The study reported information on the modification of the treatment effect by genotype status, stratified by ancestry (European vs. non-European), history of percutaneous coronary intervention (performed vs. not), and symptomatic atherothrombosis on entry into the trial (present vs. absent). In all cases, the genotype-by-treatment interaction was not statistically significant in any patient subpopulation.

The third study reporting relevant information compared conventional dual-antiplatelet therapy (aspirin plus clopidogrel) with adjunctive use of a glycoprotein IIb/IIIa inhibitor (aspirin plus clopidogrel plus abciximab) in 149 clopidogrel nonresponders (by LTA) undergoing PCI, angiography, or both.[206] Treatment-effect modification by baseline percent inhibition (≥ 21 percent vs. <21 percent) was assessed for the outcome of periprocedural myocardial infarction. An interaction test indicated that effect modification was not statistically significant (p=0.35); the reported data did not allow for the calculation of treatment-effect size stratified by baseline platelet reactivity.

The fourth study evaluated the interaction effect of baseline platelet reactivity and treatment, in a crossover RCT comparing dual antiplatelet therapy (aspirin plus clopidogrel) versus triple therapy (dual therapy plus cilostazol), stratified by diabetes status.[278] We performed a test for interaction comparing the mean difference (between treatments) among the four groups defined by diabetes status (present vs. absent) and high on-clopidogrel platelet reactivity (present vs. absent). The p-value was 0.356, suggesting that the treatment effect is not statistically significantly different between the four groups.

Information on the risk of bias of these studies is summarized in the preceding section, because they were also included in Key Question 3a. We caution that studies did not use any procedure to adjust for multiple statistical testing in their subgroup analyses of effect modification.

Key Question 4. What are the potential adverse effects or harms from genetic or phenotypic testing per se or from test-directed treatments?

Key Question 4 aimed to address the potential harms of test-guided treatment as well as the harms of the testing process itself.

Harms of Test-Directed Treatment

For harms of test-directed treatment, Table 40 summarizes the number of studies and adverse events or harms assessed for each of the designs we reviewed for Key Question 4. We discuss studies belonging to each of three designs—studies of test-and-treat strategies, studies of treatment-effect modification, and studies with test-based selection—separately for genetic testing (for CYP2C19 variants) and for phenotypic testing (of platelet reactivity). (Please see the Methods section for more information.)

Table 40. Number of studies relevant to Key Question 4 and harms assessed, by study design and test used

Study Design	Genetic Testing for CYP2C19 Variants	Phenotypic Testing for Platelet Reactivity
Comparative studies of test-and-treat strategies	1 RCT (bleeding events)	7 (6 RCTs + 1 NRCS; bleeding events)
RCTs of treatment-effect modification by test results	6 (bleeding events)	2 (bleeding events and treatment discontinuations)
RCTs with test-based selection	1 (bleeding and non-bleeding events)	12 (bleeding events, treatment discontinuations, non-bleeding events)

Abbreviations: NRCS = nonrandomized comparative study; RCT = randomized controlled trial.
See the Methods section for details on the relevant study designs.

Genetic Testing for CYP2C19 Variants

Studies of Test-and-Treat Strategies

We identified a single study comparing testing for CYP2C19 variants against a no-testing strategy to guide treatment decisionmaking.[86] The study monitored major and minor bleeding (using the TIMI classification) over 30 days of followup. Detailed information regarding the study design and patient population enrolled is provided in the corresponding section under Key Question 3. Briefly, the study assigned patients to a genotype-guided strategy (whereby *2 carriers were treated with prasugrel and non-carriers were treated with clopidogrel-based dual antiplatelet treatment) or to a control treatment strategy (whereby all patients received clopidogrel-based dual antiplatelet treatment).

All patients who underwent PCI were included in the analysis of safety outcomes. The frequency of minor and major bleeding was not different between the study groups: 5 (6 percent) of 91 patients in the genotype-guided group versus 2 (2 percent) of 96 in the control treatment group experienced TIMI minor bleeding (p=0.269); two (2.2 percent) patients in the genotype-guided group versus one (1 percent) in the control treatment group (p=0.613) experienced TIMI major bleeding.

Results regarding the risk of bias assessment for this study are presented in Appendix F and discussed under Key Question 3.

Studies of Treatment-Effect Modification by CYP2C19 Genotype Status

Six studies (reported in five publications[85,99,104,109,258,260]) provided information on treatment-effect modification of bleeding outcomes by CYP2C19 status. Five were based on large randomized trials of clopidogrel-based therapy that included more than 1000 patients in their genetic substudies. Of these, one study enrolled patients with non–ST-elevation acute coronary syndromes, one enrolled those with acute coronary syndromes undergoing PCI, one involved patients with ST-elevation or non–ST-elevation acute coronary syndromes,[104] one enrolled a mixed population of patients with manifest atherothrombotic disease (coronary, cerebrovascular, and peripheral artery disease) along with individuals at high risk for developing atherothrombotic disease,[85] and one enrolled persons with atrial fibrillation who were not appropriate candidates for vitamin K–antagonist treatment.[109] The sixth study was a small genetic substudy of 126 patients with myocardial infarction who were randomized to either aspirin plus high-dose maintenance clopidogrel or to triple-antiplatelet therapy (aspirin, clopidogrel, and cilostazol).[260]

With a followup of only 30 days, the study reported that no major bleeding events by TIMI criteria were observed in either group. Details about the selection criteria, patient characteristics, and study design are under Key Question 3a results.

Results from the five larger studies comparing the effect of alternative treatment strategies (stratified by CYP2C19 genotype) on safety outcomes (in all five studies, bleeding events) are summarized in Table 41. The test for interaction (i.e., a test for heterogeneity of treatment effects across genotype groups) was not statistically significant for the reported comparisons. This indicates that the impact of the compared treatments on bleeding events was not significantly different across patient groups defined by CYP2C19 genotype.

Table 41. Bleeding events in studies of treatment-effect modification by CYP2C19 genotype status

Author Year Country PMID Study name (if available)	Outcome Definition (timing)	Subgroup defined by genotype	Treatment group	Number with outcome/total number within phenotype-treatment group	Comparison between treatments, within genotype groups ES (95% CI); p-value [statistical test]	Comparison of treatment effects across genotype groups
Pare[109]* 2010 Multinational 20979470 CURE	Major bleeding (definition NR)	Poor metabolizers	Dual antiplatelet therapy	0/61	NA	p=0.64
			Aspirin monotherapy	1/55		
		Intermediate metabolizers	Dual antiplatelet therapy	19/437	HR=1.61 (95% CI, 0.79 to 3.28) [Cox proportional hazards model; adjusted for age, sex, ancestry]	
			Aspirin monotherapy	13/442		
		Extensive metabolizers	Dual antiplatelet therapy	42/1033	HR=1.43 (95% CI, 0.89 to 2.30) [Cox proportional hazards model; adjusted for age, sex, ancestry]	
			Aspirin monotherapy	29/987		
		Ultra metabolizers	Dual antiplatelet therapy	39/847	HR=1.19 (95% CI, 0.74 to 1.91) [Cox proportional hazards model; adjusted for age, sex, ancestry]	
			Aspirin monotherapy	31/826		
		Unknown metabolizers	Dual antiplatelet therapy	2/152	HR=1.77 (95% CI, 0.15 to 20.33) [Cox proportional hazards model; adjusted for age, sex, ancestry]	
			Aspirin monotherapy	1/176		

232

Table 41. Bleeding events in studies of treatment-effect modification by CYP2C19 genotype status (continued)

Author Year Country PMID Study name (if available)	Outcome Definition (timing)	Subgroup defined by genotype	Treatment group	Number with outcome/total number within phenotype-treatment group	Comparison between treatments, within genotype groups ES [95% CI]; p-value [statistical test]	Comparison of treatment effects across genotype groups
Pare[109] 2010 Multinational 20979470 ACTIVE A	Major hemorrhage=overt bleeding requiring transfusion of at least 2 units of blood or any overt bleeding meeting the criteria for severe hemorrhage	Poor metabolizers	Dual antiplatelet therapy	0/9	NA	p=0.08
			Aspirin monotherapy	2/12		
		Intermediate metabolizers	Dual antiplatelet therapy	10/93	HR=5.84 (95% CI, 1.26 to 27.06) [Cox proportional hazards model; adjusted for age, sex]	
			Aspirin monotherapy	2/92		
		Extensive metabolizers	Dual antiplatelet therapy	10/199	HR=0.91 (95% CI, 0.38 to 2.18) [Cox proportional hazards model; adjusted for age, sex]	
			Aspirin monotherapy	11/235		
		Ultra metabolizers	Dual antiplatelet therapy	8/222	HR=1.24 (95% CI, 0.43 to 3.59) [Cox proportional hazards model; adjusted for age, sex]	
			Aspirin monotherapy	6/200		
		Unknown metabolizers	Dual antiplatelet therapy	4/37	HR=1.84 (95% CI, 0.34 to 10.08) [Cox proportional hazards model; adjusted for age, sex]	
			Aspirin monotherapy	2/35		

Table 41. Bleeding events in studies of treatment-effect modification by CYP2C19 genotype status (continued)

Author Year Country PMID Study name (if available)	Outcome Definition (timing)	Subgroup defined by genotype	Treatment group	Number with outcome/total number within phenotype-treatment group	Comparison between treatments, within genotype groups ES (95% CI); p-value [statistical test]	Comparison of treatment effects across genotype groups
Mega[99,258]† 2009 Multinational 19106084 19414633 TRITON-TIMI 38	Safety outcome=major or minor bleeding (TIMI criteria); analysis for this outcome was performed on an "as-treated" basis	Carriers of a reduced function allele	Clopidogrel + aspirin	11/393	OR=0.66 (95% CI, 0.30 to 1.42) [calculated values]	p=0.73 [calculated from z-test between odds ratios]
			Prasugrel + aspirin	17/405		
		Noncarriers	Clopidogrel + aspirin	30/1061	OR=0.77 (95% CI, 0.48 to 1.26) [calculated values]	
			Prasugrel + aspirin	38/1047		
Kim[260] 2011 S. Korea 21511217 ACCELAMI2C19	Major bleeding events (based on TIMI criteria)	Carriers	Triple therapy (adjunctive cilostazol)	0/39	OR not estimable	NA
			High-maintenance dose clopidogrel	0/38		
		Noncarriers	Triple therapy (adjunctive cilostazol)	0/25		
			High-maintenance dose clopidogrel	0/24		
Wallentin[104] 2010 Multinational 20801498 PLATO	Major bleeding	Any CYP2C19 LOF allele (*2–*8)	Ticagrelor + aspirin	149/1380	HR =1.04 (95% CI, 0.82 to 1.30) [Cox regression with adjustment for ethnic group, sex, use of PPI, aspirin dose, smoking status, and diabetes]	0.60
			Clopidogrel+ aspirin	143/1380		

Table 41. Bleeding events in studies of treatment-effect modification by CYP2C19 genotype status (continued)

Author Year Country PMID Study name (if available)	Outcome Definition (timing)	Subgroup defined by genotype	Treatment group	Number with outcome/total number within phenotype-treatment group	Comparison between treatments, within genotype groups ES (95% CI); p-value [statistical test]	Comparison of treatment effects across genotype groups
		No CYP2C19 LOF allele (*1 or *17)	Ticagrelor + aspirin	331/3547	HR =0.96 (95% CI, 0.83 to 1.12) [Cox regression with adjustment for ethnic group, sex, use of PPI, aspirin dose, smoking status, and diabetes]	
			Clopidogrel+ aspirin	340/3506		
		No CYP2C19 LOF or GOF allele (*1)	Ticagrelor + aspirin	176/1846	HR =1.12 (95% CI, 0.90 to 1.38) [Cox regression with adjustment for ethnic group, sex, use of PPI, aspirin dose, smoking status, and diabetes]	0.19
			Clopidogrel+ aspirin	161/1856		
		Any CYP2C19 LOF allele (*2–*8) but no GOF allele (not *17)	Ticagrelor + aspirin	108/1011	HR =1.03 (95% CI, 0.79 to 1.34) [Cox regression with adjustment for ethnic group, sex, use of PPI, aspirin dose, smoking status, and diabetes]	
			Clopidogrel+ aspirin	108/1053		
		Any CYP2C19 GOF allele (*17)	Ticagrelor + aspirin	196/2070	HR =0.86 (95% CI, 0.71 to 1.05) [Cox regression with adjustment for ethnic group, sex, use of PPI, aspirin dose, smoking status, and diabetes]	
			Clopidogrel+ aspirin	214/1977		
	Major bleeding not related to CABG	Any CYP2C19 LOF allele (*2–*8)	Ticagrelor + aspirin	56/1380	HR =1.39 (95% CI, 0.93 to 2.08) [Cox regression with adjustment for ethnic group, sex, use of PPI, aspirin dose, smoking status, and diabetes]	0.31
			Clopidogrel+ aspirin	41/1380		
		No CYP2C19 LOF allele (*1 or *17)	Ticagrelor + aspirin	121/3547	HR =1.08 (95% CI, 0.84 to 1.40) [Cox regression with adjustment for ethnic group, sex, use of PPI, aspirin dose, smoking status, and diabetes]	

235

Table 41. Bleeding events in studies of treatment-effect modification by CYP2C19 genotype status (continued)

Author Year Country PMID Study name (if available)	Outcome Definition (timing)	Subgroup defined by genotype	Treatment group	Number with outcome/total number within phenotype-treatment group	Comparison between treatments, within genotype groups ES (95% CI); p-value [statistical test]	Comparison of treatment effects across genotype groups
			Clopidogrel+ aspirin	110/3506		
	Major bleeding related to CABG	Any CYP2C19 LOF allele (*2–*8)	Ticagrelor + aspirin	96/1380	HR =0.87 (95% CI, 0.66 to 1.14) [Cox regression with adjustment for ethnic group, sex, use of PPI, aspirin dose, smoking status, and diabetes]	0.93
			Clopidogrel+ aspirin	107/1380		
		No CYP2C19 LOF allele (*1 or *17)	Ticagrelor + aspirin	218/3547	HR =0.88 (95% CI, 0.73 to 1.05) [Cox regression with adjustment for ethnic group, sex, use of PPI, aspirin dose, smoking status, and diabetes]	
			Clopidogrel+ aspirin	246/3506		

236

Table 41. Bleeding events in studies of treatment-effect modification by CYP2C19 genotype status (continued)

Author Year Country PMID Study name (if available)	Outcome Definition (timing)	Subgroup defined by genotype	Treatment group	Number with outcome/total number within phenotype-treatment group	Comparison between treatments, within genotype groups ES (95% CI); p-value [statistical test]	Comparison of treatment effects across genotype groups
Bhatt[85] 2012 Multinational 22450429 CHARISMA	Major bleed (GUSTO criteria)	Poor metabolizers	Clopidogrel + aspirin	0/52	NA	0.055
			Aspirin + placebo	1/48		
		Intermediate metabolizers	Clopidogrel + aspirin	22/458	HR=5.32 (95% CI, 1.83 to 15.44) [Cox regression with adjustment for age, sex, inclusion criteria (symptomatic vs. asymptomatic), use of statins, use of calcium channel blockers, and cigarette usage]	
			Aspirin + placebo	4/445		
		Extensive metabolizers	Clopidogrel + aspirin	34/886	HR=1.31 (95% CI, 0.80 to 2.15) [Cox regression with adjustment for age, sex, inclusion criteria (symptomatic vs. asymptomatic), use of statins, use of calcium channel blockers, and cigarette usage]	
			Aspirin + placebo	30/920		
		Ultra metabolizers	Clopidogrel + aspirin	26/716	HR=1.54 (95% CI, 0.84 to 2.84) [Cox regression with adjustment for age, sex, inclusion criteria (symptomatic vs. asymptomatic), use of statins, use of calcium channel blockers, and cigarette usage]	
			Aspirin + placebo	17/715		
		Unknown metabolizers	Clopidogrel + aspirin	6/156	HR=1.40 (95% CI, 0.39 to 4.99) [Cox regression with adjustment for age, sex, inclusion criteria (symptomatic vs. asymptomatic), use of statins, use of calcium channel blockers, and cigarette usage]	
			Aspirin + placebo	4/145		

237

Table 41. Bleeding events in studies of treatment-effect modification by CYP2C19 genotype status (continued)

Author Year Country PMID Study name (if available)	Outcome Definition (timing)	Subgroup defined by genotype	Treatment group	Number with outcome/total number within phenotype-treatment group	Comparison between treatments, within genotype groups ES (95% CI); p-value [statistical test]	Comparison of treatment effects across genotype groups
	All bleeds (GUSTO criteria)	Poor metabolizers	Clopidogrel + aspirin	11/52	HR=1.63 (95% CI, 0.62 to 4.27) [Cox regression with adjustment for age, sex, inclusion criteria (symptomatic vs. asymptomatic), use of statins, use of calcium channel blockers, and cigarette usage]	0.195
			Aspirin + placebo	7/48		
		Intermediate metabolizers	Clopidogrel + aspirin	174/458	HR=1.83 (95% CI, 1.44 to 2.33) [Cox regression with adjustment for age, sex, inclusion criteria (symptomatic vs. asymptomatic), use of statins, use of calcium channel blockers, and cigarette usage]	
			Aspirin + placebo	106/445		
		Extensive metabolizers	Clopidogrel + aspirin	369/886	HR=2.21 (95% CI, 1.87 to 2.62) [Cox regression with adjustment for age, sex, inclusion criteria (symptomatic vs. asymptomatic), use of statins, use of calcium channel blockers, and cigarette usage]	
			Aspirin + placebo	210/920		
		Ultra metabolizers	Clopidogrel + aspirin	312/716	HR=2.45 (95% CI, 2.02 to 2.96) [Cox regression with adjustment for age, sex, inclusion criteria (symptomatic vs. asymptomatic), use of statins, use of calcium channel blockers, and cigarette usage]	
				156/715		
		Unknown metabolizers	Clopidogrel + aspirin	55/156	HR=1.65 (95% CI, 1.08 to 2.52) [Cox regression with adjustment for age, sex, inclusion criteria (symptomatic vs. asymptomatic), use of statins, use of calcium channel blockers, and cigarette usage]	
			Aspirin + placebo	36/145		

Abbreviations: ACTIVE A Trial = Atrial Fibrillation Clopidogrel Trial with Irbesartan for Prevention of Vascular Events A trial; CABG = coronary artery bypass grafting; GOF = gain-of-function; GUSTO = Global Utilization of Streptokinase and Tissue Plasminogen Activator for Occluded Coronary Arteries; HR = hazard ratio; LOF = loss-of-function; NA = not applicable; NR = not reported; OR = odds ratio; PLATO = PLATelet inhibition and patient Outcomes trial; PPI = proton-pump inhibitors; TIMI = Thrombolysis In Myocardial Infarction; TRITON-TIMI 38 = Trial to Assess Improvement in Therapeutic Outcomes by Optimizing Platelet Inhibition With Prasugrel–Thrombolysis In Myocardial Infarction 38.

*The authors reported extensive subgroup and sensitivity analyses across different genotype groupings and after including or excluding subgroups of patients by race or ethnicity. The results relevant to treatment effect heterogeneity from these analyses are presented in the text of this section.

†Patients with genotypes of "unclear" functional significance were excluded.

239

Because of the large differences in populations included, treatments compared, and exposure and outcome definitions among studies reporting on treatment-effect modification by CYP2C19 variants, we did not perform a meta-analysis. For purposes of illustration, we used the counts reported in the studies to compare the treatment effect among genotype-defined groups, under a dominant and a recessive model. Figure 40 presents odds ratios for the treatment effect within each genotype subgroup and relative odds ratios comparing the treatment effect across genotype groups. This relative treatment effect is equivalent to a test of genotype × treatment interaction (see Table 41 for detailed results on treatment-effect heterogeneity by genotype status). Regardless of the genetic model, estimates of effect were generally imprecise because of the relatively low event rate in all trials. Estimates under the recessive model were even less precise, owing to the low number of individuals homozygous for loss-of-function alleles in the study populations.

Figure 40. Bleeding events in large randomized trials reporting information on effect modification by CYP2C19 variants

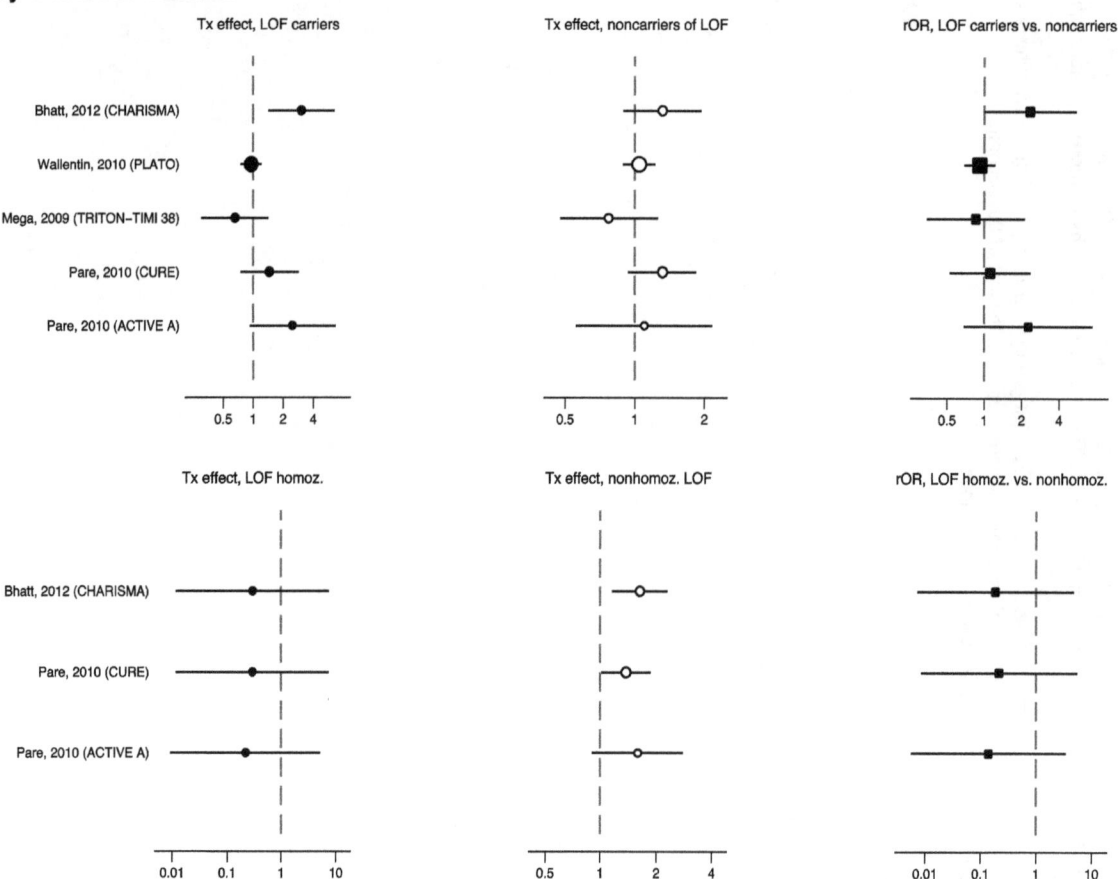

Abbreviations: ACTIVE A = Atrial Fibrillation Clopidogrel Trial with Irbesartan for Prevention of Vascular Events A; CHARISMA = Clopidogrel for High Atherothrombotic Risk and Ischemic Stabilization, Management, and Avoidance; CURE = Clopidogrel in Unstable Angina to Prevent Recurrent Events trial; PLATO = PLATelet inhibition and patient Outcomes trial; TRITON-TIMI 38 = Trial to Assess Improvement in Therapeutic Outcomes by Optimizing Platelet Inhibition with Prasugrel–Thrombolysis in Myocardial Infarction; Tx = treatment.
The top set of panels presents forest plots for treatment effects (odds ratios) on bleeding outcomes among carriers of at least one loss-of-function (LOF) allele (top left panel); treatment effects among noncarriers of LOF alleles (top middle panel); and relative effects (relative odds ratios [rOR]) comparing the treatment effect among LOF carriers and LOF noncarriers (top right panel). The bottom set of panels presents forest plots of treatment effects on bleeding outcomes among homozygotes for two LOF alleles (bottom left panel); treatment effects among non-homozygotes of LOF alleles (bottom middle panel); and relative effects comparing the treatment effect among homozygotes and non-homozygotes of LOF alleles (bottom right panel). Two studies did

not provide adequate data for the comparisons of homozygotes and non-homozygotes. The CURE, CHARISMA, and ACTIVE A trials compared aspirin plus clopidogrel versus aspirin monotherapy; the TRITON-TIMI 38 trial compared aspirin plus clopidogrel versus aspirin plus prasugrel; the PLATO trial compared aspirin plus clopidogrel versus aspirin plus ticagrelor. Point estimates for treatment effects are shown as black circles (carriers) or white circles (noncarriers); point estimates for relative treatment effects are shown as black squares. For all symbols, size is inversely proportional to the standard error of each estimate. Horizontal extending lines denote 95% confidence intervals for all estimates. Vertical dashed lines denote no effect. Please see Table 41 for definitions of the genotype categories and outcomes reported by each study. References to individual studies are provided in Table 5.

Studies With Genetic Test–Based Selection of Patients

One study, the ELEVATE-TIMI 56 trial,[87] selected patients on the basis of CYP2C19 genotype to compare different clopidogrel doses. As discussed in the corresponding section of Key Question 3, the study genotyped patients on chronic clopidogrel therapy for the presence of CYP2C19 *2 alleles; patients with at least one *2 alleles were randomized to various sequences of clopidogrel at doses of 75, 150, 225, or 300 mg daily (each for approximately 2 weeks). Non-carriers were randomized to clopidogrel 75 or 150 mg daily (each dose for two periods of approximately 2 weeks).

There were no TIMI major or minor bleeding events. Among CYP2C19 *2 noncarriers, no patients taking the 75 mg dose and five patients taking the 150 mg dose had bleeding requiring medical attention. Among carriers, a bleeding event requiring medical attention occurred in one patient in each of the following dosing regimens: 75, 225, and 300 mg. Finally, no adverse events or serious adverse events that were not prespecified end points occurred at a frequency greater than 3 percent per treatment group, and there were no significant differences in hematologic, gastrointestinal, or musculoskeletal disorders in CYP2C19*2 carriers across different clopidogrel doses.

Assessment of Risk of Bias of Individual Studies

The ELEVATE-TIMI 56 study was also included in Key Question 3a.[87] As such, detailed information on the 17 risk-of-bias items we assessed is not presented here but in the preceding section.

Phenotypic Testing for Platelet Reactivity

Studies of Test-and-Treat Strategies

Seven studies[270-276] comparing alternative test-and-treat strategies provided information on harms of test-directed treatment. The study design, patient characteristics, and phenotypic assays used in these studies have been presented in Tables 25–27 under Key Question 3a. Briefly, the studies randomized patients into groups receiving antiplatelet treatment guided by phenotypic testing or into groups receiving standard-dose clopidogrel therapy. Four of the studies used the VASP assay to monitor response and modify treatment accordingly; one study used the VerifyNow P2Y12 assay, and two studies used the Multiplate analyzer. Six of the studies were RCTs and one was a nonrandomized comparative study. No study identified a statistically significant difference between any study arms in the risk of bleeding events (Figure 41). Outcome definitions and frequency of bleeding events are given in Table 42. The studies had short followup durations (1 year in one study; 6 months in another; and 30 days in the remaining five) and few events were observed, particularly severe or major bleeding outcomes. Consequently, data were sparse and CIs around effect estimates were wide, indicating substantial uncertainty.

Table 42. Bleeding events in studies of test-and-treat strategies using phenotypic testing of platelet reactivity

Author Year Country PMID Study Name (if available)	Treatment Group Sample Size	Outcome Definition	Time Point	No. with Outcome (%)	Comparative Metric	95% CI	p-value [statistical test]
Wang[270] 2011 China 21538380	VASP-guided treatment N=150	TIMI major bleeding: intracranial bleeding, or clinically overt bleeding associated with a decrease in hemoglobin of 50 g/L	1 yr	0 (0%)	Not estimable	Not estimable	p>0.99* [unclear]
	Control N=156			0 (0%)			
	VASP-guided treatment N=150	TIMI minor bleeding	1 yr	19 (12.7%)	OR=0.76 (calculated)	0.40 to 1.45 (calculated)	p=0.06† [unclear]
	Control N=156			25 (16.6%)			
Bonello[271] 2009 France 19101221	VASP-guided treatment N=215	TIMI major bleeding	30 d	2 (0.9%)	OR=1.00 (calculated)	0.14 to 7.13 (calculated)	p>0.99 [Fisher exact test]
	Control N=214			2 (0.9%)			
	VASP-guided treatment N=215	TIMI minor bleeding	30 d	6 (2.8%)	OR=1.51 (calculated)	0.42 to 5.42 (calculated)	p=0.8 [chi-square]
	Control N=214			4 (1.9%)			
Bonello[272] 2008 France 18387444	VASP-guided treatment N=78	TIMI major bleeding: intracranial bleeding, or clinically overt bleeding associated with a decrease in hemoglobin of 5 g/dL	30 d	1 (1.3%)	OR=1.08 (calculated)	0.07 to 17.53 (calculated)	p>0.99 [Fisher exact test; calculated]
	Control N=84			1 (1.2%)			
	VASP-guided treatment N=78	TIMI minor bleeding	30 d	2 (2.6%)	OR=0.71 (calculated)	0.12 to 4.37 (calculated)	p>0.99 [Fisher exact test; calculated]
	Control N=84			3 (3.6%)			

Table 42. Bleeding events in studies of test-and-treat strategies using phenotypic testing of platelet reactivity (continued)

Author Year Country PMID Study Name (if available)	Treatment Group Sample Size	Outcome Definition	Time Point	No. with Outcome (%)	Comparative Metric	95% CI	p-value [statistical test]
Tousek[273] 2011 Czech Republic 21663983	VerifyNow-guided treatment N=30	TIMI major or minor bleeding	6 mo	2 (6.7%)	OR=1.00 (calculated)	0.13 to 7.60 (calculated)	p>0.99 [Fisher exact test; calculated]
	Control N=30			2 (6.7%)			
Aleil[274] 2008 France 19463377 VASP-02	VASP-guided treatment N=95 (93 included in analyses)	Major bleeding=intracranial bleeding or decrease in hemoglobin requiring transfusion	30 d	0 (0%)	Not defined	Not defined	NA
	Control N=58			0 (0%)			
	VASP-guided treatment N=95 (93 included in analyses)	Minor bleed=increase in skin bleeding, appearance of epistaxis, gum bleeding about which the patient complains	30 d	17 (18%)	OR=0.96 (calculated)	0.41 to 2.22 (calculated)	p=0.92 [chi-square test; calculated]
	Control N=58			11 (19%)			
Hazarbasanov[275] 2012 Bulgaria 22249353	Multiplate analyzer-guided treatment N=97	TIMI major bleeding	30 d (adverse events were monitored during "the intensified therapy" period)	1 (1%)	OR=2.97 (calculated)	0.12 to 73.79 (calculated)	p>0.99 (Fisher exact test; calculated)
	Control N=95			0 (0%)			
	Multiplate analyzer-guided treatment N=97	TIMI minor bleeding	30 d (adverse events were monitored during "the intensified therapy" period)	0 (0%)	Not estimable	Not estimable	NA

243

Table 42. Bleeding events in studies of test-and-treat strategies using phenotypic testing of platelet reactivity (continued)

Author Year Country PMID Study Name (if available)	Treatment Group Sample Size	Outcome Definition	Time Point	No. with Outcome (%)	Comparative Metric	95% CI	p-value [statistical test]
	Control N=95			0 (0%)			
Siller-Matula[276] 2012 Austria 22656044 MADONNA	Multiplate analyzer-guided treatment N=403	TIMI major bleeding	30 d	4 (1%)	OR=3.95 (calculated)	0.44 to 35.50 (calculated)	p=0.186 [unclear statistical test] p=0.373 [two-sided Fisher exact test; calculated]
	Control N=395			1 (<1%)			

Abbreviations: CI = confidence interval; d = days; mo = months; NA = not applicable; NR = not reported; OR = odds ratio; PCI = percutaneous coronary intervention; TIMI = Thrombolysis in Myocardial Infarction; VASP = vasodilator-stimulated phosphoprotein; yr = year.

"Calculated" indicates that the result was not reported by the article's authors; rather, we derived the result from reported raw data.

*It is unclear how the reported p-value of 1.0 was calculated. The p-value here is nonestimable by the chi-square test or Fisher exact test.

†Although P = 0.06 was the reported p-value, recalculation using a chi-square test gives a p-value of 0.403 and recalculation using the Fisher exact test gives a p-value of 0.420. It is unclear how the reported p-value was calculated.

244

Figure 41. Bleeding events in studies of test-and-treat strategies using phenotypic testing of platelet reactivity

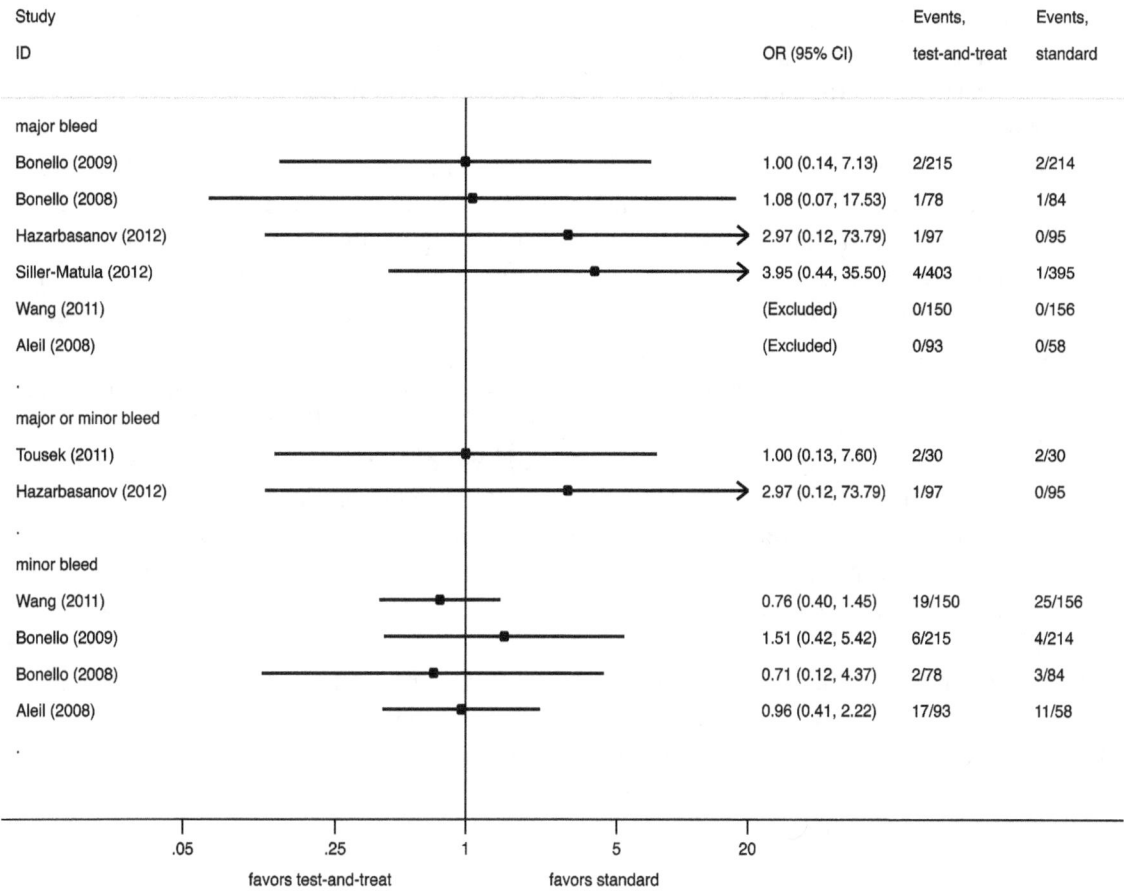

Abbreviations: CI = confidence interval; OR = odds ratio. See Table 33 for details on the strategies compared and the definitions of outcomes employed in each study.

Studies of Treatment-Effect Modification by Baseline Platelet Reactivity

Two studies provided information on treatment-effect modification by baseline on-clopidogrel platelet reactivity.[242,277] The first study reported that no treatment discontinuations, non–CABG-related major bleeding events (by Thrombolysis in Myocardial Infarction [TIMI] criteria), or severe or life-threatening bleeding events (by GUSTO [Global Utilization of Streptokinase and Tissue Plasminogen Activator for Occluded Coronary Arteries] criteria) were observed during the trial. Additional information on minor bleeding events or deaths (one death, due to cancer) was not stratified by baseline reactivity status.[277]

The second study did not identify statistically significant effect modification by baseline low platelet reactivity (defined as ≤188 arbitrary units × minute) of the relative effect of abciximab plus heparin versus bivalirudin in patients undergoing PCI on dual antiplatelet therapy (calculated P for interaction = 0.184). However, the relative odds ratio for major bleeding according to TIMI criteria was extreme (OR=13.98) with very wide confidence intervals (95%

CI 0.28 to 686.8) suggesting that the number of events (n=6) and followup duration (30 days) was not adequate to reach meaningful conclusions.[242]

Studies With Phenotypic-Test–Based Selection of Patients

Of the 14 studies that reported results from randomized trials with phenotypic testing–based patient selection, 12 reported information on treatment-related harms.[181,203,206,216,242,247,279-281,285,287,290] Detailed information about the study design, patient characteristics, and assays used in these studies is presented under Key Question 3a.

Only 2 of the 14 studies (the GRAVITAS[203] and the TRIGGER-PCI[284] trial) included more than 100 randomized patients. The large randomized GRAVITAS trial compared high-dose clopidogrel (in 1,109 patients) versus standard-dose clopidogrel (in 1,105 patients); all the patients had high on-clopidogrel platelet reactivity at baseline as measured by the VerifyNow P2Y12 assay. The study found no statistically significant difference between the two treatment groups for any bleeding event (hazard ratio for high-dose vs. standard-dose therapy, 1.19; 95% CI 0.93, 1.53) (P=0.18) after 6 months of followup. The TRIGGER-PCI trial compared prasugrel (in 212 patients) versus standard dose clopidogrel (in 211 patients); all patients had high on-clopidogrel platelet reactivity at baseline as measured by the VerifyNow P2Y12 assay. The primary safety endpoint of the trial (non-CABG TIMI criteria major bleeding) was not statistically significantly different between the two groups at 6 months of followup (OR=3.03; 95% CI, 0.31 to 29.26 [p=0.34, by our calculation]). Of note, the TRIGGER-PCI trial was terminated early for futility, on the basis of "lower than expected incidence of the primary endpoint."

The remaining 12 studies had smaller sample sizes (ranging from 21 to 159 patients) and generally had shorted followup durations (<1 month in 6 of the 12 studies) and generally reported low rates of events. Results from all studies are summarized in Table 43.

Table 43. Key findings of studies with phenotypic test–based selection of patients reporting information on harms

Author Year Country PMID Study Name (if available)	Treatment Groups (sample size)	Followup Duration	Summary of Findings
Price[203] 2011 Multinational 21406646 GRAVITAS	*High-dose clopidogrel (n=1109):* total first day dose 600 mg, followed by a maintenance dose of 150 mg/d for 6 mo *Standard-dose clopidogrel (n=1105):* loading dose of placebo, followed by a dose of 75 mg/d + a placebo tablet	6 mo	Randomized comparison*. Severe or moderate bleeding events (GUSTO criteria): HR=0.59 (95% CI, 0.31 to 1.11); p=0.10 Any bleeding: HR=1.19 (95% CI, 0.93 to 1.53); p=0.18
Valgimigli[206]† 2009 Italy 19528337 3T/2R	*IIb/IIIa inhibitor group (n=68, clopidogrel-only nonresponders):* tirofiban 50 mL diluted in 200 mL of 0.9% NaCl solution *Placebo group (n=79, clopidogrel-only nonresponders):* 50 mL of 0.9% NaCl was injected in 200 mL of 0.9% NaCl solution by an unblinded research study nurse (all other personnel were blinded to treatment assignment).	1 mo	No major bleeding events occurred in the study.
Cuisset[279] 2008 France 19463379	*IIb/IIIa inhibitor group (n=74):* systematic administration of abciximab to all patient *Conventional treatment group (n=75):* use of IIb/IIIa agonists left at the discretion of physicians	1 mo	No patients had a major bleeding event (TIMI criteria). No patients required transfusions.
Alexopoulos[280] 2012 Greece 22789884	*Ticagrelor 90 mg, 2 x daily vs. prasugrel 10 mg/d* (crossover RCT) Total N = 44 (43 completed the study)	1 mo	No patient exhibited a major bleeding event at either treatment group. Two patients during the first period developed allergic reactions under ticagrelor, leading to study drug discontinuation in 1 of them, 4 patients (2 under prasugrel and 2 under ticagrelor) reported minimal bleeding events, 2 patients both under ticagrelor reported dyspepsia, and 4 patients (all under ticagrelor) reported a mild new-onset/worsening dyspnea.

247

Table 43. Key findings of studies with phenotypic test–based selection of patients reporting information on harms (continued)

Author Year Country PMID Study Name (if available)	Treatment Groups (sample size)	Followup Duration	Summary of Findings
Gremmel[281] 2012 Austria 21546102	*High-dose group:* 100 mg aspirin and 150 mg clopidogrel per day for 3 mo post-PCI (N=21) *Standard dose group:* aspirin 100 mg/d and clopidogrel 75 mg/d (N=23)	3 mo	No patient experienced a major bleeding event.
Alexopoulos[282] 2011 Greece 21985070	*Clopidogrel* 150 mg/d or *prasugrel* 10 mg/d (crossover RCT) Total N = 21	1 mo	One patient during the pre-crossover period and another one during the post-crossover period experienced a minor bleeding event, both while receiving prasugrel.
Alexopoulos[283] 2011 Greece 21982667	*Clopidogrel* 150 mg/d or *prasugrel* 10 mg/d (crossover RCT) Total N = 28	1 mo	2 patients discontinued the study drug during the post-crossover period, due to gastrointestinal and genitourinary bleeding, while receiving clopidogrel and prasugrel respectively.
Ari[216] 2012 Turkey EFFICIENT 21239075	*High-dose clopidogrel:* clopidogrel 150 mg/d for 1 mo + aspirin (100 mg/d) (N=47) *Standard-dose clopidogrel:* clopidogrel 75 mg/d for 1 mo + aspirin (100 mg/d) (N = 47)	6 mo	*TIMI major bleeding:* 1 event in the high-dose group vs. 0 in the standard-dose group; absolute risk difference = 2.1% (95% CI, 5.5 to 11.1); p=0.32 [reported results]; OR=3.07 (95% CI, 0.12 to 77.17); p=0.50 [calculated] *TIMI minor bleeding:* 3 events in the high-dose group vs. 1 in the standard-dose group; absolute risk difference = 4.3% (95% CI, –2.0 to 15.1); p=0.30 [reported results] ; OR=3.14 (95% CI, 0.31 to 31.30); p=0.33 [calculated]
Trenk[284] 2012 Multinational (North America and Europe) 22520250 TRIGGER-PCI	*Prasugrel + placebo:* prasugrel (60 mg) loading dose within 9 h after administration of the non-study-related clopidogrel maintenance dose (75 mg), followed by maintenance treatment of prasugrel 10 mg/d + placebo, starting the day after the loading dose of the study drug (N=212; 136 completed the study) *Clopidogrel + placebo:* placebo loading dose within 9 h after administration of the non-study-related clopidogrel maintenance dose (75 mg), followed by maintenance treatment of clopidogrel (75 mg) + placebo, starting the day after the loading dose of the study drug (N=211; 137 completed the study)	6 mo	*Non-CABG TIMI major bleeding:* 3 events in the prasugrel group vs. 1 events in the clopidogrel group; OR=3.03 (95% CI, 0.31 to 29.26); p=0.34 *Non-CABG TIMI fatal bleeding:* 0 events in the prasugrel group vs. 0 events in the clopidogrel group; OR and p-values not estimable *Non-CABG TIMI life-threatening bleeding:* 0 events in the prasugrel group vs. 1 events in the clopidogrel group; OR=0.33 (95% CI, 0.01 to 8.19); p=0.50 *Non-CABG TIMI major or minor bleeding:* 3 events in the prasugrel group vs. 2 events in the clopidogrel group; OR=1.51 (95% CI, 0.25 to 9.11); p=0.66 *Non-CABG TIMI major, minor, or minimal bleeding:* 6 events in the prasugrel group vs. 4 events in the clopidogrel group; OR=1.52 (95% CI, 0.42 to 5.45); p=0.53

248

Table 43. Key findings of studies with phenotypic test-based selection of patients reporting information on harms (continued)

Author Year Country PMID Study Name (if available)	Treatment Groups (sample size)	Followup Duration	Summary of Findings
Aradi[181] 2012 Hungary 21902692 DOSER	*High-dose clopidogrel:* clopidogrel maintenance 150 mg/d for 1 mo. After 28 days, all patients returned to 75 mg maintenance dose of clopidogrel until 1 year. (N=36) *Standard dose clopidogrel:* clopidogrel maintenance at a dose of 75 mg/d for 1 mo (N=38)	1 mo (for adverse events)	During the 4-week period, 1 TIMI major bleeding event occurred in the high-dose clopidogrel group vs. 0 events in the standard-dose group; OR=3.25 (95% CI, 0.13 to 82.50); p=0.47
Tang[247] 2012 China 22490487	*High dose dual antiplatelet therapy:* aspirin (200 mg/d) + clopidogrel (150 mg/d) (N=30) *Standard dual antiplatelet treatment:* aspirin 100 mg/d + clopidogrel (75 mg/d) (N=30)	12 mo	No patient had intracranial hemorrhage. The gastrointestinal hemorrhage rate in the standard dose group was 0% vs. 3.3% in the high-dose group.
Alexopoulos[285] 2011 Greece 21511219	*Prasugrel* 10 mg/d or *clopidogrel* 150 mg/d (crossover RCT) Total N=71	2 mo	During the pre-crossover period, 1 patient allocated to clopidogrel had TIMI major bleeding and was excluded from analysis. During the post-crossover period, 1 patient had TIMI major bleeding and 1 experienced a minor bleeding (both allocated to clopidogrel). 3 patients (allocated to prasugrel) experienced minor bleeding events.

Abbreviations: ACS = acute coronary syndrome; CABG = coronary artery bypass grafting; CI = confidence interval; CV = cardiovascular; d = day; GUSTO = Global Utilization of Streptokinase and Tissue Plasminogen Activator for Occluded Coronary Arteries; HR = hazard ratio; LTA = light-transmission aggregometry; MI = myocardial infarction; mo = month; OR = odds ratio; PCI = percutaneous coronary intervention; PRI = platelet reactivity index; RCT = randomized controlled trial; TIMI = Thrombolysis In Myocardial Infarction.

*Detailed results on the comparison of patients with high versus low platelet reactivity receiving standard dose clopidogrel (i.e., the nonrandomized comparison) has been summarized in the report's section on Key Question 2b.

†Outcome data were extracted only for patients with poor response to clopidogrel or clopidogrel and aspirin (i.e., we did not extract data on patients who were poor responders to aspirin alone).

249

Combined Testing for CYP2C19 Variants and Phenotypic Testing To Guide Antiplatelet Treatment

Of the four studies[287-290] providing information on phenotypic test-based treatment strategies that also provided information on the CYP2C19 genotype of participants, none reported data on treatment related harms stratified by treatment group and genotype status. As such, the interaction of genotype status and treatment could not be assessed.

Assessment of Risk of Bias of Individual Studies

All studies addressing Key Question 4 also addressed Key Question 3a. As such, detailed information on the 17 risk-of-bias items we assessed are not presented here, but rather, in the preceding section.

Harms of Testing Per Se

We found no studies reporting on the harms of the testing process for CYP2C19 genotyping or measuring platelet reactivity in the populations of interest. A review of the extensive literature on potential harms of prognostic or predictive testing in general (potential for discrimination, privacy concerns, or other ethical, legal, or social issues) was considered beyond the scope of this review. Regarding platelet reactivity testing, in many patients (e.g., those undergoing PCI), blood samples can be obtained as part of standard procedures (e.g., after placement of the arterial sheath). In such cases, obtaining samples for analysis would not be expected to cause additional harm.

One study[272] comparing VASP-guided therapy with standard clopidogrel dosing in the PCI setting noted that patients in the test-guided arm had a longer time from clopidogrel loading to PCI than patients in the non–test-guided treatment arm (means, 26 ± 3 hours vs. 65 ± 24 hours; $p<0.001$). The delay was due to the need for repeat testing and treatment modification until a predefined reactivity threshold was reached in the test-guided group. It is unclear whether this delay resulted in harm to patients.

Discussion

Antiplatelet therapy is used for a number of ischemic cardiovascular conditions. Clopidogrel is among the most commonly prescribed antiplatelet drugs. It is used extensively in the interventional management of coronary artery disease and the treatment and secondary prevention of acute coronary syndromes.[291] Furthermore, it is used for the management of patients undergoing neurointervention (with stent placement), for the prevention of stroke in patients with atrial fibrillation who are not candidates for vitamin K antagonist therapy, and for the management of selected patients with peripheral arterial disease. Response to clopidogrel therapy—as assessed by *ex vivo* studies of platelet function— is variable among patients and over time (within a patient). Some patients experience little suppression of platelet reactivity (despite being compliant to treatment) while others experience more profound suppression that may increase their risk of bleeding. Given the availability of several therapeutic options for antiplatelet treatment (e.g., increasing the loading or daily maintenance dose of clopidogrel or using adjunctive or replacement therapies such as prasugrel, ticagrelor, or cilostazol), there is interest in reliably identifying patients who are less likely to respond to standard clopidogrel treatment, as well as those who are most likely to respond to alternative treatments. This report reviewed the evidence of the effectiveness and comparative effectiveness of two types of tests that have been extensively evaluated as biomarkers for outcome prognosis for patients receiving clopidogrel therapy and as biomarkers of treatment response: genetic testing for CYP2C19 variants and phenotypic testing for on-clopidogrel platelet reactivity.

Key Findings and Assessment of the Strength of Evidence

Table 44 presents a summary of the report's key findings for each Key Question. When appropriate, results are presented separately for each of the populations and outcomes of interest. We did not assess the strength of evidence for evidence on analytic validity (because analytic validity is a prerequisite for the clinical use of the tests and because no framework exists for assessing the strength of evidence for analytic validity studies) or for studies exclusively assessing platelet reactivity as an outcome (because platelet reactivity measurements during followup are not usually performed as part of clinical care and because platelet reactivity is not a patient-relevant outcome). Instead, we focus here on the body of evidence pertaining to predictive effects, treatment decisionmaking, and harms as related to patient-relevant clinical outcomes. Please see the Methods section for a detailed discussion of our approach to rating the strength of evidence.

251

Table 44. Key findings from this review and assessment of strength of evidence

Key Question	Population	Test/Assay	Outcome	SOE Summary and Comments
1a: What it the analytic validity of tests for genotyping CYP2C19 variants?	NA	Genotyping for any CYP2C19 variant	NA	SOE = NA • Few studies provided information on analytic validity specifically using samples obtained from patient populations relevant to this review. • When available, data were limited to test–retest reliability or inter-assay agreement. • There was limited information comparing the validity of different genetic testing assays. • However, it is generally accepted that the analytic validity of genotyping assays is robust.
1b: What is the predictive value of genetic testing for CYP2C19 variants?	Ischemic heart disease	Genotyping for LOF CYP2C19 variants	Stent thrombosis	SOE = Moderate • Meta-analysis of 17 studies found a statistically significant association under a dominant model. • RR=1.52 (95% CI 1.17 to 1.97) • There was little evidence of heterogeneity (I^2=0%); but the test for small-study effects was statistically significant. • Results under additive and recessive models were consistent with a positive association and produced larger effect sizes; however, these analyses were based on a small subset of the available studies. • There was some concern about selective outcome reporting. • Studies reported few outcome events and the summary estimate was imprecise.
			MACE	SOE = Moderate • Meta-analysis of 25 studies found a statistically significant association under a dominant model. • RR=1.20 (95% CI 1.04 to 1.39). • There was some evidence of heterogeneity (I^2=31%). • Results under additive and recessive models were consistent with a positive association and produced larger effect sizes; however, these analyses were based on a small subset of the available studies. • The test for small study effects was statistically significant.
			Cardiovascular mortality	SOE = Low • Meta-analysis of 7 studies found a statistically significant association under a dominant model. • RR=1.98 (95% CI 1.13 to 3.46) • There was no evidence of heterogeneity (I^2=0%). The summary estimate was imprecise. • The test for small study effects was not statistically significant. There was some concern about selective outcome reporting.

252

Table 44. Key findings from this review and assessment of strength of evidence (continued)

Key Question	Population	Test/Assay	Outcome	SOE Summary and Comments
			All other clinical outcomes	SOE = Insufficient • Few studies reported information for noncomposite clinical outcomes other than stent thrombosis. • There was substantial concern about selective outcome reporting. • Study-specific and meta-analysis estimates (when performed) indicated substantial uncertainty.
		Genotyping for GOF CYP2C19 variants	MACE	SOE = Low • Meta-analysis of 7 studies found a statistically significant protective effect (for carriers vs. noncarriers). • RR=0.82 (95% CI 0.74 to 0.92) • There was substantial concern about selective outcome reporting.
			All other clinical outcomes	SOE = Insufficient • Few studies provided relevant information. • There was substantial concern about selective outcome reporting. • Study-specific and meta-analysis estimates (when performed) indicated substantial uncertainty.
	Other patient groups who are candidates for clopidogrel therapy	Genotyping for any CYP2C19 variants	All clinical outcomes	SOE = Insufficient • Only few (often a single) study was available for patient population other than those with ischemic heart disease; • Some of the studies did not report information on clinical outcomes.

253

Table 44. Key findings from this review and assessment of strength of evidence (continued)

Key Question	Population	Test/Assay	Outcome	SOE Summary and Comments
1c: What factors affect the predictive value of genetic testing for CYP2C19 variants?	All patient populations	Genotyping for any CYP2C19 variants	All clinical outcomes	SOE = Insufficient • 20 studies provided information on effect modification; a single study reported a statistically significant interaction effect on the prognostic performance of CYP2C19 variants for a clinical outcome. • No factor was assessed by more than 5 studies, giving rise to concerns about selective outcome reporting. • In meta-regression analyses (using study-level factors as covariates) we found some evidence of effect modification by ethnicity (East Asians vs. White populations) for MACE and stent thrombosis. However, this result is based on comparisons across studies (which may be confounded by other study characteristics) and was not corroborated by within-study analyses. Confidence intervals for all interaction effects were wide for all genotype–outcome pairs assessed and only few studies in East Asian populations were available. • Estimates of effect-modification by study-level variables are susceptible to confounding by other study-level characteristics
2a: What is the analytic validity of tests for on-clopidogrel platelet reactivity?	NA	All assays used to measure on-clopidogrel platelet reactivity	NA	SOE = NA • Few studies reported information on analytic sensitivity and specificity, possibly reflecting the research community's belief that there is no good reference standard assay for platelet reactivity. • Agreement ranged from poor to moderate and was variable between tests. • The highest agreement was observed between applications of the same assay with different concentrations of agonists, rather than between different assays.
2b: What is the predictive ability of phenotypic testing for platelet reactivity?	Ischemic heart disease	LTA	All-cause mortality	SOE = Low • 13 studies using heterogeneous methods to define increased reactivity were available. • These studies support an association between increased platelet reactivity measured by LTA and mortality. • There was some concern about selective outcome reporting.
			Cardiovascular mortality	SOE = Low • 9 studies using heterogeneous methods to define increased reactivity were available. • Studies provided evidence of an association between increased reactivity and cardiovascular mortality; however, clinical heterogeneity precluded firm conclusions. • There was some concern about selective outcome reporting.
			Acute coronary syndromes	SOE = Low • 18 studies using heterogeneous methods to define increased reactivity were available. • Studies often found statistically significant associations between increased reactivity as measured by LTA and clinical events; however, clinical heterogeneity did not allow for stronger conclusions.

254

Table 44. Key findings from this review and assessment of strength of evidence (continued)

Key Question	Population	Test/Assay	Outcome	Summary and Comments
				• There was some concern about selective outcome reporting.
			Stent thrombosis	SOE = Low • 19 studies using heterogeneous methods to define increased reactivity were available. • Studies often found statistically significant associations between increased reactivity as measured by LTA and clinical events; however, clinical heterogeneity did not allow for stronger conclusions. • There was some concern about selective outcome reporting.
			Stroke	SOE = Low (for lack of association) • 12 studies using heterogeneous methods to define increased reactivity were available. • Studies generally did not report statistically significant associations between increased reactivity as measured by LTA and clinical events; however, clinical heterogeneity did not allow for stronger conclusions or quantitative synthesis to increase precision.
			MACE	SOE = Low • 37 studies using heterogeneous methods to define increased reactivity were available. • The majority of reviewed studies suggested a statistically significant association between increased platelet reactivity measured by LTA and composite cardiovascular events. • Definitions of composite outcomes where often heterogeneous.
			All other clinical outcomes	SOE = Insufficient • Clinical and population heterogeneity or small number of studies limited our ability to draw conclusions.
		VerifyNow	All-cause mortality	SOE = Low (for lack of association) • 10 studies were available. Meta-analysis of 4 studies did not find an association between increased reactivity measured by VerifyNow and all-cause mortality. • RR=1.21 (95% CI 0.83 to 1.76) • The summary estimate was imprecise and 95% CI did not rule out clinically meaningful effects.
			Cardiovascular mortality	SOE = Moderate • 7 studies were available. Meta-analysis of 4 studies found a statistically significant association with little evidence of heterogeneity. • RR=2.50 (95% CI 1.28 to 4.87) • The CI of the summary estimate indicated substantial uncertainty. • There was some concern about selective outcome reporting.
			Acute coronary syndromes	SOE = Low • 19 studies using heterogeneous methods to define increased reactivity were available. • Studies generally suggested an association between increased reactivity as measured by VerifyNow and acute coronary syndromes, both periprocedurally and during longer followup.

255

Table 44. Key findings from this review and assessment of strength of evidence (continued)

Key Question	Population	Test/Assay	Outcome	SOE Summary and Comments
			Stent thrombosis	SOE = Low (for lack of association) • 15 studies were available. Meta-analysis of 6 studies did not find an association between reactivity measured by VerifyNow and stent thrombosis. • RR=1.67 (95% CI 0.80 to 3.47) • There was some evidence of heterogeneity (I^2=37%) and the CI of the summary estimate indicated substantial uncertainty. • Studies not included in the meta-analysis generally produced non-significant results. • There was some concern about selective outcome reporting. • The test for small-study effects was statistically significant.
			MACE	SOE = Moderate • 24 studies were available. Meta-analysis of 13 studies identified a statistically significant association. • RR=2.48 (95% CI 1.85 to 3.32) • There was moderate statistical heterogeneity (I^2=44 percent) and studies used fairly similar definitions of increased reactivity. • The test for small-study effects was statistically significant.
			Bleeding events (major and all levels of severity combined)	SOE = Low (for lack of association) • 13 studies were available. • Meta-analysis of 4 studies with data on any bleeding event did not find an association between increased reactivity measured by VerifyNow. • RR=1.09 (95% CI 0.88 to 1.36). There was little evidence of heterogeneity (I^2=0 percent). • Meta-analysis of 4 studies with data on major bleeding events did not find an association between increased reactivity measured by VerifyNow. • RR=0.85 (95% CI 0.32, 2.25). There was evidence of moderate heterogeneity (I^2=57 percent). • For major bleeding events the summary estimate was imprecise and the 95% CI did not rule out clinically meaningful effects.
			All other clinical outcomes	SOE = Insufficient • Clinical heterogeneity or small number of studies limited our ability to draw conclusions

Table 44. Key findings from this review and assessment of strength of evidence (continued)

Key Question	Population	Test/Assay	Outcome	SOE Summary and Comments
		VASP assay	Cardiovascular mortality	SOE = Insufficient • 6 studies were available. Meta-analysis of 4 studies did not identify a statistically significant association. • RR=2.42 (95% CI 0.86 to 6.82) • Although the test for heterogeneity was nonsignificant, point estimates from individual studies ranged from protective effects to strong harmful effects. • The meta-analytic summary point estimate was far from the null and its CI was wide (imprecise). • Clinically significant effects could not be ruled out.
			Acute coronary syndromes	SOE = Low (for lack of association) • 6 studies were available. Meta-analysis of 3 studies did not identify a statistically significant association. • RR=1.47 (95% CI 0.77 to 2.79) • The test for heterogeneity was non-significant but point estimates from individual studies were highly variable. • The meta-analytic summary point estimate was far from the null and its CI was wide (imprecise). • Clinically significant effects could not be ruled out.
			Stent thrombosis	SOE = Low • 10 studies were available. Meta-analysis of 4 studies identified a statistically significant association. • RR=3.37 (95% CI 1.59 to 7.11) • There was little evidence of statistical heterogeneity and the 4 studies used fairly similar definitions of increased reactivity. • The summary estimate was imprecise but the lower bound was consistent with a 59% increase in risk in the high-reactivity group. • There was some concern about selective outcome reporting.
			MACE	SOE = Low • 8 studies were available. Meta-analysis of 6 studies identified a statistically significant association. • RR=2.57 (95% CI 1.21 to 5.47) • There was evidence of statistical heterogeneity. • The summary estimate was imprecise but the lower bound was consistent with a 21% increase in risk in the high-reactivity group. • There was some concern about selective outcome reporting.
			All other clinical outcomes	SOE = Insufficient • Few studies reported information. • Clinical heterogeneity or small number of studies limited our ability to draw conclusions.
		PFA-100	MACE	SOE = Low

257

Table 44. Key findings from this review and assessment of strength of evidence (continued)

Key Question	Population	Test/Assay	Outcome	SOE Summary and Comments
				• 7 of the 9 studies on this assay reporting information on composite clinical outcomes produced statistically significant results indicating an association between increased reactivity and adverse outcomes.
				• Heterogeneity in the methods used to define increased reactivity precluded definitive conclusions; however, studies generally indicated an association between increase platelet reactivity as measured by the PFA-100 assay and composite clinical outcomes.
			All other clinical outcomes	SOE = Insufficient
				• Few of the available studies reported information on other outcomes.
				• There was concern about selective outcome reporting.
		All other assays	All clinical outcomes	SOE = Insufficient
				• Few studies were available.
				• When ≥2 studies were available for the same outcome they used heterogeneous metrics or thresholds to define increased reactivity or used different agonists for ex vivo stimulation of platelets.
	Other patient groups who are candidates for clopidogrel therapy	All assays used to measure on-clopidogrel platelet reactivity	All clinical outcomes	SOE = Insufficient
				• Only 6 studies, using diverse assays to measure reactivity, were available in clinically heterogeneous populations.
				• Studies were fairly small.

258

Table 44. Key findings from this review and assessment of strength of evidence (continued)

Key Question	Population	Test/Assay	Outcome	SOE Summary and Comments
2c: What factors affect the predictive value of phenotypic testing for platelet reactivity?	All patient populations	All assays used to measure on-clopidogrel platelet reactivity	All clinical outcomes	SOE = Insufficient • 7 studies provided information on effect modification; no factor was assessed by more than 3 studies. • Effect modification by study-level factors could not be assessed for most assay–outcome pairs; when such analysis was possible (for VerifyNow MACE), results indicated substantial uncertainty.
3a: What is the comparative effectiveness of alternative test-and-treat strategies	Ischemic heart disease	Genetic testing for CYP2C19 variants or phenotypic testing for platelet reactivity (all assays assessed)	All clinical outcomes	SOE = Insufficient • 1 RCT of testing vs. no testing was identified; the study had short duration and a small sample size; no events were observed in the two groups during the study period. • 3 studies provided information on treatment effect modification for clinical outcomes (and reported at least one outcome event) • 1 study randomized patients selected on the basis of genotype status into different clopidogrel doses; no conclusions could be drawn regarding clinical outcomes because of the short duration and small sample size of the study. • Studies compared different antiplatelet treatments and produced heterogeneous results. • Study-specific estimates were imprecise.
		Phenotypic testing for platelet reactivity	All clinical outcomes	SOE = Insufficient • The 6 RCTs of testing strategies were small, had different designs, and produced extreme results with considerable statistical uncertainty. • 1 NRCS was judged to be at high-risk of bias on the basis of study design (patients in each of the two compared arms were enrolled at different centers). • 3 studies of effect modification were identified; studies evaluated heterogeneous interventions and used different methods to assess reactivity. • Studies of test-based patient selection assessed different treatments, enrolled heterogeneous patient populations, and did not provide robust evidence on clinical outcomes.
	Atrial fibrillation	Genetic testing for CYP2C19 variants or phenotypic testing for platelet reactivity (all assays assessed)	All clinical outcomes	SOE = Insufficient • Only one study providing information on effect modification by CYP2C19 status was identified. • The study did not find evidence of effect modification by genotype status but there was considerable statistical uncertainty in the study estimates.

259

Table 44. Key findings from this review and assessment of strength of evidence (continued)

Key Question	Population	Test/Assay	Outcome	SOE Summary and Comments
		Phenotypic testing for platelet reactivity	All clinical outcomes	SOE = Insufficient • No studies were identified.
	Other patient populations	Genetic testing for CYP2C19 variants or phenotypic testing for platelet reactivity (all assays assessed)	All clinical outcomes	SOE = Insufficient • 1 study provided information on treatment effect modification in a mixed population of • patients with atherothrombotic disease (cardiovascular, cerebrovascular, or peripheral arterial) along with asymptomatic individuals at risk for atherothrombotic disease • The study did not provide robust evidence of effect modification.
		Phenotypic testing for platelet reactivity	All clinical outcomes	SOE = Insufficient • No studies were identified.

Table 44. Key findings from this review and assessment of strength of evidence (continued)

Key Question	Population	Test/Assay	Outcome	SOE Summary and Comments
3b: What factors modify the comparative effectiveness of alternative test-and-treat strategies?	All patient populations	Genetic testing for CYP2C19 variants or phenotypic testing for platelet reactivity (all assays assessed)	All clinical outcomes	SOE = Insufficient • 4 studies provided information on effect modification; each assessed different effect modifiers; no statistically significant interactions were reported.
4: What are the harms of testing? What are the harms of test-directed treatment?	All patient populations	Genetic testing for CYP2C19 variants	All clinical outcomes	SOE = Insufficient • 1 RCT of testing vs. no testing was identified; the study had short duration and a small sample size; few events were observed in the two groups during the study period. • 5 studies assessed treatment effect modification by genotype status (and reported at least one outcome event). • One study randomized patients selected on the basis of genotype status; it did not provide robust evidence regarding harms due to the relatively small sample size and short followup. • Studies compared different antiplatelet treatments and had heterogeneous results. • No studies provided direct information on the harms of testing per se.
		Phenotypic testing for platelet reactivity (all assays assessed)	All clinical outcomes	SOE = Insufficient • The 6 randomized studies of testing strategies were small, had different designs, and produced extreme results with considerable statistical uncertainty (and in some cases simply did not report any outcome events). • 1 NRCS was judged to be at high-risk of bias on the basis of study design (patients in each of the two compared arms were enrolled at different centers). • 2 studies of effect modification were identified; in one study safety outcomes either did not occur (regardless of reactivity status) or results were not stratified by reactivity group; the second study did not identify a significant effect but had short term followup and reported very few outcome events to allow any robust conclusions to be drawn. • Studies of test-based patient selection assessed different treatments.

Abbreviations: CI = confidence interval; GOF = gain-of-function; LOF = loss-of-function; MACE = major adverse cardiovascular events; NA = not applicable; RR = relative risk; SOE = strength of evidence.

261

Analytic Validity

Overall, we found limited evidence on the analytic validity of CYP2C19 genotyping assays in the populations of interest. However, the available studies reported almost perfect test–retest reliability and there is general consensus that genotyping methods have adequate analytic performance for clinical application (given the nature of genetic testing, we believe that supportive evidence can be drawn from the application of genetic tests to other patient populations and from the application of genotyping methods to other genes).

In contrast, numerous studies on the analytic validity of assays for measuring platelet reactivity in the populations of interest were available. Platelet reactivity can be affected by environmental exposures (e.g., drugs received by the patient) and patient characteristics (e.g., patients with diabetes have higher reactivity than nondiabetic individuals) and is variable within a person over time. Many of the studies we reviewed performed inappropriate analyses for comparing measurements obtained by reactivity assays, and often did not report information adequate to allow for a complete evaluation of their experimental design and analyses. In the subset of studies using appropriate designs and analyses to assess agreement or analytic performance, tests considered as "analytic gold standards" in some publications were considered as index tests (with measurement error that cannot be ignored) in other publications, indicating the lack of consensus on the optimal method for reactivity measurement. In the studies we reviewed, assays had low to moderate levels of interassay agreement. Agreement was generally higher between applications of the same assay across different concentrations of agonists (e.g., LTA with 5 μM ADP concentration vs. 20 μM) than between different assays. The Working Group on High On-Treatment Platelet Reactivity identified the lack of a universally accepted reference assay as a key reason for the limited implementation of platelet reactivity testing in clinical settings.[38]

Predictive Value of Genetic and Phenotypic Testing for Patients on Clopidogrel-Based Antiplatelet Therapy

Studies assessing the predictive value of CYP2C19 variants and platelet reactivity for patients receiving clopidogrel-based antiplatelet therapy represented the majority of the studies included in this report. It is interesting to compare our findings with previous systematic reviews and meta-analyses assessing CYP2C19 polymorphisms (Table 45) and those assessing assays for measuring platelet reactivity (Table 46).

Genetic Testing for CYP2C19 Variants

In our comparative effectiveness review, we have synthesized more publications than previous reviews, with generally similar findings. We found evidence supporting an association between loss-of-function CYP2C19 alleles and increased risk of stent thrombosis, cardiovascular death, and the composite of adverse cardiovascular outcomes, but not all-cause mortality. Furthermore, we found an association between gain-of-function alleles and reduced risk of MACE (composite). The strength of these findings is limited by concerns about selective reporting bias, because only a subset of the available studies contributed results to the polymorphism–outcome pairs of interest. Furthermore, studies reported on a relatively limited number of events, leading to substantial uncertainty in their effect-size estimates. In addition, data were reported almost exclusively under a dominant genetic model (carriers of at least one allele vs. noncarriers). Analyses under alternative genetic models (recessive and additive) were possible only for a minority of the included studies. Generally, results for the association of loss-of-function alleles with MACE and stent thrombosis under these alternative models were consistent with analyses under a dominant model and had larger effect sizes. The true underlying genetic model remains unknown; the reported data precluded further analyses to address this issue with regards to clinical outcomes. Further, studies did not genotype the same CYP2C19 alleles—for example, loss-of-function alleles other than *2 were not commonly genotyped. However, most loss-of-function variants other than *2 are relatively rare and as such we believe that any effect of exposure misclassification due to incomplete genotyping is likely to be limited. Finally, we found some evidence of statistically significant small-study effects for the two outcomes assessed by most studies (MACE and stent thrombosis). The interpretation of this result is complicated by the fact that statistically significant results of tests for small study effects can be explained by different reasons (selective publication, selective outcome reporting in published papers, real differences between smaller and larger studies, or chance).[62] Nonetheless, the presence of small study effects weakens our confidence in the summary estimates and is reflected, among other factors, in the strength of evidence.

Generally, regarding the prognostic effects of CYP2C19 genotype status, existing systematic reviews have reached similar conclusions to ours, both in magnitude and direction. Also consistent with our findings, previous analyses have suggested that selective outcome reporting and publication bias may have affected meta-analytic estimates.[20,41]

Table 45. Results of systematic reviews assessing the effect of CYP2C19 variants on clinical outcomes among patients receiving clopidogrel treatment

Author Year PMID	No. of Studies	Selection Criteria	Outcome [no. of studies/events]: Effect Size
Holmes[41] 2011 22203539	32	Articles reporting original data without language restriction	*Carriers of at least one CYP2C19 LOF allele vs. noncarriers* MACE [24 studies]: RR=1.18 (95% CI, 1.09 to 1.28) MI-fatal and nonfatal [9 studies]: RR=1.37 (95% CI, 1.13 to 1.65) MI-nonfatal [3 studies]: RR=1.48 (95% CI, 1.05 to 2.07) Stent thrombosis [14 studies]: RR=1.75 (95% CI, 1.50 to 2.03) Stroke-fatal and nonfatal [4 studies]: RR=1.98 (95% CI, 0.77 to 5.09) Bleeding-all [3 studies]: RR=0.84 (95% CI, 0.75, 0.94) Bleeding-severe [4 studies]: RR=1.07 (95% CI, 0.92 to 1.25)
Liu[292] 2011 21794898	20	Articles, conference abstracts and presentation slides; no language restriction	*Carriers of at least one CYP2C19 LOF allele vs. noncarriers* Stent thrombosis [18 studies]: OR=2.58 (95% CI, 1.77 to 3.77) MACE [18 studies]: OR=1.26 (95% CI, 1.06 to 1.50) *Carriers of at least one CYP2C19 GOF allele versus noncarriers* MACE [6 studies]: OR=0.82 (95% CI, 0.69 to 0.98)

Table 45. Results of systematic reviews assessing the effect of CYP2C19 variants on clinical outcomes among patients receiving clopidogrel treatment (continued)

Author Year PMID	No. of Studies	Selection Criteria	Outcome [no. of studies/events]: Effect Size
Bauer[20] 2011 21816733	15	Observational studies and clinical trials; no language restriction	*Carriers of at least one CYP2C19 LOF allele vs. noncarriers* MACE [12 studies]: OR=1.11 (95% CI, 0.89 to 1.39) Stent thrombosis [9 studies]: OR=1.77 (95% CI, 1.31 to 2.40) *Carriers of at least one CYP2C19 GOF allele vs. noncarriers* MACE [5 studies]: OR=0.93 (95% CI, 0.75 to 1.14) Stent thrombosis [3 studies]: OR=0.99 (95% CI, 0.60 to 1.62)
Zabalza[293] 2012 21693476	13	Case–control or prospective cohort; English language	*Carriers of at least one CYP2C19 LOF allele vs. noncarriers* MACE [11 studies]: HR=1.23 (95% CI, 0.97 to 1.55) ST [7 studies]: HR=2.24 (95% CI, 1.52 to 3.30) *Carriers of at least one CYP2C19 GOF allele vs. noncarriers* MACE [4 studies]: HR=0.75 (95% CI, 0.66 to 0.87) Major bleeding [4 studies]: HR=1.26 (95% CI, 1.05 to 1.50)
Hulot[40] 2010 20620727	10	Original epidemiological studies; no language restriction	MACE [10 studies, 1003 events]: OR=1.29 (95% CI, 1.12 to 1.49) Stent thrombosis [4 studies]: OR=3.45 (95% CI, 2.14 to 5.57) Mortality [5 studies]: OR=1.79 (95% CI, 1.10 to 2.91)
Mega[294] 2010 20978260	9	Prospective cohort studies or clopidogrel-treated arms from RCTs; summary data for meta-analysis were provided by the primary investigators	*Carriers of at least one CYP2C19 LOF allele vs. noncarriers* MACE [9 studies]: HR=1.57 (95% CI, 1.13 to 2.16) Stent thrombosis [6 studies]: HR=2.81 (95% CI, 1.81 to 4.37) Cardiovascular death [9 studies]: HR=1.84 (95% CI, 1.03 to 3.28) Nonfatal MI [9 studies]: HR=1.45 (95% CI, 1.09 to 1.92) Nonfatal stroke [9 studies]: HR=1.73 (95% CI, 0.68 to 4.38)
Jin[295] 2011 20845077	8	Prospective cohort studies; English language only	*Carriers of at least one CYP2C19 LOF allele vs. noncarriers* Adverse clinical events [8 studies]: OR=1.46 (95% CI, 1.01 to 2.13) Cardiac mortality [5 studies]: OR=2.07 (95% CI, 1.22 to 3.52) MI [5 studies]: OR=1.69 (95% CI, 1.09 to 2.61) ST [5 studies]: OR=3.81 (95% CI, 2.27 to 6.40)
Li[296] 2012 22123356	8	Randomized or cohort studies; no information on language reported	*Carriers of at least one CYP2C19 GOF allele vs. noncarriers* MACE [8 studies]: OR=0.86 (95% CI, 0.76 to 0.97) ST [4 studies]: OR=0.92 (95% CI, 0.51 to 1.75) Death [3 studies]: OR=1.23 (95% CI, 0.77, 1.95) Bleeding [4 studies in CAD]: OR=1.25 (195% CI,.07 to 1.47) Bleeding [6 studies, including non-CAP populations]: OR=1.20 (95% CI, 0.88 to 1.66)

Table 45. Results of systematic reviews assessing the effect of CYP2C19 variants on clinical outcomes among patients receiving clopidogrel treatment (continued)

Author Year PMID	No. of Studies	Selection Criteria	Outcome [no. of studies/events]: Effect Size
Sofi[297] 2011 20351750	7	Prospective studies; no language restriction	*Carriers of at least one CYP2C19 LOF allele vs. noncarriers* Cardiovascular events [7 studies]: RR=1.96 (95% CI, 1.14 to 3.37) ST [4 studies]: RR=3.82 (95% CI, 2.23 to 6.54)
Yamaguchi[298] 2012 22757746	7	Prospective observational studies or RCTs; English language only	*Carriers of at least one CYP2C19 *2 allele vs. noncarriers* All-cause death [7 studies]: OR 2.00 (95% CI, 1.22 to 3.27) MI [6 studies]: OR=3.07 (95% CI, 2.19 to 4.31) ST [6 studies]: OR=3.26 (95% CI, 1.63 to 6.51) Stroke [3 studies]: OR=1.99 (95% CI, 0.74 to 5.31)

Abbreviations: CI = confidence interval; CAD = coronary artery disease; GOF = gain-of-function; HR = hazard ratio; LOF = loss-of-function; MACE = major adverse cardiovascular events; MI = myocardial infarction OR = odds ratio; RCT = randomized controlled trial; RR = relative risk; ST = stent thrombosis.

Effect-size values higher than 1 indicate a detrimental effect (increased frequency of outcomes) among patients carrying the LOF allele. Not all studies reported all outcomes. Reviews are listed by number of included studies contributing to analyses of clinical outcomes, then chronologically. When available, meta-analysis results are from analyses using random effects models. For consistency, data are presented only from dominant genetic models.

Phenotypic Testing for Platelet Reactivity

A large number of studies assessed the prognostic value of various assays for measuring platelet reactivity, mostly in patients with ischemic heart disease. Studies used different assays, definitions, and cutoff values to define increased platelet reactivity. Cutoff values were often identified through analyses of receiver-operating-characteristic curves conducted on the same datasets used to assess the phenotypic test's predictive ability, suggesting that estimates of predictive performance (i.e., estimates of the prediction error) may be overly optimistic. Similar to the situation with genetic testing for CYP2C19 variants, only a subset of the studies evaluating each assay contributed data to each of the outcomes of interest, raising concerns about selective outcome reporting.

Compared to previous systematic reviews, our review includes a much larger number of studies and considers multiple assays assessing on-clopidogrel platelet reactivity using agonists to stimulate platelets ex vivo. In contrast to previous meta-analyses, our review does not combine results across different assays (i.e., across tests using different measurement principles), different agonist concentrations, or different calculation methods or cutoff values for defining high reactivity. We believe that this choice is supported by our review of analytic validity that found low-to-moderate agreement between different assays. We found statistically significant associations between platelet reactivity as measured by various assays (particularly LTA, VerifyNow P2Y12, and the VASP assay) and adverse cardiovascular outcomes. Of note, our analyses include almost double the number of studies included in a recently published meta-analysis of individual data on the VerifyNow assay.[299] Despite differences in selection criteria and analysis methods, our findings were similar, identifying a fairly strong association between platelet reactivity measured by this assay and ischemic events.

Table 46. Results of systematic reviews assessing the predictive ability of phenotypic testing on clinical outcomes among patients receiving clopidogrel treatment

Author Year PMID	No. of Studies	Selection Criteria	Outcome [no. of studies/events]: Effect Size (95% CI)
Snoep[300] 2007 17643570	25	Prospective cohort or case–control studies, and RCTs; no language restriction	*Clopidogrel resistance vs. nonresistance* MACE [9 studies] OR=8.0 (95% CI, 3.36 to 19.05) Subacute ST [3 studies] OR=7.02 (95% CI, 0.63 to 79.01) Composite endpoint of clinical ischemic events [4 studies]: OR=12.02 (95% CI, 5.91 to 24.42) Myonecrosis (elevated CK-MB levels) [1 study]: OR=2.20 (95% CI, 0.93 to 5.22)
Aradi[301] 2010 20826265	20	Observational studies; no language restriction	*High vs. normal on-clopidogrel platelet reactivity* Nonfatal MI [11 studies]: OR=3.00 (95% CI, 2.26 to 3.99) ST [11 studies]: OR=4.14 (95% CI, 2.74 to 6.25) Composite ischemic events [17 studies]: OR=4.95 (95% CI, 3.34 to 7.34) CV death [11 studies]: OR=3.35 (95% CI, 2.39 to 4.70)
Combescure[302] 2010 20156305	15	Prospective cohort or RCTs; no language restriction	*Clopidogrel nonresponder vs. responder* Recurrent ischemic events [15 studies]: RR=3.53 (95% CI, 2.39 to 5.20) *ADP cutoff >65% for clopidogrel nonresponse* Recurrent ischemic events [3 studies]: RR=5.8 (95% CI, 3.2 to 10.3) *ADP lower cutoff for clopidogrel nonresponse* Recurrent ischemic events [7 studies]: RR=2.9 (95% CI, 2.2 to 3.7)
Sofi[303] 2010 20135063	14	Prospective cohort studies; no language restriction	*Clopidogrel responder vs. nonresponder* MACE [14 studies]: OR=5.67 (95% CI, 2.97 to 10.84)
Yamaguchi[298] 2012 22757746	8	Prospective observational studies or RCTs; English language only	*High on-treatment platelet reactivity vs. normal on-treatment platelet reactivity* MACE [8 studies]: OR=3.03 (95% CI, 2.32 to 3.96) All-cause death [5 studies]: OR=1.11 (95% CI, 0.70 to 1.77) MI [3 studies]: OR=1.37 (95% CI, 0.67 to 2.77) ST [5 studies]: OR=2.65 (95% CI, 1.46 to 4.84)
Brar[299] 2011 22032704	6	Individual patient data meta-analysis of studies of the VerifyNow P2Y12 assay; no language restriction	*PRU ≥230 vs. <230* Composite primary endpoint [6 studies]: HR=2.10 (95% CI, 1.62 to 2.73) Death [6 studies]: HR=1.66 (95% CI, 1.03 to 2.68) MI [6 studies]: HR=2.04 (95% CI, 1.51 to 2.76) Stent thrombosis [6 studies]: HR=3.11 (95% CI, 1.50 to 6.46)

Abbreviations: CI = confidence interval; CK-MB = creatine kinase (MB fraction); HR = hazard ratio; MACE = major adverse cardiovascular events; MI = myocardial infarction; OR = odds ratio; PRU = platelet reactivity unit; RCT = randomized controlled trial; RR = relative risk; ST = stent thrombosis.

Effect size values higher than 1 indicate a detrimental effect (increased frequency of outcomes) among patients with increased on-clopidogrel platelet reactivity. Not all studies reported all outcomes. Reviews are listed by the number of included studies. When available, meta-analysis results are from analyses using random effects models.

Comparisons Between Alternative Phenotypic Tests and Between Genetic and Phenotypic Testing

We found that directly comparative studies of test performance (defined as studies assessing the prognostic value of two or more tests on the same patient population) were generally rare and almost universally did not perform analyses (or report data) to inform about the relative predictive ability of tests. A qualitative comparison of point estimates and CIs from the available studies suggested that the tests assessed had comparable predictive performance. However, confidence intervals were wide and overlapping, precluding any definitive conclusion. Our findings regarding the comparison of genetic testing for CYP2C19 variants and phenotypic testing for platelet reactivity were similarly inconclusive.

Use of Testing To Guide Treatment Decisionmaking

To our knowledge, this is the first review to comprehensively evaluate the use of genetic and phenotypic testing for guiding antiplatelet therapy with a focus on patient-relevant benefits and harms. Only a small subset of the reviewed studies directly tested the link between test-based therapy and outcomes. Ideally, directly comparative studies of test-guided treatment versus no testing (or alternative testing strategies) would be used to inform clinical decisions on the benefits and harms of testing. However, because such studies are rarely available, we also considered studies of effect modification based on RCTs of non–test based treatments as well as RCTs of non–test-based therapies using the tests of interest to select "nonresponsive" patients (e.g., patients with high on-clopidogrel reactivity at baseline).

Genetic Testing for CYP2C19 Variants

The single directly comparative study of testing versus no-testing for *2 alleles did not provide information regarding clinical outcomes and had short followup. We also reviewed several studies assessing effect modification by CYP2C19 variants; of these, 5 were based on large RCTs comparing antiplatelet treatments within patient groups defined by CYP2C19 genotype. To our knowledge, only one previously published review evaluated such studies of effect modification by CYP2C19 variants and quantitatively synthesized relevant data from large randomized trials. The authors concluded that there is "no clinically significant interaction of CYP2C19 genotype with the association of clopidogrel therapy and cardiovascular events."[41] On the basis of population and treatment heterogeneity, we refrained from quantitatively synthesizing studies of effect modification. Given that the drugs compared have different mechanisms of action, it is plausible that that the true interaction effects (treatment × CYP2C19 genotype) being estimated in the studies may have different magnitudes or directions. However, none of the four studies provided strong evidence that the CYP2C19 genotype modifies the effectiveness of clopidogrel therapy. Despite the studies having included several thousand randomized participants, CIs for relative treatment effects (by genotype status) were fairly wide (with the exception of the CI for the PLATO study) and we could not rule out clinically meaningful differences with regard to relative treatment effectiveness.

Currently, the United States FDA-approved label for clopidogrel[j] states that poor metabolizers (as identified by CYP2C19 genotype) treated with clopidogrel "exhibit higher cardiovascular event rates following myocardial infarction than do patients with normal CYP2C19 function." The label also states that CYP2C19 genotyping "can be used as an aid in determining therapeutic strategy", and that alternative treatment strategies should be considered "in patients identified as CYP2C19 poor metabolizers." Our review of observational (mostly cohort) studies identified evidence to support the association between loss-of-function CYP2C19 variants and increased rates of some cardiovascular events. At the same time, there was

---

[j]Available at http://products.sanofi.us/PLAVIX/PLAVIX.html; last accessed May 10, 2012.

insufficient evidence of antiplatelet treatment effect modification by genotype status. However, the studies investigating treatment effect modification were not specifically designed to assess treatment-genotype interactions, did not have adequate statistical power to detect such effects, and may have been susceptible to selection or survivor bias that could explain the null effects.

Phenotypic Testing for Platelet Reactivity

Regarding phenotypic testing for platelet reactivity, we identified a small number of comparative studies (6 RCTs and 1 NRCS) evaluating alternative test-and-treatment strategies. The studies were generally small and produced extreme results (with very wide CIs) for all clinical outcomes reported (both benefits and harms). Furthermore, studies had heterogeneous designs (e.g., they differed in the number of measurements performed for monitoring and in the treatment modifications applied for nonresponding patients) and relatively short followup periods (all less than 1 year). In addition, we identified only three studies evaluating different treatments that also provided information on effect modification by baseline platelet reactivity. These studies did not provide compelling evidence of effect modification by baseline platelet reactivity. Finally, although we identified a number of studies selecting patients on the basis of high baseline platelet reactivity and then randomizing them into non–test based comparator groups, these studies are informative about the value of testing to guide treatment selection only if it is assumed that the randomized treatments have the same effect (or at least a relative effect known with certainty) in patients with low baseline platelet reactivity. Overall, we believe there is insufficient evidence to support (or refute) the use of use of phenotypic testing for platelet reactivity to guide antiplatelet treatment selection. Our findings do support current clinical practice guidelines, which in general do not advocate the use of phenotypic testing for platelet reactivity for guiding choice of treatment.

Modifiers of the Impact of Test Results

We found limited evidence that patient-level characteristics, disease features, cointerventions (including PPIs), or system-level factors impact the predictive effect of genetic or phenotypic tests of interest. No modifier was assessed in more than a few studies for any test–outcome pair of interest to this review. Even when considering information across studies (meta-regression) we did not identify convincing evidence that study-level characteristic modify the prognostic effect of genetic testing (meta-regression analyses were undertaken for CYP2C19 variants only, owing to the small number of available studies for other outcomes). Nonetheless, these analyses provided some indication that the association between loss-of-function alleles with MACE and stent thrombosis is modified by ethnicity, with East Asians experiencing a stronger harmful effect. This is particularly interesting given the reported higher frequency of loss-of-function alleles in East Asian populations. These findings should be investigated further to ensure that this is a true effect and not due to the small number of studies in East Asian populations of confounding by other study-level factors

Harms of Testing and Test-Directed Treatment

Direct evidence on the harms of test-directed treatment was reported by a limited number of comparative studies. Although the studies did not raise concerns about an increased rate of harms, they were generally small and had followup periods too short to permit conclusions. We found no evidence on harms of testing per se, possibly reflecting the fact that testing procedures, both for genetic and phenotypic testing, are associated with minimal physical harm (e.g., minor complications of phlebotomy to obtain blood samples). Other potential harms of testing—unnecessary exposure to higher-risk treatment or ethical and social issues, such as discrimination on the basis of genetic information and the possibility that the prognostic value of genetic information may be overestimated by patients[304]—were not considered in the studies we reviewed.

Applicability

The vast majority of included studies enrolled patients with ischemic heart disease (acute or chronic coronary disease represented almost all available studies for all Key Questions). Other populations who are potential candidates for antiplatelet therapy (e.g., patients with cerebrovascular disease, peripheral arterial disease, or atrial fibrillation) were included in a minority of studies only. This imbalance is not unexpected, given that clopidogrel's primary indications pertain to ischemic heart disease. However, it is probably not prudent to extrapolate findings from studies of ischemic heart disease to other patient populations. Given that a large number of studies included patients undergoing PCI, applicability may also be limited in noninterventional settings.

Particularly for genetic testing for CYP2C19 variants, patient race or ethnicity may be an important effect modifier, because the prevalence of variant alleles is substantially different among racial and ethnic groups (e.g., *2 variants are much more common in East Asian populations than others). We found limited evidence that prognostic effects were different in subgroup and meta-regression analysis by ethnicity (East Asian versus white); more evidence is needed for patient populations underrepresented in this review (e.g., blacks) and to validate our findings.

The majority of studies were conducted in tertiary (usually academic) medical centers. Studies of treatment-effect modification by CYP2C19 genotype were based on large randomized trials, and findings may not be generalizable to everyday care settings. Because patient information on preexisting vascular disease in studies of predictive effects was generally incompletely reported, it is unclear whether patients in the included studies are representative of those seen in clinical practice. Nonetheless, the distribution of risk factors for ischemic vascular disease (male sex, hyperlipidemia, diabetes, hypertension, smoking, etc.) appeared to be representative of contemporary patient populations, and the majority of studies were conducted in recent years.

Implications for Clinical and Policy Decisionmaking

Despite the large literature on the use of genetic testing of CYP2C19 variants and phenotypic testing of platelet reactivity for predicting outcomes in patients receiving clopidogrel-based therapy, studies provided limited information on the value added by these tests over ascertainment of conventional risk factors in the populations of interest (e.g., clinical or laboratory information or disease-specific predictive scores). Furthermore, there was little comparative evidence that could be used to identify the most informative test or combination of tests for predicting clinical outcomes. This and other limitations of the existing literature may reduce the potential for clinical application of the tests reviewed herein as prognostic markers for patients on clopidogrel-based antiplatelet therapy. The available evidence was even more limited regarding the use of either type of testing to guide the choice of antiplatelet therapy.

Additional research seems warranted for both genetic and phenotypic tests. Genetic testing methods appear to be fairly standardized and reliable so new research can focus on clinical outcomes. In contrast, phenotypic testing with platelet reactivity can be done using a number of different assays and principles of measurement. Identifying the optimal assay, agonist concentration, and reactivity cutoff values for predicting clinical events is a significant challenge for future research. This challenge needs to be addressed in order to prioritize which reactivity assays should be evaluated as methods for guiding treatment choice.

Limitations of the Evidence

On the basis of the large number of reviewed studies, we believe that the evidence regarding genetic testing for CYP2C19 variants and phenotypic testing for platelet reactivity (for guiding antiplatelet treatment and predicting outcomes in patients who receive it) is limited in the following ways:

- Despite the large number of available studies providing information on analytic validity, *most studies used inappropriate statistical methods to assess inter-assay agreement*. Few studies accounted for the lack of a perfect reference standard test (no "gold" standard) and the statistical analyses used where often inappropriate for assessing agreement.

- *Lack of comparative studies of alternative testing strategies evaluating the relative predictive ability of the tests of interest*. No studies reported valid direct comparisons between the tests of interest in terms of prognostic performance; studies either assessed a single test or simply provided information on test performance separately for each test applied to the study population.

- *Lack of separation of development ("training") and assessment ("test") samples when developing prognostic markers*. Many studies of phenotypic tests used receiver-operating-characteristic methods to define an "optimal" cutoff value of reactivity (typically, one that maximized the sum of sensitivity and specificity), without using any methods to limit overfitting.[305] In most cases these cutoffs were then applied to the same population sample that was used to derive them, in order to calculate predictive performance. This approach leads to overly optimistic estimates of test performance (i.e., inflated sensitivity and specificity) that are unlikely to generalize to the target population.[306]

- *Selective outcome reporting was a concern for the association between test results and several clinical outcomes*. Most studies reported information on composite clinical outcomes but often did not provide results for the component clinical events.

- *Uncertainty about the genetic model for CYP2C19 variants*. Poor reporting of primary study results precluded the assessment of alternative genetic models (i.e., results were often reported only for collapsed genotype categories).

- *Heterogeneity in exposure definitions and uncertainty about the underlying genetic model for CYP2C19 variants*. Our ability to synthesize findings across studies was limited by the use of heterogeneous methods to define exposure status. This was particularly true for studies of platelet reactivity assays because of the large variability in measurement methods (existence of multiple assays) and in cutoff values for defining positive results (among studies using the same assay). Heterogeneity of exposure definitions was also present in studies of CYP2C19 variants, because studies genotyped different subsets of known CYP2C19 alleles (e.g., loss-of-function alleles other than *2 were not commonly genotyped). Furthermore, with few exceptions, data were reported in a way that only allowed for analyses under a dominant genetic model (carriers vs. noncarriers), which may not be the true genetic model.

- *Paucity of studies evaluating the impact of test-guided treatment selection on the basis of the tests of interest.* The literature we reviewed included few studies directly comparing alternative testing strategies or assessing effect modification by test results. Available studies were small, had short followup periods, or did not report information on clinical outcomes. The five large studies reporting information on treatment effect modification by CYP2C19 status based on RCTs of antiplatelet regimens were conducted in heterogeneous populations, compared different treatment regimens, and had several design limitations. No studies used quantitative methods to assess the intermediate outcomes of impact of testing on predictive probabilities or treatment decisions.
- *The number of studies providing information on treatment effect modification by CYP2C19 genotype status or baseline on-clopidogrel platelet reactivity was limited.* Investigations based on completed randomized trials (repurposed RCTs) were not powered to detect treatment effect modification and were susceptible to selection bias because included patients represented only a minority of the populations included in the parent trials.

Ongoing Research

A search on May 3, 2012, in the ClinicalTrials.gov registry identified 173 potentially relevant records. After full text review, 28 records of studies that can be expected to provide information relevant to Key Questions 3 and 4 of this report were identified. Appendix G summarizes information from these studies. None of these studies provided results in the ClinicalTrials.gov database at the time of this search.

Evidence Gaps

Table 47 summarizes the evidence gaps with regards to the five Key Questions of this systematic review.

Table 47. Evidence gaps

Key Question	Category	Evidence Gap
1. Analytic validity and predictive value of genetic testing for CYP2C19 variants	Population	• The analytic validity of alternative assays for measuring platelet reactivity has not been established. • Studies of the prognostic value of CYP2C19 variants were almost exclusively limited to patients with ischemic heart disease. Additional evidence is needed on the predictive value of tests in other patient populations who are candidates for antiplatelet therapy.
	Intervention and exposure definition	• Additional studies comprehensively genotyping CYP2C19 variants (i.e., genotyping all variants prevalent in the population of interest) and reporting on long-term clinical outcomes are needed. • Combinations of types of tests (e.g., genetic and phenotypic testing) or combinations of genetic tests were rarely assessed. • Research to identify the most likely genetic model for CYP2C19 variants is needed. Approaches combining clinical data along with pharmacodynamic and pharmacogenetic information would probably be most informative.
	Comparator	• No studies reported valid direct comparisons of the prognostic value of different tests (e.g., comparisons between genetic vs. phenotypic testing, or among alternative phenotypic tests) were available.
	Outcome	• Many studies assessed platelet reactivity exclusively and clinical outcomes were often reported only as composites. More data on individual clinical outcomes is needed.
2. Analytic validity and predictive value of phenotypic testing for platelet reactivity	Population	• Evidence on the analytic validity and predictive value for populations other than those with ischemic heart disease was limited.
	Intervention and exposure definition	• No single assay for measuring platelet reactivity can be considered a "gold standard" test. • Combinations of tests (e.g., genetic and phenotypic testing) or combinations of genetic tests were rarely assessed.
	Comparator	• No studies reporting valid direct comparisons the predictive value of different tests were available.
	Outcome	• Studies reporting clinical outcomes often reported only composite outcomes (without providing information on the component outcomes separately).
3. Use of testing to guide treatment choice	General evidence gap	• Directly comparative studies of alternative test strategies using phenotypic tests were few and had short followup durations and heterogeneous designs. • A single randomized study with short followup compared genetic testing for CYP2C19 variants versus no testing. • Studies of effect modification were few, pertained to heterogeneous populations, reported information on intermediate outcomes only, or compared different antiplatelet treatments. These studies were based on well-conducted randomized efficacy trials but were not specifically designed to detect effect modification and may have been susceptible to selection (survivor) bias.
4. Harms of testing or test-directed treatment	General evidence gap	• Few studies provided direct comparative information on the impact of alternative test-and-treat strategies on patient safety. • No studies on the harms of testing per se were identified. • More evidence is needed regarding monitoring strategies that involve repeat testing that may lead to delays in invasive interventional procedures.

Future Research

This review has identified substantial gaps in the literature on genetic testing for CYP2C19 variants and phenotypic testing for platelet reactivity, both as biomarkers of future outcomes among patients who are receiving clopidogrel therapy and—more importantly—as tests for guiding treatment selection for patients who are candidates for antiplatelet treatment. We believe that the following evidence gaps may represent fruitful areas for future research (i.e., that they represent areas in need of future research):

- *Analytic validity of phenotypic testing:* Future studies using rigorous methods to inform the analytic validity of tests for measuring platelet reactivity are needed, particularly with regard to test–retest reliability, interassay agreement, and analytic performance. Ideally studies should evaluate multiple assays applied to the same samples, enroll a large number of patients, and be conducted in a multilaboratory setting. The existing genotypic assays are considered robust; however, studies of CYP2C19 assays should report details of their genotyping quality control methods.[307]

- *Prognostic accuracy, with a focus on comparative prognostic performance:* Although we identified several studies reporting on the prognostic value of the tests of interest, studies had several limitations in their design and analysis methods (see the Limitations of the Evidence Base section above). Thus, large-scale prospective studies of the tests of interest are needed to derive reliable estimates of prognostic performance. Because the major source of costs for conducting such studies stems from the need to follow up with large numbers of individuals over time, it may be worthwhile to perform measurements of on-clopidogrel platelet reactivity at baseline using multiple assays as well as obtain genetic material for genotyping CYP2C19 variants or other emerging genetic biomarkers. Such a design would provide information on multiple tests simultaneously; for conducting informative direct comparisons between assays, however, such studies would have to be large. This is because the results of different reactivity assays are correlated (although interassay agreement is not perfect, correlations higher than 0.5 were common in the reviewed studies). Studies of CYP2C19 variants need to assess all polymorphisms with adequate prevalence in the populations of interest; considerations should also be given to genotyping other genes involved in clopidogrel metabolism (e.g., ABCB1 or PON1) and the assessment of gene–gene interactions. Studies will need to predefine cutoff values and genotype groupings and compare the classification performance of individual tests, as well as the reclassification performance of each assay compared to established clinical risk scores or results of other assays.[308-313] Complete data for all outcomes assessed should be reported.

- *Direct comparisons of methods for test-guided treatment selection:* Even if the prognostic value of tests were established, this information is often inadequate as a basis for treatment decisionmaking. Once the prognostic performance of the tests of interest is established, the most promising tests could be prioritized for assessment in directly comparative studies of testing versus no testing. Such studies can provide unconfounded estimates of the relative benefits and harms of the compared strategies. However, randomized comparisons of alternative testing strategies are costly and time consuming. Furthermore, recruitment may be challenging or impossible if one of the treatment groups is standard clopidogrel-based therapy, in view of the current FDA-approved labeling and recent results from studies using pharmacodynamic endpoints. Still, such designs may be appropriate when comparing antiplatelet therapies other than standard clopidogrel dosing (including high-dose clopidogrel treatment). For example, one design that may be particularly appealing for the tests of interest to this review is the use of a test in all patients who are candidates for antiplatelet treatment, followed by randomization of only test-"positive patients to receive one of several different treatments. This design can provide information on the relative harms and benefits of a treatment among patients whose treatment would be expected to change on the basis of test results. A third comparator arm of standard treatment in the test-negative patients can be included as an additional (nonrandomized) "control" group (such an approach was taken by the randomized GRAVITAS trial, and some smaller studies, considered under Key Questions 2 and 3 of this report). A more detailed discussion of efficient biomarker study designs and the conditions under which they can lead to increases in statistical power are out of the scope of this report but have been discussed extensively elsewhere (e.g., Scher et al. 2011,[314] Simon 2010[315]). When experimental studies are not considered logistically or ethically feasible, observational data may be useful, especially given that CYP2C19 testing is not universally implemented.

- *"Repurposing" completed randomized trials to assess effect modification:* An alternative to direct comparative studies of testing strategies is to assess effect modification by genotype status by repurposing already completed randomized trials, in which the drugs of interest were tested against a suitable comparator, by genotyping samples from enrollees. Results of genetic analyses can be associated with the prospectively recorded clinical outcomes.[48,49] Although this approach did not provide definitive answers in this review due to limitations of the existing studies, future repurposed trials could yield more informative results if they are properly planned. Such planning must include a strategy for obtaining samples from all participants (or a random sample thereof), acquiring specimens prior to treatment, and using appropriate methods to control for multiple testing. When randomized trials are not available for repurposing, a similar approach can be implemented in the setting of registries linking DNA information to electronic health records. Patients receiving different antiplatelet therapies in whom the choice of treatment has not been based on CYP2C19 status, but for whom material for genotyping is available, are candidates for such research.

- *Monitoring of platelet reactivity to guide treatment:* Strategies of monitoring platelet reactivity can be conceptualized as "dynamic treatment regimes"[316-318] (i.e., rules for sequential decisionmaking based on the evolution of reactivity measurements over time; obviously such methods are not applicable to CYP2C19 testing). Such approaches formalize the process of choosing between competing monitoring strategies, based on expected responses to treatment and related intermediate and long-term outcomes, using appropriate statistical models. Compared to standard research methods (e.g., directly comparing two monitoring strategies in a parallel-group study), dynamic treatment modeling may be better at identifying the optimal monitoring regime while accounting for multiple monitoring visits and the fact that treatment decisions at each visit are determined by the measurements (e.g., platelet reactivity, other laboratory measurements, etc.) obtained in previous visits. Indeed, statistical methods exist that can use observational or randomized study data to determine the factors that should be considered as triggers for intervention, as well as the optimal cutoff values of these factors. These approaches may increase the efficiency of future research because it is impossible to conduct randomized trials comparing all alternative test-and-treat strategies for different assays, thresholds of reactivity, and alternative therapeutic interventions.

Conclusions

In summary, we found limited evidence on the analytic validity of genetic testing for platelet reactivity. However, using evidence from other populations and genetic variants, we believe that the available assays for CYP2C19 genotyping have adequate technical test performance. In contrast, we found a large body of evidence on the analytic validity of assays for measuring platelet reactivity, suggesting that interassay agreement is only poor to moderate. No phenotypic assays can be considered a "gold standard" test.

We found some evidence supporting a significant association between loss-of-function CYP2C19 variants and increased risk of stent thrombosis, cardiovascular mortality, and MACE. We also found a significant association between gain-of-function alleles and reduced risk of MACE. The interpretation of these associations should be cautious, given the potential for selective reporting and small-study effects to have affected study results. Furthermore, the applicability of findings to patient populations other than those with ischemic coronary artery disease (particularly those undergoing revascularization procedures) was limited. We also found evidence supporting an association between high on-clopidogrel platelet reactivity as measured by various assays (particularly LTA, VerifyNow P2Y12, and the VASP assay) and adverse cardiovascular events. Our confidence in these findings is limited by the relatively small number of studies available for each test–outcome combination, the potential for selective outcome reporting, and the common lack of separation between the populations used to derive test thresholds of optimal predictive value and those used to assess predictive value at these thresholds.

The evidence on the use of testing to guide treatment choice was insufficient. A single randomized trial of CYP2C19 testing versus no-testing provided limited evidence on clinical outcomes. Sub-analyses of five well done randomized controlled trials generally did not find strong evidence of effect modification by CYP2C19 status; however, concern for selection bias and the heterogeneity of patient populations and treatments rendered the evidence inconclusive. Similarly, the short follow-up periods and low numbers of outcome events in trials of platelet reactivity-guided treatment versus standard antiplatelet therapy did not offer a firm base for conclusions. No studies comparing alternative testing strategies were identified.

Additional research is needed to better establish the prognostic value and clinical utility for treatment decisionmaking, both for genetic testing for CYP2C19 variants and phenotypic testing for platelet reactivity, focusing on standardizing testing methods and assessing the relative impact of testing strategies on patient-relevant clinical outcomes in large, well-conducted clinical trials.

References

1. Kamath S, Blann AD, Lip GYH. Platelets and atrial fibrillation. European Heart Journal 2001 Dec 1;22(24):2233-42.

2. Writing Group, Roger VrL, Go AS, et al. Executive Summary: Heart Disease and Stroke Statistics 2012 Update. Circulation 2012 Jan 3;125(1):188-97.

3. Keenan NL, Shaw KM. Coronary heart disease and stroke deaths - United States, 2006. MMWR Surveill Summ 2011 Jan 14;60 Suppl:62-66.

4. Squizzato A, Keller T, Romualdi E, et al. Clopidogrel plus aspirin versus aspirin alone for preventing cardiovascular disease. Cochrane Database Syst Rev 2011 Jan(1):CD005158.

5. Writing Committee, Levine GN, Bates ER, et al. 2011 ACCF/AHA/SCAI Guideline for Percutaneous Coronary Intervention. Circulation 2011 Dec 6;124(23):e574-e651.

6. Bowry AD, Brookhart MA, Choudhry NK. Meta-analysis of the efficacy and safety of clopidogrel plus aspirin as compared to antiplatelet monotherapy for the prevention of vascular events. Am J Cardiol 2008 Apr 1;101(7):960-66.

7. Sabatine MS, Hamdalla HN, Mehta SR, et al. Efficacy and safety of clopidogrel pretreatment before percutaneous coronary intervention with and without glycoprotein IIb/IIIa inhibitor use. Am Heart J 2008 May;155(5):910-17.

8. Sudlow CL, Mason G, Maurice JB, et al. Thienopyridine derivatives versus aspirin for preventing stroke and other serious vascular events in high vascular risk patients. Cochrane Database Syst Rev 2009 Oct 7(4):CD001246.

9. Collaborative meta-analysis of randomised trials of antiplatelet therapy for prevention of death, myocardial infarction, and stroke in high risk patients. 2002.

10. Effect of Clopidogrel Added to Aspirin in Patients with Atrial Fibrillation. N Engl J Med 2009 May 14;360(20):2066-78. PMID: doi: 10.1056/NEJMoa0901301.

11. Bellemain-Appaix A, Brieger D, Beygui F, et al. New P2Y12 Inhibitors Versus Clopidogrel in Percutaneous Coronary Intervention: A Meta-Analysis. Journal of the American College of Cardiology 2010 Nov 2;56(19):1542-51. PMID: doi: 10.1016/j.jacc.2010.07.012.

12. Wallentin L, Becker RC, Budaj A, et al. Ticagrelor versus clopidogrel in patients with acute coronary syndromes. N Engl J Med 2009 Sep 10;361(11):1045-57.

13. Wiviott SD, Braunwald E, McCabe CH, et al. Prasugrel versus clopidogrel in patients with acute coronary syndromes. N Engl J Med 2007 Nov 15;357(20):2001-15.

14. Navarese EP, Verdoia M, Schaffer A, et al. Ischaemic and bleeding complications with new, compared to standard, ADP-antagonist regimens in acute coronary syndromes: a meta-analysis of randomized trials. QJM 2011 Jul 1;104(7):561-69.

15. Geiger J, Brich J, Honig-Liedl P, et al. Specific impairment of human platelet P2Y(AC) ADP receptor-mediated signaling by the antiplatelet drug clopidogrel. Arterioscler Thromb Vasc Biol 1999 Aug;19(8):2007-11.

16. Kazui M, Nishiya Y, Ishizuka T, et al. Identification of the human cytochrome P450 enzymes involved in the two oxidative steps in the bioactivation of clopidogrel to its pharmacologically active metabolite. Drug Metab Dispos 2010 Jan;38(1):92-99.

17. Anderson CD, Biffi A, Greenberg SM, et al. Personalized approaches to clopidogrel therapy: are we there yet? Stroke 2010 Dec;41(12):2997-3002.

18. Ma TK, Lam YY, Tan VP, et al. Impact of genetic and acquired alteration in cytochrome P450 system on pharmacologic and clinical response to clopidogrel. Pharmacol Ther 2010 Feb;125(2):249-59.

19. Li-Wan-Po A, Girard T, Farndon P, et al. Pharmacogenetics of CYP2C19: functional and clinical implications of a new variant CYP2C19*17. Br J Clin Pharmacol 2010 Mar;69(3):222-30.

20. Bauer T, Bouman HJ, van Werkum JW, et al. Impact of CYP2C19 variant genotypes on clinical efficacy of antiplatelet treatment with clopidogrel: systematic review and meta-analysis. BMJ 2011;343:d4588.

21. Scholz I, Oberwittler H, Riedel KD, et al. Pharmacokinetics, metabolism and bioavailability of the triazole antifungal agent voriconazole in relation to CYP2C19 genotype. Br J Clin Pharmacol 2009 Dec;68(6):906-15.

22. Yoo HD, Cho HY, Lee YB. Population pharmacokinetic analysis of cilostazol in healthy subjects with genetic polymorphisms of CYP3A5, CYP2C19 and ABCB1. Br J Clin Pharmacol 2010 Jan;69(1):27-37.

23. Yasui-Furukori N, Takahata T, Nakagami T, et al. Different inhibitory effect of fluvoxamine on omeprazole metabolism between CYP2C19 genotypes. Br J Clin Pharmacol 2004 Apr;57(4):487-94.

24. Minelli C, Thompson JR, Abrams KR, et al. Bayesian implementation of a genetic model-free approach to the meta-analysis of genetic association studies. Stat Med 2005 Dec 30;24(24):3845-61.

25. Chang MH, Lindegren ML, Butler MA, et al. Prevalence in the United States of selected candidate gene variants: Third National Health and Nutrition Examination Survey, 1991-1994. Am J Epidemiol 2009 Jan 1;169(1):54-66.

26. Chan MY, Tan K, Tan HC, et al. CYP2C19 and PON1 polymorphisms regulating clopidogrel bioactivation in Chinese, Malay and Indian subjects. Pharmacogenomics 2012 Apr;13(5):533-42.

27. Yin SJ, Ni YB, Wang SM, et al. Differences in genotype and allele frequency distributions of polymorphic drug metabolizing enzymes CYP2C19 and CYP2D6 in mainland Chinese Mongolian, Hui and Han populations. J Clin Pharm Ther 2012 Jun;37(3):364-69.

28. Veiga MI, Asimus S, Ferreira PE, et al. Pharmacogenomics of CYP2A6, CYP2B6, CYP2C19, CYP2D6, CYP3A4, CYP3A5 and MDR1 in Vietnam. Eur J Clin Pharmacol 2009 Apr;65(4):355-63.

29. Shuldiner AR, O'Connell JR, Bliden KP, et al. Association of cytochrome P450 2C19 genotype with the antiplatelet effect and clinical efficacy of clopidogrel therapy. JAMA 2009 Aug 26;302(8):849-57.

30. Harrison P, Frelinger AL, III, Furman MI, et al. Measuring antiplatelet drug effects in the laboratory. Thromb Res 2007;120(3):323-36.

31. Gurbel PA, Tantry US. Drug insight: Clopidogrel nonresponsiveness. Nat Clin Pract Cardiovasc Med 2006 Jul;3(7):387-95.

32. Ben-Dor I, Kleiman NS, Lev E. Assessment, mechanisms, and clinical implication of variability in platelet response to aspirin and clopidogrel therapy. Am J Cardiol 2009 Jul 15;104(2):227-33.

33. Favaloro EJ. Clinical utility of the PFA-100. Semin Thromb Hemost 2008 Nov;34(8):709-33.

34. Hayward CP, Harrison P, Cattaneo M, et al. Platelet function analyzer (PFA)-100 closure time in the evaluation of platelet disorders and platelet function. J Thromb Haemost 2006 Feb;4(2):312-19.

35. Jilma B. Platelet function analyzer (PFA-100): a tool to quantify congenital or acquired platelet dysfunction. J Lab Clin Med 2001 Sep;138(3):152-63.

36. van Werkum JW, Harmsze AM, Elsenberg EH, et al. The use of the VerifyNow system to monitor antiplatelet therapy: a review of the current evidence. Platelets 2008 Nov;19(7):479-88.

37. Price MJ. Bedside evaluation of thienopyridine antiplatelet therapy. Circulation 2009 May 19;119(19):2625-32.

38. Bonello L, Tantry US, Marcucci R, et al. Consensus and future directions on the definition of high on-treatment platelet reactivity to adenosine diphosphate. J Am Coll Cardiol 2010 Sep 14;56(12):919-33.

39. Tantry US, Kereiakes DJ, Gurbel PA. Clopidogrel and proton pump inhibitors: influence of pharmacological interactions on clinical outcomes and mechanistic explanations. JACC Cardiovasc Interv 2011 Apr;4(4):365-80.

40. Hulot JS, Collet JP, Silvain J, et al. Cardiovascular risk in clopidogrel-treated patients according to cytochrome P450 2C19*2 loss-of-function allele or proton pump inhibitor coadministration: a systematic meta-analysis. J Am Coll Cardiol 2010 Jul 6;56(2):134-43.

41. Holmes MV, Perel P, Shah T, et al. CYP2C19 Genotype, Clopidogrel Metabolism, Platelet Function, and Cardiovascular Events. JAMA: The Journal of the American Medical Association 2011 Dec 28;306(24):2704-14.

42. Krishna V, Diamond GA, Kaul S. Do platelet function testing and genotyping improve outcome in patients treated with antithrombotic agents?: the role of platelet reactivity and genotype testing in the prevention of atherothrombotic cardiovascular events remains unproven. Circulation 2012 Mar 13;125(10):1288-303.

43. Gurbel PA, Tantry US. Do platelet function testing and genotyping improve outcome in patients treated with antithrombotic agents?: platelet function testing and genotyping improve outcome in patients treated with antithrombotic agents. Circulation 2012 Mar 13;125(10):1276-87.

44. Scott SA, Sangkuhl K, Gardner EE, et al. Clinical Pharmacogenetics Implementation Consortium guidelines for cytochrome P450-2C19 (CYP2C19) genotype and clopidogrel therapy. Clin Pharmacol Ther 2011 Aug;90(2):328-32.

45. Eikelboom JW, Hirsh J, Spencer FA, et al. Antiplatelet drugs: Antithrombotic Therapy and Prevention of Thrombosis, 9th ed: American College of Chest Physicians Evidence-Based Clinical Practice Guidelines. Chest 2012 Feb;141(2 Suppl):e89S-119S.

46. Moher D, Liberati A, Tetzlaff J, et al. Preferred Reporting Items for Systematic Reviews and Meta-Analyses: The PRISMA Statement. PLoS Med 2009 Jul 21;6(7):e1000097. PMID: doi:10.1371/journal.pmed.1000097.

47. Wallace BC, Trikalinos TA, Lau J, et al. Semi-automated screening of biomedical citations for systematic reviews. BMC Bioinformatics 2010;11:55.

48. Simon RM, Paik S, Hayes DF. Use of archived specimens in evaluation of prognostic and predictive biomarkers. J Natl Cancer Inst 2009 Nov 4;101(21):1446-52.

49. Dahabreh IJ, Terasawa T, Castaldi PJ, et al. Systematic review: Anti-epidermal growth factor receptor treatment effect modification by KRAS mutations in advanced colorectal cancer. Ann Intern Med 2011 Jan 4;154(1):37-49.

50. Kitsios GD, Kent DM. Personalised medicine: not just in our genes. BMJ 2012 Apr 3;344

51. DerSimonian R, Laird N. Meta-analysis in clinical trials. Controlled Clinical Trials 1986 Sep;7(3):177-88. PMID: doi: 10.1016/0197-2456(86)90046-2.

52. Cochran WG. The combination of estimates from different experiments. Biometrics 1954 Mar;10(1):101-29.

53. Higgins JPT, Thompson SG. Quantifying heterogeneity in a meta-analysis. Statist Med 2002;21(11):1539-58. PMID: 10.1002/sim.1186.

54. Ioannidis JP, Patsopoulos NA, Evangelou E. Uncertainty in heterogeneity estimates in meta-analyses. BMJ 2007 Nov 1;335

55. Reitsma JB, Glas AS, Rutjes AW, et al. Bivariate analysis of sensitivity and specificity produces informative summary measures in diagnostic reviews. J Clin Epidemiol 2005 Oct;58(10):982-90.

56. Hamza TH, Reitsma JB, Stijnen T. Meta-analysis of diagnostic studies: a comparison of random intercept, normal-normal, and binomial-normal bivariate summary ROC approaches. Med Decis Making 2008 Sep;28(5):639-49.

57. Pearce N. What does the odds ratio estimate in a case-control study? Int J Epidemiol 1993 Dec;22(6):1189-92.

58. Knol MJ, Vandenbroucke JP, Scott P, et al. What do case-control studies estimate? Survey of methods and assumptions in published case-control research. Am J Epidemiol 2008 Nov 1;168(9):1073-81.

59. Miettinen OS. Theoretical epidemiology: principles of occurrence research in medicine. Wiley New York; 1985.

60. Berlin JA, Santanna J, Schmid CH, et al. Individual patient- versus group-level data meta-regressions for the investigation of treatment effect modifiers: ecological bias rears its ugly head. Statist Med 2002;21(3):371-87. PMID: 10.1002/sim.1023.

61. Egger M, Davey SG, Schneider M, et al. Bias in meta-analysis detected by a simple, graphical test. BMJ 1997 Sep 13;315(7109):629-34.

62. Lau J, Ioannidis JP, Terrin N, et al. The case of the misleading funnel plot. BMJ 2006 Sep 16;333(7568):597-600.

63. Terrin N, Schmid CH, Lau J. In an empirical evaluation of the funnel plot, researchers could not visually identify publication bias. J Clin Epidemiol 2005 Sep;58(9):894-901.

64. Terrin N, Schmid CH, Lau J, et al. Adjusting for publication bias in the presence of heterogeneity. Statist Med 2003;22(13):2113-26. PMID: 10.1002/sim.1461.

65. Sterne JA, Sutton AJ, Ioannidis JP, et al. Recommendations for examining and interpreting funnel plot asymmetry in meta-analyses of randomised controlled trials. BMJ 2011;343:d4002.

66. Ioannidis JPA, Ntzani EE, Trikalinos TA, et al. Replication validity of genetic association studies. Nat Genet 2001 Nov;29(3):306-09. PMID: 10.1038/ng749.

67. Trikalinos TA, Ntzani EE, Contopoulos-Ioannidis DG, et al. Establishment of genetic associations for complex diseases is independent of early study findings. Eur J Hum Genet 2004 Jun 23;12(9):762-69.

68. Agency for Healthcare Research and Quality. Methods Reference Guide for Effectiveness and Comparative Effectiveness Reviews. Available at: www.effectivehealthcare.ahrq.gov. AHRQ Publication No 10(11)-EHC063-EF 2011

69. Viswanathan M, Ansari MT, Berkman ND, et al. Assessing the Risk of Bias of Individual Studies in Systematic Reviews of Health Care Interventions. Rockville, MD: Agency for Healthcare Research and Quality; 2012.

70. Agency for Healthcare Research and Quality. Methods Guide for Medical Test Reviews. Rockville, MD: AHRQ; 2012.

71. Whiting PF, Rutjes AWS, Westwood ME, et al. QUADAS-2: A Revised Tool for the Quality Assessment of Diagnostic Accuracy Studies. Annals of Internal Medicine 2011 Oct 18;155(8):529-36.

72. Whiting P, Rutjes AW, Reitsma JB, et al. The development of QUADAS: a tool for the quality assessment of studies of diagnostic accuracy included in systematic reviews. BMC Med Res Methodol 2003 Nov 10;3:25.

73. Whiting P, Rutjes AW, Dinnes J, et al. Development and validation of methods for assessing the quality of diagnostic accuracy studies. Health Technol Assess 2004 Jun;8(25):iii, 1-iii234.

74. Whiting PF, Weswood ME, Rutjes AWS, et al. Evaluation of QUADAS, a tool for the quality assessment of diagnostic accuracy studies. BMC Med Res Methodol 2006;6:9.

75. Higgins JPT, Douglas GA, Peter CG, et al. The Cochrane Collaboration □ÇÖs tool for assessing risk of bias in randomised trials. BMJ 2011 Oct 18;343

76. Owens DK, Lohr KN, Atkins D, et al. AHRQ series paper 5: grading the strength of a body of evidence when comparing medical interventions--agency for healthcare research and quality and the effective health-care program. J Clin Epidemiol 2010 May;63(5):513-23.

77. Atkins D, Chang SM, Gartlehner G, et al. Assessing applicability when comparing medical interventions: AHRQ and the Effective Health Care Program. J Clin Epidemiol. 2011;64:1198-207. PMID: <[31] UNIQUE ID (DOI)>.

78. Sibbing D, Stegherr J, Latz W, et al. Cytochrome P450 2C19 loss-of-function polymorphism and stent thrombosis following percutaneous coronary intervention. European Heart Journal 2009 Apr;30(8):916-22.

79. Sibbing D, Koch W, Gebhard D, et al. Cytochrome 2C19*17 allelic variant, platelet aggregation, bleeding events, and stent thrombosis in clopidogrel-treated patients with coronary stent placement. Circulation 2010 Feb 2;121(4):512-18.

80. Sibbing D, Koch W, Massberg S, et al. No association of paraoxonase-1 Q192R genotypes with platelet response to clopidogrel and risk of stent thrombosis after coronary stenting. European Heart Journal 2011 Jul;32(13):1605-13.

81. Trenk D, Hochholzer W, Fromm MF, et al. Paraoxonase-1 Q192R polymorphism and antiplatelet effects of clopidogrel in patients undergoing elective coronary stent placement. Circulation 2011 Aug 1;Cardiovascular(4):429-36.

82. Siller-Matula JM, le-Karth G, Lang IM, et al. Phenotyping vs. genotyping for prediction of clopidogrel efficacy and safety: the PEGASUS-PCI study. J Thromb Haemost 2012 Apr;10(4):529-42.

83. Namazi S, Kojuri J, Khalili A, et al. The impact of genetic polymorphisms of P2Y12, CYP3A5 and CYP2C19 on clopidogrel response variability in Iranian patients. Biochem Pharmacol 2012 Apr 1;83(7):903-08.

84. Delaney JT, Ramirez AH, Bowton E, et al. Predicting clopidogrel response using DNA samples linked to an electronic health record. Clin Pharmacol Ther 2012 Feb;91(2):257-63.

85. Bhatt DL, Pare G, Eikelboom JW, et al. The relationship between CYP2C19 polymorphisms and ischaemic and bleeding outcomes in stable outpatients: the CHARISMA genetics study. Eur Heart J 2012 Mar 26

86. Roberts JD, Wells GA, Le May MR, et al. Point-of-care genetic testing for personalisation of antiplatelet treatment (RAPID GENE): a prospective, randomised, proof-of-concept trial. Lancet 2012 May 5;379(9827):1705-11.

87. Mega JL, Hochholzer W, Frelinger AL, III, et al. Dosing clopidogrel based on CYP2C19 genotype and the effect on platelet reactivity in patients with stable cardiovascular disease. JAMA 2011 Nov 23;306(20):2221-28.

88. Campo G, Parrinello G, Ferraresi P, et al. Prospective evaluation of on-clopidogrel platelet reactivity over time in patients treated with percutaneous coronary intervention relationship with gene polymorphisms and clinical outcome. Journal of the American College of Cardiology 2011 Jun 21;57(25):2474-83.

89. Malek LA, Przyluski J, Spiewak M, et al. Cytochrome P450 2C19 polymorphism, suboptimal reperfusion and all-cause mortality in patients with acute myocardial infarction. Cardiology 2010;117(2):81-87.

90. Sawada T, Shinke T, Shite J, et al. Impact of cytochrome P450 2C19*2 polymorphism on intra-stent thrombus after drug-eluting stent implantation in Japanese patients receiving clopidogrel. Circulation Journal 2010 Dec 24;75(1):99-105.

91. Tiroch KA, Sibbing D, Koch W, et al. Protective effect of the CYP2C19 *17 polymorphism with increased activation of clopidogrel on cardiovascular events. Am Heart J 2010 Sep;160(3):506-12.

92. Chen M, Liu XJ, Yan SD, et al. Association between cytochrome P450 2C19 polymorphism and clinical outcomes in Chinese patients with coronary artery disease. Atherosclerosis 2012 Jan;220(1):168-71.

93. Nishio R, Shinke T, Otake H, et al. Effect of Cytochrome P450 2C19 Polymorphism on Target Lesion Outcome After Drug-Eluting Stent Implantation in Japanese Patients Receiving Clopidogrel. Circ J 2012 Sep 25;76(10):2348-55.

94. Collet JP, Hulot JS, Pena A, et al. Cytochrome P450 2C19 polymorphism in young patients treated with clopidogrel after myocardial infarction: a cohort study. Lancet 2009 Jan 24;373(9660):309-17.

95. Giusti B, Gori AM, Marcucci R, et al. Relation of cytochrome P450 2C19 loss-of-function polymorphism to occurrence of drug-eluting coronary stent thrombosis. American Journal of Cardiology 2009 Mar 15;103(6):806-11.

96. Malek LA, Kisiel B, Spiewak M, et al. Coexisting polymorphisms of P2Y12 and CYP2C19 genes as a risk factor for persistent platelet activation with clopidogrel. Circulation Journal 2008 Jul;72(7):1165-69.

97. Yamamoto K, Hokimoto S, Chitose T, et al. Impact of CYP2C19 polymorphism on residual platelet reactivity in patients with coronary heart disease during antiplatelet therapy. Journal of Cardiology 2011 Mar;57(2):194-201.

98. Luo Y, Zhao YT, Verdo A, et al. Relationship between cytochrome P450 2C19*2 polymorphism and stent thrombosis following percutaneous coronary intervention in Chinese patients receiving clopidogrel. J Int Med Res 2011;39(5):2012-19.

99. Mega JL, Close SL, Wiviott SD, et al. Cytochrome p-450 polymorphisms and response to clopidogrel. N Engl J Med 2009 Jan 22;360(4):354-62.

100. Bonello L, Armero S, Ait MO, et al. Clopidogrel loading dose adjustment according to platelet reactivity monitoring in patients carrying the 2C19*2 loss of function polymorphism. Journal of the American College of Cardiology 2010 Nov 9;56(20):1630-36.

101. Bouman HJ, Harmsze AM, van Werkum JW, et al. Variability in on-treatment platelet reactivity explained by CYP2C19*2 genotype is modest in clopidogrel pretreated patients undergoing coronary stenting. Heart 2011 Aug;97(15):1239-44.

102. Bouman HJ, Schomig E, van Werkum JW, et al. Paraoxonase-1 is a major determinant of clopidogrel efficacy.[Erratum appears in Nat Med. 2011 Sep;17(9):1153]. Nature Medicine 2011 Jan;17(1):110-16.

103. Harmsze AM, van Werkum JW, Ten Berg JM, et al. CYP2C19*2 and CYP2C9*3 alleles are associated with stent thrombosis: a case-control study. European Heart Journal 2010 Dec;31(24):3046-53.

104. Wallentin L, James S, Storey RF, et al. Effect of CYP2C19 and ABCB1 single nucleotide polymorphisms on outcomes of treatment with ticagrelor versus clopidogrel for acute coronary syndromes: a genetic substudy of the PLATO trial. Lancet 2010 Oct 16;376(9749):1320-28. PMID: 20801498.

105. Hulot JS, Collet JP, Cayla G, et al. CYP2C19 but not PON1 genetic variants influence clopidogrel pharmacokinetics, pharmacodynamics, and clinical efficacy in post-myocardial infarction patients. Circ Cardiovasc Interv 2011 Oct 1;4(5):422-28.

106. Jaitner J, Morath T, Byrne RA, et al. No association of ABCB1 C3435T genotype with clopidogrel response or risk of stent thrombosis in patients undergoing coronary stenting. Circ Cardiovasc Interv 2012 Feb 1;5(1):82.

107. Cayla G, Hulot JS, O'Connor SA, et al. Clinical, angiographic, and genetic factors associated with early coronary stent thrombosis. JAMA 2011 Oct 26;306(16):1765-74.

108. Ono T, Kaikita K, Hokimoto S, et al. Determination of cut-off levels for on-clopidogrel platelet aggregation based on functional CYP2C19 gene variants in patients undergoing elective percutaneous coronary intervention. Thromb Res 2011 Dec;128(6):e130-e136.

109. Pare G, Mehta SR, Yusuf S, et al. Effects of CYP2C19 genotype on outcomes of clopidogrel treatment. N Engl J Med 2010 Oct 28;363(18):1704-14.

110. Simon T, Verstuyft C, Mary-Krause M, et al. Genetic determinants of response to clopidogrel and cardiovascular events. N Engl J Med 2009 Jan 22;360(4):363-75.

111. Trenk D, Hochholzer W, Fromm MF, et al. Cytochrome P450 2C19 681G>A polymorphism and high on-clopidogrel platelet reactivity associated with adverse 1-year clinical outcome of elective percutaneous coronary intervention with drug-eluting or bare-metal stents. Journal of the American College of Cardiology 2008 May 20;51(20):1925-34.

112. Rideg O, Komocsi A, Magyarlaki T, et al. Impact of genetic variants on post-clopidogrel platelet reactivity in patients after elective percutaneous coronary intervention. Pharmacogenomics 2011 Sep;12(9):1269-80.

113. Harmsze AM, van Werkum JW, Souverein PC, et al. Combined influence of proton-pump inhibitors, calcium-channel blockers and CYP2C19*2 on on-treatment platelet reactivity and on the occurrence of atherothrombotic events after percutaneous coronary intervention. J Thromb Haemost 2011 Oct;9(10):1892-901.

114. Jeong YH, Tantry US, Kim IS, et al. Effect of CYP2C19*2 and *3 loss-of-function alleles on platelet reactivity and adverse clinical events in East Asian acute myocardial infarction survivors treated with clopidogrel and aspirin. Circ Cardiovasc Interv 2011 Dec 1;4(6):585-94.

115. Tello-Montoliu A, Jover E, Marin F, et al. Influence of CYP2C19 polymorphisms in platelet reactivity and prognosis in an unselected population of non ST elevation acute coronary syndrome. Rev Esp Cardiol (Engl) 2012 Mar;65(3):219-26.

116. Teixeira R, Monteiro P, Marques G, et al. CYP2C19*2 and prognosis after an acute coronary syndrome: Insights from a Portuguese center. Rev Port Cardiol 2012 Apr;31(4):265-73.

117. Marcucci R, Giusti B, Paniccia R, et al. High on-treatment platelet reactivity by ADP and increased risk of MACE in good clopidogrel metabolizers. Platelets 2012 Mar 5

118. Wallentin L, James S, Storey RF, et al. Effect of CYP2C19 and ABCB1 single nucleotide polymorphisms on outcomes of treatment with ticagrelor versus clopidogrel for acute coronary syndromes: a genetic substudy of the PLATO trial. Lancet 2010 Oct 16;376(9749):1320-28.

119. Harmsze AM, van Werkum JW, Hackeng CM, et al. The influence of CYP2C19*2 and *17 on on-treatment platelet reactivity and bleeding events in patients undergoing elective coronary stenting. Pharmacogenet Genomics 2012 Mar;22(3):169-75.

120. Dai ZL, Chen H, Wu XY. Relationship between cytochrome P450 2C19*17 genotype distribution, platelet aggregation and bleeding risk in patients with blood stasis syndrome of coronary artery disease treated with clopidogrel. Zhong Xi Yi Jie He Xue Bao 2012 Jun;10(6):647-54.

121. Collet JP, Hulot JS, Pena A, et al. Cytochrome P450 2C19 polymorphism in young patients treated with clopidogrel after myocardial infarction: a cohort study. Lancet 2009 Jan 24;373(9660):309-17.

122. Fernando H, Bassler N, Habersberger J, et al. Randomized double-blind placebo-controlled crossover study to determine the effects of esomeprazole on inhibition of platelet function by clopidogrel. J Thromb Haemost 2011 Aug;9(8):1582-89.

123. Maeda A, Ando H, Asai T, et al. Differential impacts of CYP2C19 gene polymorphisms on the antiplatelet effects of clopidogrel and ticlopidine. Clinical Pharmacology & Therapeutics 2011 Feb;89(2):229-33.

124. Simon T, Steg PG, Gilard M, et al. Clinical events as a function of proton pump inhibitor use, clopidogrel use, and cytochrome P450 2C19 genotype in a large nationwide cohort of acute myocardial infarction: results from the French Registry of Acute ST-Elevation and Non-ST-Elevation Myocardial Infarction (FAST-MI) registry. Circulation 2011 Feb 8;123(5):474-82.

125. Harmsze A, van Werkum JW, Bouman HJ, et al. Besides CYP2C19*2, the variant allele CYP2C9*3 is associated with higher on-clopidogrel platelet reactivity in patients on dual antiplatelet therapy undergoing elective coronary stent implantation. Pharmacogenetics and Genomics 2010 Jan;20(1):18-25.

126. Liu XL, Wang ZJ, Yang Q, et al. Impact of CYP2C19 polymorphism and smoking on response to clopidogrel in patients with stable coronary artery disease. Chinese Medical Journal 2010 Nov;123(22):3178-83.

127. Kesteven GL. The coefficient of variation. Nature 1946;Oct. 12(158):520.

128. Bland JM, Altman DG. Statistical methods for assessing agreement between two methods of clinical measurement. Lancet 1986;Feb. 8;1(8476):307-10.

129. Lin LI. A concordance correlation coefficient to evaluate reproducibility. Biometrics 1989;45(1):255-68. PMID: PMID 2720055.

130. Landis JR, Koch GG. The measurement of observer agreement for categorical data. Biometrics 1977;33(1):159-74.

131. Varenhorst C, James S, Erlinge D, et al. Assessment of P2Y12 inhibition with the point-of-care device VerifyNow P2Y12 in patients treated with prasugrel or clopidogrel coadministered with aspirin. Am Heart J. 2009;157:562. PMID: <[31] UNIQUE ID (DOI)>.

132. Jeong YH, Kim IS, Choi BR, et al. The optimal threshold of high post-treatment platelet reactivity could be defined by a point-of-care VerifyNow P2Y12 assay. European Heart Journal 2008 Sep 1;29(17):2186-87.

133. Michelson AD, Frelinger AL, III, Braunwald E, et al. Pharmacodynamic assessment of platelet inhibition by prasugrel vs. clopidogrel in the TRITON-TIMI 38 trial. European Heart Journal 2009 Jul;30(14):1753-63.

134. Angiolillo DJ, Bernardo E, Sabate M, et al. Impact of platelet reactivity on cardiovascular outcomes in patients with type 2 diabetes mellitus and coronary artery disease. Journal of the American College of Cardiology 2007 Oct 16;50(16):1541-47.

135. Aradi D, Konyi A, Palinkas L, et al. Thienopyridine therapy influences late outcome after coronary stent implantation. Angiology 2008 Apr;59(2):172-78.

136. Bellemain-Appaix A, Montalescot G, Silvain J, et al. Slow response to clopidogrel predicts low response. Journal of the American College of Cardiology 2010 Feb 23;55(8):815-22.

137. Bliden KP, Dichiara J, Tantry US, et al. Increased risk in patients with high platelet aggregation receiving chronic clopidogrel therapy undergoing percutaneous coronary intervention: is the current antiplatelet therapy adequate? Journal of the American College of Cardiology 2007 Feb 13;49(6):657-66.

138. Blindt R, Stellbrink K, de TA, et al. The significance of vasodilator-stimulated phosphoprotein for risk stratification of stent thrombosis. Thrombosis & Haemostasis 2007 Dec;98(6):1329-34.

139. Breet NJ, van Werkum JW, Bouman HJ, et al. Do not adjust the platelet count in light transmittance aggregometry when predicting thrombotic events after percutaneous coronary intervention. Journal of Thrombosis & Haemostasis 2010 Oct;8(10):2326-28.

140. Breet NJ, van Werkum JW, Bouman HJ, et al. Comparison of platelet function tests in predicting clinical outcome in patients undergoing coronary stent implantation.[Erratum appears in JAMA. 2010 Apr 7;303(13):1257], [Erratum appears in JAMA. 2011 Jun 1;305(21):2174], [Erratum appears in JAMA. 2011 Jun 1;305(21):2172-3; PMID: 21562204]. JAMA 2010 Feb 24;303(8):754-62.

141. Breet NJ, van Werkum JW, Bouman HJ, et al. High on-treatment platelet reactivity to both aspirin and clopidogrel is associated with the highest risk of adverse events following percutaneous coronary intervention. Heart 2011 Jun;97(12):983-90.

142. Buonamici P, Marcucci R, Migliorini A, et al. Impact of platelet reactivity after clopidogrel administration on drug-eluting stent thrombosis. Journal of the American College of Cardiology 2007 Jun 19;49(24):2312-17.

143. Campo G, Valgimigli M, Gemmati D, et al. Poor responsiveness to clopidogrel: drug-specific or class-effect mechanism? Evidence from a clopidogrel-to-ticlopidine crossover study. Journal of the American College of Cardiology 2007 Sep 18;50(12):1132-37.

144. Cuisset T, Frere C, Quilici J, et al. High post-treatment platelet reactivity identified low-responders to dual antiplatelet therapy at increased risk of recurrent cardiovascular events after stenting for acute coronary syndrome. Journal of Thrombosis & Haemostasis 2006 Mar;4(3):542-49.

145. Cuisset T, Frere C, Quilici J, et al. Benefit of a 600-mg loading dose of clopidogrel on platelet reactivity and clinical outcomes in patients with non-ST-segment elevation acute coronary syndrome undergoing coronary stenting. J Am Coll Cardiol 2006 Oct 3;48(7):1339-45.

146. Cuisset T, Frere C, Quilici J, et al. High post-treatment platelet reactivity is associated with a high incidence of myonecrosis after stenting for non-ST elevation acute coronary syndromes. Thrombosis & Haemostasis 2007 Feb;97(2):282-87.

147. Cuisset T, Frere C, Quilici J, et al. Predictive values of post-treatment adenosine diphosphate-induced aggregation and vasodilator-stimulated phosphoprotein index for stent thrombosis after acute coronary syndrome in clopidogrel-treated patients. American Journal of Cardiology 2009 Oct 15;104(8):1078-82.

148. Cuisset T, Cayla G, Frere C, et al. Predictive value of post-treatment platelet reactivity for occurrence of post-discharge bleeding after non-ST elevation acute coronary syndrome. Shifting from antiplatelet resistance to bleeding risk assessment? Eurointervention 2009 Aug;5(3):325-29.

149. Frere C, Cuisset T, Quilici J, et al. ADP-induced platelet aggregation and platelet reactivity index VASP are good predictive markers for clinical outcomes in non-ST elevation acute coronary syndrome. Thrombosis & Haemostasis 2007 Oct;98(4):838-43.

150. Geisler T, Langer H, Wydymus M, et al. Low response to clopidogrel is associated with cardiovascular outcome after coronary stent implantation. European Heart Journal 2006 Oct;27(20):2420-25.

151. Geisler T, Grass D, Bigalke B, et al. The Residual Platelet Aggregation after Deployment of Intracoronary Stent (PREDICT) score. Journal of Thrombosis & Haemostasis 2008 Jan;6(1):54-61.

152. Geisler T, Mueller K, Aichele S, et al. Impact of inflammatory state and metabolic control on responsiveness to dual antiplatelet therapy in type 2 diabetics after PCI: prognostic relevance of residual platelet aggregability in diabetics undergoing coronary interventions.[Erratum appears in Clin Res Cardiol. 2010 Nov;99(11):769]. Clinical Research in Cardiology 2010 Nov;99(11):743-52.

153. Geisler T, Zurn C, Simonenko R, et al. Early but not late stent thrombosis is influenced by residual platelet aggregation in patients undergoing coronary interventions. European Heart Journal 2010 Jan;31(1):59-66.

154. Gori AM, Marcucci R, Paniccia R, et al. Thrombotic events in high risk patients are predicted by evaluating different pathways of platelet function. Thrombosis & Haemostasis 2008 Dec;100(6):1136-45.

155. Gori AM, Marcucci R, Migliorini A, et al. Incidence and clinical impact of dual nonresponsiveness to aspirin and clopidogrel in patients with drug-eluting stents. Journal of the American College of Cardiology 2008 Aug 26;52(9):734-39.

156. Gurbel PA, Bliden KP, Hiatt BL, et al. Clopidogrel for coronary stenting: response variability, drug resistance, and the effect of pretreatment platelet reactivity. Circulation 2003 Jun 17;107(23):2908-13.

157. Gurbel PA, Bliden KP. Durability of platelet inhibition by clopidogrel. American Journal of Cardiology 2003 May 1;91(9):1123-25.

158. Gurbel PA, Samara WM, Bliden KP. Failure of clopidogrel to reduce platelet reactivity and activation following standard dosing in elective stenting: implications for thrombotic events and restenosis. Platelets 2004 Mar;15(2):95-99.

159. Gurbel PA, Bliden KP, Guyer K, et al. Platelet reactivity in patients and recurrent events post-stenting: results of the PREPARE POST-STENTING Study. Journal of the American College of Cardiology 2005 Nov 15;46(10):1820-26.

160. Gurbel PA, Antonino MJ, Bliden KP, et al. Platelet reactivity to adenosine diphosphate and long-term ischemic event occurrence following percutaneous coronary intervention: a potential antiplatelet therapeutic target. Platelets 2008 Dec;19(8):595-604.

161. Gurbel PA, Bliden KP, Navickas IA, et al. Adenosine diphosphate-induced platelet-fibrin clot strength: a new thrombelastographic indicator of long-term poststenting ischemic events. Am Heart J 2010 Aug;160(2):346-54.

162. Gurbel PA, Bliden KP, Butler K, et al. Response to ticagrelor in clopidogrel nonresponders and responders and effect of switching therapies: the RESPOND study. Circulation 2010 Mar 16;121(10):1188-99.

163. Hochholzer W, Trenk D, Bestehorn HP, et al. Impact of the degree of peri-interventional platelet inhibition after loading with clopidogrel on early clinical outcome of elective coronary stent placement. Journal of the American College of Cardiology 2006 Nov 7;48(9):1742-50.

164. Hoshino K, Horiuchi H, Tada T, et al. Clopidogrel resistance in Japanese patients scheduled for percutaneous coronary intervention. Circulation Journal 2009 Feb;73(2):336-42.

165. Htun P, Fateh-Moghadam S, Bischofs C, et al. Low responsiveness to clopidogrel increases risk among CKD patients undergoing coronary intervention. Journal of the American Society of Nephrology 2011 Apr;22(4):627-33.

166. L'Allier PL, Ducrocq G, Pranno N, et al. Clopidogrel 600-mg double loading dose achieves stronger platelet inhibition than conventional regimens: results from the PREPAIR randomized study. Journal of the American College of Cardiology 2008 Mar 18;51(11):1066-72.

167. Liu Y, Liu N, Li W, et al. Clopidogrel response variability and its correlation with early recurrent cardiovascular events in chinese patients undergoing percutaneous coronary intervention. Pharmacology 2011;87(5-6):321-30.

168. Matetzky S, Shenkman B, Guetta V, et al. Clopidogrel resistance is associated with increased risk of recurrent atherothrombotic events in patients with acute myocardial infarction.[Erratum appears in Circulation. 2011 Oct 25;124(17):e459 Note: Bienart, Roy [corrected to Beinart, Roy]]. Circulation 2004 Jun 29;109(25):3171-75.

169. Muller I, Besta F, Schulz C, et al. Prevalence of clopidogrel non-responders among patients with stable angina pectoris scheduled for elective coronary stent placement. Thrombosis & Haemostasis 2003 May;89(5):783-87.

170. Muller K, Aichele S, Herkommer M, et al. Impact of inflammatory markers on platelet inhibition and cardiovascular outcome including stent thrombosis in patients with symptomatic coronary artery disease. Atherosclerosis 2010 Nov;213(1):256-62.

171. Obradovic SD, Antovic JP, Antonijevic NM, et al. Elevations in soluble CD40 ligand in patients with high platelet aggregability undergoing percutaneous coronary intervention. Blood Coagulation & Fibrinolysis 2009 Jun;20(4):283-89.

172. Saw J, Madsen EH, Chan S, et al. The ELAPSE (Evaluation of Long-Term Clopidogrel Antiplatelet and Systemic Anti-Inflammatory Effects) study. J Am Coll Cardiol 2008 Dec 2;52(23):1826-33.

173. Wang L, Wang X, Chen F. Clopidogrel resistance is associated with long-term thrombotic events in patients implanted with drug-eluting stents. Drugs in R & D 2010;10(4):219-24.

174. Wang ZJ, Zhou YJ, Liu YY, et al. Impact of clopidogrel resistance on thrombotic events after percutaneous coronary intervention with drug-eluting stent. Thrombosis Research 2009 May;124(1):46-51.

175. Yong G, Rankin J, Ferguson L, et al. Randomized trial comparing 600- with 300-mg loading dose of clopidogrel in patients with non-ST elevation acute coronary syndrome undergoing percutaneous coronary intervention: results of the Platelet Responsiveness to Aspirin and Clopidogrel and Troponin Increment after Coronary intervention in Acute coronary Lesions (PRACTICAL) Trial. Am Heart J 2009 Jan;157(1):60-69.

176. Gurbel PA, Bliden KP, Antonino MJ, et al. Time dependence of clopidogrel loading effect: platelet activation versus platelet aggregation. Thromb Res 2012 Jan;129(1):1-2.

177. Kalantzi KI, Dimitriou AA, Goudevenos JA, et al. The platelet hyporesponsiveness to clopidogrel in acute coronary syndrome patients treated with 75 mg/day clopidogrel may be overcome within 1 month of treatment. Platelets 2012;23(2):121-31.

178. Angiolillo DJ, Bernardo E, Zanoni M, et al. Impact of insulin receptor substrate-1 genotypes on platelet reactivity and cardiovascular outcomes in patients with type 2 diabetes mellitus and coronary artery disease. J Am Coll Cardiol 2011 Jun 28;58(1):30-39.

179. Saad AA, Ismail EA, Darwish YW, et al. Platelet function profile post-clopidogrel therapy in patients with type 2 diabetes undergoing coronary stent implantation. Clin Appl Thromb Hemost 2012 Jun;18(3):249-57.

180. Gaglia MA, Torguson R, Pakala R, et al. Correlation between light transmission aggregometry, VerifyNow P2Y12, and VASP-P platelet reactivity assays following percutaneous coronary intervention. J Interv Cardiol 2011 Dec;24(6):529-34.

181. Aradi D, Rideg O, Vorobcsuk A, et al. Justification of 150 mg clopidogrel in patients with high on-clopidogrel platelet reactivity. Eur J Clin Invest 2012 Apr;42(4):384-92.

182. Ge H, Zhou Y, Liu X, et al. Relationship between plasma inflammatory markers and platelet aggregation in patients with clopidogrel resistance after angioplasty. Angiology 2012 Jan;63(1):62-66.

183. Kim IS, Jeong YH, Kang MK, et al. Correlation of high post-treatment platelet reactivity assessed by light transmittance aggregometry and the VerifyNow P2Y12 assay. J Thromb Thrombolysis 2010 Nov;30(4):486-95.

184. Cuisset T, Frere C, Quilici J, et al. Lack of association between the 807 C/T polymorphism of glycoprotein Ia gene and post-treatment platelet reactivity after aspirin and clopidogrel in patients with acute coronary syndrome. Thrombosis & Haemostasis 2007 Feb;97(2):212-17.

185. Linnemann B, Schwonberg J, Toennes SW, et al. Variability of residual platelet function despite clopidogrel treatment in patients with peripheral arterial occlusive disease. Atherosclerosis 2010 Apr;209(2):504-09.

186. Reny JL, Berdague P, Poncet A, et al. Antiplatelet drug response status does not predict recurrent ischemic events in stable cardiovascular patients: results of the Antiplatelet Drug Resistances and Ischemic Events study. Circulation 2012 Jun 26;125(25):3201-10.

187. Campo G, Fileti L, de CN, et al. Long-term clinical outcome based on aspirin and clopidogrel responsiveness status after elective percutaneous coronary intervention: a 3T/2R (tailoring treatment with tirofiban in patients showing resistance to aspirin and/or resistance to clopidogrel) trial substudy. Journal of the American College of Cardiology 2010 Oct 26;56(18):1447-55.

188. Cotton JM, Worrall AM, Hobson AR, et al. Individualised assessment of response to clopidogrel in patients presenting with acute coronary syndromes: a role for short thrombelastography?.[Erratum appears in Cardiovasc Ther. 2010 Aug;28(4):254 Note: Rajendra, R [corrected to Raghuraman, R P]]. Cardiovascular therapeutics 2010 Jun;28(3):139-46.

189. Cuisset T, Hamilos M, Sarma J, et al. Relation of low response to clopidogrel assessed with point-of-care assay to periprocedural myonecrosis in patients undergoing elective coronary stenting for stable angina pectoris. American Journal of Cardiology 2008 Jun 15;101(12):1700-03.

190. de Miguel CA, Cuellas RC, Diego NA, et al. Post-treatment platelet reactivity predicts long-term adverse events better than the response to clopidogrel in patients with non-ST-segment elevation acute coronary syndrome. Revista Espanola de Cardiologia 2009 Feb;62(2):126-35.

191. Gladding P, Webster M, Zeng I, et al. The pharmacogenetics and pharmacodynamics of clopidogrel response: an analysis from the PRINC (Plavix Response in Coronary Intervention) trial. Jacc: Cardiovascular Interventions 2008 Dec;1(6):620-27.

192. Huczek Z, Filipiak KJ, Kochman J, et al. Medium on-treatment platelet reactivity to ADP is favorable in patients with acute coronary syndromes undergoing coronary stenting. Platelets 2011;22(7):521-29.

193. Kim BK, Oh SJ, Yoon SJ, et al. A randomized study assessing the effects of pretreatment with cilostazol on periprocedural myonecrosis after percutaneous coronary intervention. Yonsei Medical Journal 2011 Sep;52(5):717-26.

194. Ko YG, Suh JW, Kim BH, et al. Comparison of 2 point-of-care platelet function tests, VerifyNow Assay and Multiple Electrode Platelet Aggregometry, for predicting early clinical outcomes in patients undergoing percutaneous coronary intervention. Am Heart J 2011 Feb;161(2):383-90.

195. Lee K, Lee SW, Lee JW, et al. The significance of clopidogrel low-responsiveness on stent thrombosis and cardiac death assessed by the verifynow p(2)y(12) assay in patients with acute coronary syndrome within 6 months after drug-eluting stent implantation. Sunhwangi 2009 Dec;39(12):512-18.

196. Mangiacapra F, Patti G, Peace A, et al. Comparison of platelet reactivity and periprocedural outcomes in patients with versus without diabetes mellitus and treated with clopidogrel and percutaneous coronary intervention. American Journal of Cardiology 2010 Sep 1;106(5):619-23.

197. Mangiacapra F, Barbato E, Patti G, et al. Point-of-care assessment of platelet reactivity after clopidogrel to predict myonecrosis in patients undergoing percutaneous coronary intervention. Jacc: Cardiovascular Interventions 2010 Mar;3(3):318-23.

198. Mangiacapra F, De BB, Muller O, et al. High residual platelet reactivity after clopidogrel: extent of coronary atherosclerosis and periprocedural myocardial infarction in patients with stable angina undergoing percutaneous coronary intervention. Jacc: Cardiovascular Interventions 2010 Jan;3(1):35-40.

199. Marcucci R, Gori AM, Paniccia R, et al. Cardiovascular death and nonfatal myocardial infarction in acute coronary syndrome patients receiving coronary stenting are predicted by residual platelet reactivity to ADP detected by a point-of-care assay: a 12-month follow-up. Circulation 2009 Jan 20;119(2):237-42.

200. Patti G, Nusca A, Mangiacapra F, et al. Point-of-care measurement of clopidogrel responsiveness predicts clinical outcome in patients undergoing percutaneous coronary intervention results of the ARMYDA-PRO (Antiplatelet therapy for Reduction of MYocardial Damage during Angioplasty-Platelet Reactivity Predicts Outcome) study. Journal of the American College of Cardiology 2008 Sep 30;52(14):1128-33.

201. Patti G, Pasceri V, Vizzi V, et al. Usefulness of platelet response to clopidogrel by point-of-care testing to predict bleeding outcomes in patients undergoing percutaneous coronary intervention (from the Antiplatelet Therapy for Reduction of Myocardial Damage During Angioplasty-Bleeding Study). American Journal of Cardiology 2011 Apr 1;107(7):995-1000.

202. Price MJ, Endemann S, Gollapudi RR, et al. Prognostic significance of post-clopidogrel platelet reactivity assessed by a point-of-care assay on thrombotic events after drug-eluting stent implantation. European Heart Journal 2008 Apr;29(8):992-1000.

203. Price MJ, Berger PB, Teirstein PS, et al. Standard- vs high-dose clopidogrel based on platelet function testing after percutaneous coronary intervention: the GRAVITAS randomized trial.[Erratum appears in JAMA. 2011 Jun 1;305(21);2174 Note: Stillablower, Michael E [corrected to Stillabower, Michael E]]. JAMA 2011 Mar 16;305(11):1097-105.

287

204. Saw J, Densem C, Walsh S, et al. The effects of aspirin and clopidogrel response on myonecrosis after percutaneous coronary intervention: a BRIEF-PCI (Brief Infusion of Intravenous Eptifibatide Following Successful Percutaneous Coronary Intervention) trial substudy. JACC Cardiovasc Interv 2008 Dec;1(6):654-59.

205. Suh JW, Lee SP, Park KW, et al. Multicenter randomized trial evaluating the efficacy of cilostazol on ischemic vascular complications after drug-eluting stent implantation for coronary heart disease: results of the CILON-T (influence of CILostazol-based triple antiplatelet therapy ON ischemic complication after drug-eluting stenT implantation) trial. Journal of the American College of Cardiology 2011 Jan 18;57(3):280-89.

206. Valgimigli M, Campo G, de CN, et al. Intensifying platelet inhibition with tirofiban in poor responders to aspirin, clopidogrel, or both agents undergoing elective coronary intervention: results from the double-blind, prospective, randomized Tailoring Treatment with Tirofiban in Patients Showing Resistance to Aspirin and/or Resistance to Clopidogrel study. Circulation 2009 Jun 30;119(25):3215-22.

207. Vavuranakis M, Vrachatis DA, Papaioannou TG, et al. Residual platelet reactivity after clopidogrel loading in patients with ST-elevation myocardial infarction undergoing an unexpectedly delayed primary percutaneous coronary intervention. -Impact on intracoronary thrombus burden and myocardial perfusion-. Circ J 2011;75(9):2105-12.

208. Price MJ, Angiolillo DJ, Teirstein PS, et al. Platelet reactivity and cardiovascular outcomes after percutaneous coronary intervention: a time-dependent analysis of the Gauging Responsiveness with a VerifyNow P2Y12 assay: Impact on Thrombosis and Safety (GRAVITAS) trial. Circulation 2011 Sep 6;124(10):1132-37.

209. Mangiacapra F, Patti G, Barbato E, et al. A therapeutic window for platelet reactivity for patients undergoing elective percutaneous coronary intervention: results of the ARMYDA-PROVE (Antiplatelet therapy for Reduction of MYocardial Damage during Angioplasty-Platelet Reactivity for Outcome Validation Effort) study. JACC Cardiovasc Interv 2012 Mar;5(3):281-89.

210. Park KW, Jeon KH, Kang SH, et al. Clinical outcomes of high on-treatment platelet reactivity in Koreans receiving elective percutaneous coronary intervention (from results of the CROSS VERIFY study). Am J Cardiol 2011 Dec 1;108(11):1556-63.

211. Park DW, Lee SW, Yun SC, et al. A point-of-care platelet function assay and C-reactive protein for prediction of major cardiovascular events after drug-eluting stent implantation. J Am Coll Cardiol 2011 Dec 13;58(25):2630-39.

212. Jin HY, Yang TH, Kim DI, et al. High post-clopidogrel platelet reactivity assessed by a point-of-care assay predicts long-term clinical outcomes in patients with ST-segment elevation myocardial infarction who underwent primary coronary stenting. Int J Cardiol 2012 Jun 9

213. Yu LH, Kim MH, Zhang HZ, et al. Impact of platelet function test on platelet responsiveness and clinical outcome after coronary stent implantation: platelet responsiveness and clinical outcome. Korean Circ J 2012 Jun;42(6):382-89.

214. Saraf S, Christopoulos C, Salha IB, et al. Impaired endogenous thrombolysis in acute coronary syndrome patients predicts cardiovascular death and nonfatal myocardial infarction. J Am Coll Cardiol 2010 May 11;55(19):2107-15.

215. Codner P, Vaduganathan M, Rechavia E, et al. Clopidogrel response up to six months after acute myocardial infarction. Am J Cardiol 2012 Aug 1;110(3):321-25.

216. Ari H, Ozkan H, Karacinar A, et al. The EFFect of hIgh-dose ClopIdogrel treatmENT in patients with clopidogrel resistance (The EFFICIENT Trial). Int J Cardiol 2012 Jun 14;157(3):374-80.

217. Ryu DS, Hong CK, Sim YS, et al. Anti-platelet drug resistance in the prediction of thromboembolic complications after neurointervention. Journal of Korean Neurosurgical Society 2010 Oct;48(4):319-24.

218. Kang HS, Kwon BJ, Kim JE, et al. Preinterventional clopidogrel response variability for coil embolization of intracranial aneurysms: clinical implications. AJNR Am J Neuroradiol 2010 Aug;31(7):1206-10.

219. Drazin D, Choulakian A, Nuno M, et al. Body weight: a risk factor for subtherapeutic antithrombotic therapy in neurovascular stenting. J Neurointerv Surg 2011 Jun;3(2):177-81.

220. Bjelland TW, Hjertner O, Klepstad P, et al. Antiplatelet effect of clopidogrel is reduced in patients treated with therapeutic hypothermia after cardiac arrest. Resuscitation 2010 Dec;81(12):1627-31.

221. Bonello L, Paganelli F, rpin-Bornet M, et al. Vasodilator-stimulated phosphoprotein phosphorylation analysis prior to percutaneous coronary intervention for exclusion of postprocedural major adverse cardiovascular events. Journal of Thrombosis & Haemostasis 2007 Aug;5(8):1630-36.

222. Djukanovic N, Todorovic Z, Grdinic A, et al. Thienopyridine resistance among patients undergoing intracoronary stent implantation and treated with dual antiplatelet therapy: assessment of some modifying factors. Journal of Pharmacological Sciences 2008 Aug;107(4):451-55.

223. El Ghannudi S, Ohlmann P, Meyer N, et al. Impact of P2Y12 inhibition by clopidogrel on cardiovascular mortality in unselected patients treated by percutaneous coronary angioplasty: a prospective registry. Jacc: Cardiovascular Interventions 2010 Jun;3(6):648-56.

224. El Ghannudi S, Ohlmann P, Jesel L, et al. Impaired inhibition of P2Y(12) by clopidogrel is a major determinant of cardiac death in diabetes mellitus patients treated by percutaneous coronary intervention. Atherosclerosis 2011 Aug;217(2):465-72.

225. Freynhofer MK, Brozovic I, Bruno V, et al. Multiple electrode aggregometry and vasodilator stimulated phosphoprotein-phosphorylation assay in clinical routine for prediction of postprocedural major adverse cardiovascular events. Thrombosis & Haemostasis 2011 Aug;106(2):230-39.

226. Kalantzi KI, Dimitriou AA, Milionis HJ, et al. Clopidogrel differentially affects platelet-mediated thrombosis and inflammatory response in patients with acute coronary syndromes. Journal of Thrombosis & Haemostasis 2011 Apr;9(4):875-78.

227. Morel O, El GS, Jesel L, et al. Cardiovascular mortality in chronic kidney disease patients undergoing percutaneous coronary intervention is mainly related to impaired P2Y12 inhibition by clopidogrel. Journal of the American College of Cardiology 2011 Jan 25;57(4):399-408.

228. Palmerini T, Barozzi C, Tomasi L, et al. A randomised study comparing the antiplatelet and antiinflammatory effect of clopidogrel 150 mg/day versus 75 mg/day in patients with ST-segment elevation acute myocardial infarction and poor responsiveness to clopidogrel: results from the DOUBLE study. Thrombosis Research 2010 Apr;125(4):309-14.

229. Schafer A, Flierl U, Kossler J, et al. Early determination of clopidogrel responsiveness by platelet reactivity indexidentifies patients at risk for cardiovascular events after myocardial infarction. Thrombosis & Haemostasis 2011 Jul;106(1):141-48.

230. Siller-Matula JM, Haberl K, Prillinger K, et al. The effect of antiplatelet drugs clopidogrel and aspirin is less immediately after stent implantation. Thromb Res 2009 Apr;123(6):874-80.

231. Siller-Matula JM, Christ G, Lang IM, et al. Multiple electrode aggregometry predicts stent thrombosis better than the vasodilator-stimulated phosphoprotein phosphorylation assay. Journal of Thrombosis & Haemostasis 2010 Feb;8(2):351-59.

232. Tselepis AD, Tsoumani ME, Kalantzi KI, et al. Influence of high-density lipoprotein and paraoxonase-1 on platelet reactivity in patients with acute coronary syndromes receiving clopidogrel therapy. J Thromb Haemost 2011 Dec;9(12):2371-78.

233. Cuisset T, Quilici J, Grosdidier C, et al. Comparison of platelet reactivity and clopidogrel response in patients </= 75 Years Versus > 75 years undergoing percutaneous coronary intervention for non-ST-segment elevation acute coronary syndrome. Am J Cardiol 2011 Nov 15;108(10):1411-16.

234. Eshtehardi P, Windecker S, Cook S, et al. Dual low response to acetylsalicylic acid and clopidogrel is associated with myonecrosis and stent thrombosis after coronary stent implantation. Am Heart J 2010 May;159(5):891-98.

235. Ivandic BT, Sausemuth M, Ibrahim H, et al. Dual antiplatelet drug resistance is a risk factor for cardiovascular events after percutaneous coronary intervention. Clinical Chemistry 2009 Jun;55(6):1171-76.

236. Schulz S, Sibbing D, Braun S, et al. Platelet response to clopidogrel and restenosis in patients treated predominantly with drug-eluting stents. Am Heart J 2010 Aug;160(2):355-61.

237. Sibbing D, Braun S, Morath T, et al. Platelet reactivity after clopidogrel treatment assessed with point-of-care analysis and early drug-eluting stent thrombosis. Journal of the American College of Cardiology 2009 Mar 10;53(10):849-56.

238. Sibbing D, Schulz S, Braun S, et al. Antiplatelet effects of clopidogrel and bleeding in patients undergoing coronary stent placement. Journal of Thrombosis & Haemostasis 2010 Feb;8(2):250-56.

239. Sibbing D, Steinhubl SR, Schulz S, et al. Platelet aggregation and its association with stent thrombosis and bleeding in clopidogrel-treated patients: initial evidence of a therapeutic window. Journal of the American College of Cardiology 2010 Jul 20;56(4):317-18.

240. Sibbing D, Morath T, Braun S, et al. Clopidogrel response status assessed with Multiplate point-of-care analysis and the incidence and timing of stent thrombosis over six months following coronary stenting. Thrombosis & Haemostasis 2010 Jan;103(1):151-59.

241. Gerotziafas GT, Zarifis J, Bandi A, et al. Description of response to aspirin and clopidogrel in outpatients with coronary artery disease using multiple electrode impedance aggregometry. Clin Appl Thromb Hemost 2012 Jul;18(4):356-63.

242. Sibbing D, Bernlochner I, Schulz S, et al. Prognostic value of a high on-clopidogrel treatment platelet reactivity in bivalirudin versus abciximab treated non-ST-segment elevation myocardial infarction patients. ISAR-REACT 4 (Intracoronary Stenting and Antithrombotic Regimen: Rapid Early Action for Coronary Treatment-4) platelet substudy. J Am Coll Cardiol 2012 Jul 31;60(5):369-77.

243. Johnston LR, Larsen PD, La Flamme AC, et al. Suboptimal response to clopidogrel and the effect of prasugrel in acute coronary syndromes. Int J Cardiol 2012 Mar 31

244. Siller-Matula JM, le-Karth G, Christ G, et al. Dual non-responsiveness to antiplatelet treatment is a stronger predictor of cardiac adverse events than isolated non-responsiveness to clopidogrel or aspirin. Int J Cardiol 2012 Feb 1

245. Muller-Schunk S, Linn J, Peters N, et al. Monitoring of clopidogrel-related platelet inhibition: correlation of nonresponse with clinical outcome in supra-aortic stenting. Ajnr: American Journal of Neuroradiology 2008 Apr;29(4):786-91.

246. Kwak YL, Kim JC, Choi YS, et al. Clopidogrel responsiveness regardless of the discontinuation date predicts increased blood loss and transfusion requirement after off-pump coronary artery bypass graft surgery. Journal of the American College of Cardiology 2010 Dec 7;56(24):1994-2002.

247. Tang FK, Lin LJ, Hua N, et al. Earlier application of loading doses of aspirin and clopidogrel decreases rate of recurrent cardiovascular ischemic events for patients undergoing percutaneous coronary intervention. Chin Med J (Engl) 2012 Feb;125(4):631-38.

248. Malek LA, Spiewak M, Filipiak KJ, et al. Persistent platelet activation is related to very early cardiovascular events in patients with acute coronary syndromes. Kardiologia Polska 2007 Jan 12;65(1):40-45.

249. Foussas SG, Zairis MN, Patsourakos NG, et al. The impact of oral antiplatelet responsiveness on the long-term prognosis after coronary stenting. Am Heart J 2007 Oct;154(4):676-81.

250. Smit JJ, van Werkum JW, ten BJ, et al. Prehospital triple antiplatelet therapy in patients with acute ST elevation myocardial infarction leads to better platelet aggregation inhibition and clinical outcome than dual antiplatelet therapy. Heart 2010 Nov;96(22):1815-20.

251. Huczek Z, Filipiak KJ, Kochman J, et al. Prognostic significance of platelet function in the early phase of ST-elevation myocardial infarction treated with primary angioplasty. Med Sci Monit 2008 Mar;14(3):CR144-CR151.

252. Moerenhout CM, Claeys MJ, Haine S, et al. Clinical relevance of clopidogrel unresponsiveness during elective coronary stenting: experience with the point-of-care platelet function assay-100 C/ADP. Am Heart J 2010 Mar;159(3):434-38.

253. Chiu FC, Wang TD, Lee JK, et al. Residual platelet reactivity after aspirin and clopidogrel treatment predicts 2-year major cardiovascular events in patients undergoing percutaneous coronary intervention. Eur J Intern Med 2011 Oct;22(5):471-77.

254. Dziewierz A, Dudek D, Heba G, et al. Inter-individual variability in response to clopidogrel in patients with coronary artery disease. Kardiologia Polska 118 20;62(2):108-17.

255. Lindvall G, Sartipy U, Bjessmo S, et al. Aprotinin reduces the antiplatelet effect of clopidogrel. Interactive Cardiovascular & Thoracic Surgery 2009 Aug;9(2):178-81.

256. Lakkis NM, George S, Thomas E, et al. Use of ICHOR-platelet works to assess platelet function in patients treated with GP IIb/IIIa inhibitors. Catheter Cardiovasc Interv 2001 Jul;53(3):346-51.

257. Mobley JE, Bresee SJ, Wortham DC, et al. Frequency of nonresponse antiplatelet activity of clopidogrel during pretreatment for cardiac catheterization. American Journal of Cardiology 2004 Feb 15;93(4):456-58.

258. Mega JL, Close SL, Wiviott SD, et al. Cytochrome P450 genetic polymorphisms and the response to prasugrel: relationship to pharmacokinetic, pharmacodynamic, and clinical outcomes. Circulation 2009 May 19;119(19):2553-60.

259. Mega JL, Close SL, Wiviott SD, et al. Genetic variants in ABCB1 and CYP2C19 and cardiovascular outcomes after treatment with clopidogrel and prasugrel in the TRITON-TIMI 38 trial: a pharmacogenetic analysis. Lancet 2010 Oct 16;376(9749):1312-19.

260. Kim IS, Jeong YH, Park Y, et al. Platelet inhibition by adjunctive cilostazol versus high maintenance-dose clopidogrel in patients with acute myocardial infarction according to cytochrome P450 2C19 genotype. Jacc: Cardiovascular Interventions 2011 Apr;4(4):381-91.

261. Varenhorst C, James S, Erlinge D, et al. Genetic variation of CYP2C19 affects both pharmacokinetic and pharmacodynamic responses to clopidogrel but not prasugrel in aspirin-treated patients with coronary artery disease. Eur Heart J 2009 Jul;30(14):1744-52. PMID: 19429918.

262. Tantry US, Bliden KP, Wei C, et al. First analysis of the relation between CYP2C19 genotype and pharmacodynamics in patients treated with ticagrelor versus clopidogrel: the ONSET/OFFSET and RESPOND genotype studies. Circulation 2010 Dec;Cardiovascular(6):556-66.

263. Hwang SJ, Jeong YH, Kim IS, et al. Cytochrome 2C19 polymorphism and response to adjunctive cilostazol versus high maintenance-dose clopidogrel in patients undergoing percutaneous coronary intervention. Circulation: Cardiovascular Interventions 2010 Oct;3(5):450-59.

264. Park KW, Park JJ, Lee SP, et al. Cilostazol attenuates on-treatment platelet reactivity in patients with CYP2C19 loss of function alleles receiving dual antiplatelet therapy: a genetic substudy of the CILON-T randomised controlled trial. Heart 2011 Apr;97(8):641-47.

265. Collet JP, Hulot JS, Anzaha G, et al. High doses of clopidogrel to overcome genetic resistance: the randomized crossover CLOVIS-2 (Clopidogrel and Response Variability Investigation Study 2). JACC Cardiovasc Interv 2011 Apr;4(4):392-402.

266. Taubert D, von Beckerath N, Grimberg G, et al. Impact of P-glycoprotein on clopidogrel absorption. Clin Pharmacol Ther 2006 Nov;80(5):486-501.

267. Wallentin L, Varenhorst C, James S, et al. Prasugrel achieves greater and faster P2Y12receptor-mediated platelet inhibition than clopidogrel due to more efficient generation of its active metabolite in aspirin-treated patients with coronary artery disease. European Heart Journal 2008 Jan 1;29(1):21-30.

268. Gurbel PA, Bliden KP, Butler K, et al. Randomized double-blind assessment of the ONSET and OFFSET of the antiplatelet effects of ticagrelor versus clopidogrel in patients with stable coronary artery disease: the ONSET/OFFSET study. Circulation 2009 Dec 22;120(25):2577-85.

269. Gladding P, Webster M, Zeng I, et al. The Antiplatelet Effect of Higher Loading and Maintenance Dose Regimens of Clopidogrel: The PRINC (Plavix Response in Coronary Intervention) Trial. Jacc: Cardiovascular Interventions 2008 Dec;1(6):612-19. PMID: doi: 10.1016/j.jcin.2008.09.005.

270. Wang XD, Zhang DF, Zhuang SW, et al. Modifying clopidogrel maintenance doses according to vasodilator-stimulated phosphoprotein phosphorylation index improves clinical outcome in patients with clopidogrel resistance. Clinical Cardiology 2011 May;34(5):332-38.

271. Bonello L, Camoin-Jau L, Armero S, et al. Tailored clopidogrel loading dose according to platelet reactivity monitoring to prevent acute and subacute stent thrombosis. American Journal of Cardiology 2009 Jan 1;103(1):5-10.

272. Bonello L, Camoin-Jau L, Arques S, et al. Adjusted clopidogrel loading doses according to vasodilator-stimulated phosphoprotein phosphorylation index decrease rate of major adverse cardiovascular events in patients with clopidogrel resistance: a multicenter randomized prospective study. Journal of the American College of Cardiology 2008 Apr 8;51(14):1404-11.

273. Tousek P, Osmancik P, Paulu P, et al. Clopidogrel up-titration versus standard dose in patients with high residual platelet reactivity after percutaneous coronary intervention: a single-center pilot randomised study. International Journal of Cardiology 2011 Jul 15;150(2):231-32.

274. Aleil B, Jacquemin L, De PF, et al. Clopidogrel 150 mg/day to overcome low responsiveness in patients undergoing elective percutaneous coronary intervention: results from the VASP-02 (Vasodilator-Stimulated Phosphoprotein-02) randomized study. Jacc: Cardiovascular Interventions 2008 Dec;1(6):631-38.

275. Hazarbasanov D, Velchev V, Finkov B, et al. Tailoring clopidogrel dose according to multiple electrode aggregometry decreases the rate of ischemic complications after percutaneous coronary intervention. J Thromb Thrombolysis 2012 Jul;34(1):85-90. PMID: 10.1007/s11239-012-0684-z [doi].

276. Siller-Matula JM, Francesconi M, Dechant C, et al. Personalized antiplatelet treatment after percutaneous coronary intervention: The MADONNA study. Int J Cardiol 2012 May 30 PMID: S0167-5273(12)00651-1 [pii];10.1016/j.ijcard.2012.05.040 [doi].

277. Montalescot G, Sideris G, Cohen R, et al. Prasugrel compared with high-dose clopidogrel in acute coronary syndrome. The randomised, double-blind ACAPULCO study. Thrombosis & Haemostasis 2010 Jan;103(1):213-23.

278. Capranzano P, Ferreiro JL, Ueno M, et al. Pharmacodynamic effects of adjunctive cilostazol therapy in patients with coronary artery disease on dual antiplatelet therapy: Impact of high on-treatment platelet reactivity and diabetes mellitus status. Catheter Cardiovasc Interv 2012 Mar 19 PMID: 10.1002/ccd.24416 [doi].

279. Cuisset T, Frere C, Quilici J, et al. Glycoprotein IIb/IIIa inhibitors improve outcome after coronary stenting in clopidogrel nonresponders: a prospective, randomized study. Jacc: Cardiovascular Interventions 2008 Dec;1(6):649-53.

280. Alexopoulos D, Galati A, Xanthopoulou I, et al. Ticagrelor versus prasugrel in acute coronary syndrome patients with high on-clopidogrel platelet reactivity following percutaneous coronary intervention: a pharmacodynamic study. J Am Coll Cardiol 2012 Jul 17;60(3):193-99. PMID: S0735-1097(12)01508-2 [pii];10.1016/j.jacc.2012.03.050 [doi].

281. Gremmel T, Steiner S, Seidinger D, et al. A high maintenance dose increases the inhibitory response to clopidogrel in patients with high on-treatment residual platelet reactivity. Int J Cardiol 2012 Oct 4;160(2):109-13. PMID: S0167-5273(11)00348-2 [pii];10.1016/j.ijcard.2011.04.001 [doi].

282. Alexopoulos D, Panagiotou A, Xanthopoulou I, et al. Antiplatelet effects of prasugrel vs. double clopidogrel in patients on hemodialysis and with high on-treatment platelet reactivity. J Thromb Haemost 2011 Dec;9(12):2379-85. PMID: 10.1111/j.1538-7836.2011.04531.x [doi].

283. Alexopoulos D, Xanthopoulou I, Davlouros P, et al. Prasugrel overcomes high on-clopidogrel platelet reactivity in chronic coronary artery disease patients more effectively than high dose (150 mg) clopidogrel. Am Heart J 2011 Oct;162(4):733-39. PMID: S0002-8703(11)00570-9 [pii];10.1016/j.ahj.2011.07.026 [doi].

284. Trenk D, Stone GW, Gawaz M, et al. A randomized trial of prasugrel versus clopidogrel in patients with high platelet reactivity on clopidogrel after elective percutaneous coronary intervention with implantation of drug-eluting stents: results of the TRIGGER-PCI (Testing Platelet Reactivity In Patients Undergoing Elective Stent Placement on Clopidogrel to Guide Alternative Therapy With Prasugrel) study. J Am Coll Cardiol 2012 Jun 12;59(24):2159-64. PMID: S0735-1097(12)00978-3 [pii];10.1016/j.jacc.2012.02.026 [doi].

285. Alexopoulos D, Dimitropoulos G, Davlouros P, et al. Prasugrel overcomes high on-clopidogrel platelet reactivity post-stenting more effectively than high-dose (150-mg) clopidogrel: the importance of CYP2C19*2 genotyping. JACC Cardiovasc Interv 2011 Apr;4(4):403-10. PMID: S1936-8798(11)00134-8 [pii];10.1016/j.jcin.2010.12.011 [doi].

286. Thygesen K, Alpert JS, White HD, et al. Universal Definition of Myocardial Infarction. Circulation 2007 Nov 27;116(22):2634-53.

287. Alexopoulos D, Panagiotou A, Xanthopoulou I, et al. Antiplatelet effects of prasugrel vs. double clopidogrel in patients on hemodialysis and with high on-treatment platelet reactivity. J Thromb Haemost 2011 Dec;9(12):2379-85. PMID: 10.1111/j.1538-7836.2011.04531.x [doi].

288. Aleil B, Leon C, Cazenave JP, et al. CYP2C19*2 polymorphism is not the sole determinant of the response to clopidogrel: implications for its monitoring. J Thromb Haemost 2009 Oct;7(10):1747-49.

289. Price MJ, Murray SS, Angiolillo DJ, et al. Influence of genetic polymorphisms on the effect of high- and standard-dose clopidogrel after percutaneous coronary intervention: the GIFT (Genotype Information and Functional Testing) study. J Am Coll Cardiol 2012 May 29;59(22):1928-37.

290. Alexopoulos D, Dimitropoulos G, Davlouros P, et al. Prasugrel overcomes high on-clopidogrel platelet reactivity post-stenting more effectively than high-dose (150-mg) clopidogrel: the importance of CYP2C19*2 genotyping. JACC Cardiovasc Interv 2011 Apr;4(4):403-10.

291. Holmes DR, Jr., Dehmer GJ, Kaul S, et al. ACCF/AHA clopidogrel clinical alert: approaches to the FDA "boxed warning": a report of the American College of Cardiology Foundation Task Force on clinical expert consensus documents and the American Heart Association endorsed by the Society for Cardiovascular Angiography and Interventions and the Society of Thoracic Surgeons. J Am Coll Cardiol 2010 Jul;56(4):321-41.

292. Liu YP, Hao PP, Zhang MX, et al. Association of genetic variants in CYP2C19 and adverse clinical outcomes after treatment with clopidogrel: an updated meta-analysis. Thromb Res 2011 Dec;128(6):593-94.

293. Zabalza M, Subirana I, Sala J, et al. Meta-analyses of the association between cytochrome CYP2C19 loss- and gain-of-function polymorphisms and cardiovascular outcomes in patients with coronary artery disease treated with clopidogrel. Heart 2012 Jan;98(2):100-08.

294. Mega JL, Simon T, Collet JP, et al. Reduced-function CYP2C19 genotype and risk of adverse clinical outcomes among patients treated with clopidogrel predominantly for PCI: a meta-analysis. JAMA 2010 Oct 27;304(16):1821-30.

295. Jin B, Ni HC, Shen W, et al. Cytochrome P450 2C19 polymorphism is associated with poor clinical outcomes in coronary artery disease patients treated with clopidogrel. Mol Biol Rep 2011 Mar;38(3):1697-702.

296. Li Y, Tang HL, Hu YF, et al. The gain-of-function variant allele CYP2C19*17: a double-edged sword between thrombosis and bleeding in clopidogrel-treated patients. J Thromb Haemost 2012 Feb;10(2):199-206.

297. Sofi F, Giusti B, Marcucci R, et al. Cytochrome P450 2C19*2 polymorphism and cardiovascular recurrences in patients taking clopidogrel: a meta-analysis. Pharmacogenomics J 2011 Jun;11(3):199-206.

298. Yamaguchi Y, Abe T, Sato Y, et al. Effects of VerifyNow P2Y12 test and CYP2C19*2 testing on clinical outcomes of patients with cardiovascular disease: A systematic review and meta-analysis. Platelets 2012 Jul 3 PMID: 10.3109/09537104.2012.700969 [doi].

299. Brar SS, ten Berg J, Marcucci R, et al. Impact of Platelet Reactivity on Clinical Outcomes After Percutaneous Coronary Intervention: A Collaborative Meta-Analysis of Individual Participant Data. Journal of the American College of Cardiology 2011 Nov 1;58(19):1945-54. PMID: doi: 10.1016/j.jacc.2011.06.059.

300. Snoep JD, Hovens MM, Eikenboom JC, et al. Clopidogrel nonresponsiveness in patients undergoing percutaneous coronary intervention with stenting: a systematic review and meta-analysis. Am Heart J 2007 Aug;154(2):221-31.

301. Aradi D, Komocsi A, Vorobcsuk A, et al. Prognostic significance of high on-clopidogrel platelet reactivity after percutaneous coronary intervention: systematic review and meta-analysis. Am Heart J 2010 Sep;160(3):543-51.

302. Combescure C, Fontana P, Mallouk N, et al. Clinical implications of clopidogrel non-response in cardiovascular patients: a systematic review and meta-analysis. J Thromb Haemost 2010 May;8(5):923-33.

303. Sofi F, Marcucci R, Gori AM, et al. Clopidogrel non-responsiveness and risk of cardiovascular morbidity. An updated meta-analysis. Thromb Haemost 2010 Apr;103(4):841-48.

304. Burke W. Genetic Testing. N Engl J Med 2002 Dec 5;347(23):1867-75. PMID: doi: 10.1056/NEJMoa012113.

305. Baker SG. The Central Role of Receiver Operating Characteristic (ROC) Curves in Evaluating Tests for the Early Detection of Cancer. Journal of the National Cancer Institute 2003 Apr 2;95(7):511-15.

306. Castaldi PJ, Dahabreh IJ, Ioannidis JPA. An empirical assessment of validation practices for molecular classifiers. Briefings in Bioinformatics 2011 May 1;12(3):189-202.

307. Ransohoff DF. Rules of evidence for cancer molecular-marker discovery and validation. Nat Rev Cancer 2004 Apr;4(4):309-14. PMID: 10.1038/nrc1322.

308. Tzoulaki I, Liberopoulos G, Ioannidis JPA. Assessment of Claims of Improved Prediction Beyond the Framingham Risk Score. JAMA: The Journal of the American Medical Association 2009 Dec 2;302(21):2345-52.

309. Macaskill P, Walter SD, Irwig L, et al. Assessing the gain in diagnostic performance when combining two diagnostic tests. Statist Med 2002;21(17):2527-46. PMID: 10.1002/sim.1227.

310. Pencina MJ, D'Agostino RB, Steyerberg EW. Extensions of net reclassification improvement calculations to measure usefulness of new biomarkers. Statist Med 2011;30(1):11-21. PMID: 10.1002/sim.4085.

311. Pencina MJ, D' Agostino RB, D' Agostino RB, et al. Evaluating the added predictive ability of a new marker: From area under the ROC curve to reclassification and beyond. Statist Med 2008;27(2):157-72. PMID: 10.1002/sim.2929.

312. Steyerberg EW, Pencina MJ, Lingsma HF, et al. Assessing the incremental value of diagnostic and prognostic markers: a review and illustration. European Journal of Clinical Investigation 2012;42(2):216-28. PMID: 10.1111/j.1365-2362.2011.02562.x.

313. Pencina MJ, D'Agostino RB, Vasan RS. Statistical methods for assessment of added usefulness of new biomarkers. Clin Chem Lab Med 2010 Dec;48(12):1703-11.

314. Scher HI, Nasso SF, Rubin EH, et al. Adaptive Clinical Trial Designs for Simultaneous Testing of Matched Diagnostics and Therapeutics. Clinical Cancer Research 2011 Nov 1;17(21):6634-40.

315. Simon R. Clinical trial designs for evaluating the medical utility of prognostic and predictive biomarkers in oncology. Per Med 2010;7(1):33-47.

316. Cain LE, Robins JM, Lanoy E, et al. When to start treatment? A systematic approach to the comparison of dynamic regimes using observational data. Int J Biostat 2010;6(2):18.

317. Hernan MA, Lanoy E, Costagliola D, et al. Comparison of Dynamic Treatment Regimes via Inverse Probability Weighting. Basic & Clinical Pharmacology & Toxicology 2006;98(3):237-42. PMID: 10.1111/j.1742-7843.2006.pto_329.x.

318. Orellana L, Rotnitzky A, Robins JM. Dynamic regime marginal structural mean models for estimation of optimal dynamic treatment regimes, Part I: main content. Int J Biostat 2010;6(2):8.

Acronyms

ACTIVE A trial	Atrial Fibrillation Clopidogrel Trial with Irbesartan for Prevention of Vascular Events A trial
ACS	Acute coronary syndromes
ADP	Adenosine diphosphate
AHRQ	Agency for Healthcare Research and Quality
CABG	Coronary artery bypass graft
CHARISMA trial	Clopidogrel for High Atherothrombotic Risk and Ischemic Stabilization, Management and Avoidance trial
CI	Confidence interval
CURE trial	Clopidogrel in Unstable Angina to Prevent Recurrent Events trial
EGAPP	Evaluation of Genomic Applications in Practice and Prevention
EPC	Evidence-based Practice Center
FDA	U.S. Food and Drug Administration
GOF	Gain-of-function
GRAVITAS trial	Gauging Responsiveness with a VerifyNow Assay—Impact on Thrombosis and Safety trial
GUSTO criteria	Global Utilization of Streptokinase and Tissue Plasminogen Activator for Occluded Coronary Arteries criteria
HuGENet	Human Genome Epidemiology Network
ISAR-REACT 4 trial	Intracoronary Stenting and Antithrombotic Regimen: Rapid Early Action for Coronary Treatment 4 trial
LOF	Loss-of-function
LTA	Light-transmission aggregometry
MACE	Major adverse cardiovascular events
OR	Odds ratio
PCI	Percutaneous coronary intervention
PCR	Polymerase chain reaction
PFA	Platelet Function Analyzer
PPI	Proton pump inhibitor
PRI	Platelet reactivity index
PRU	Platelet reactivity units
PLATO trial	PLATelet inhibition and patient Outcomes trial
QUADAS-2	Quality Assessment of Diagnostic Accuracy Studies 2
RCT	Randomized Controlled Trial
RFLP	Restriction fragment length polymorphism
rOR	Relative odds ratio
RR	Relative risk
SIP	Scientific information packets
SRC	Scientific resource center
ST	Stent thrombosis
TEP	Technical Expert Panel
TOO	Task Order Officer
TRIGGER-PCI	Testing Platelet Reactivity In Patients Undergoing Elective Stent Placement on Clopidogrel to Guide Alternative Therapy With Prasugre

TRITON-TIMI 38   Trial to Assess Improvement in Therapeutic Outcomes by trial Optimizing Platelet Inhibition With Prasugrel–Thrombolysis In Myocardial Infarction 38

VASP   Vasodilator-stimulated phosphoprotein

www.ingramcontent.com/pod-product-compliance
Lightning Source LLC
Chambersburg PA
CBHW080633180526
45168CB00008B/3158